Back Pain

John Perrier was born in 1967 and grew up and was educated in Brisbane. He is a Bachelor of Physiotherapy of the University of Queensland and is a Member of the Australian Physiotherapy Association. He is founder and President of PhysioWorks, which has 14 centres throughout Australia, and has treated over 20,000 cases of spinal pain. He is married with two children and lives in Brisbane.

Back Pain

How to Get Rid of It
Forever

John Perrier

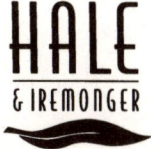

© John Perrier, 1999

This book is copyright. Apart from any fair dealing for the purposes of study, research, criticism, review, or as otherwise permitted under the Copyright Act, no part may be reproduced by any process without written permission. Inquiries should be made to the publisher.

First published in 1999

Typeset by
Midland Typesetters Pty Ltd
Maryborough, Victoria 3465

Printed and bound by
Griffin Press, Pty Ltd
Netley, SA

For the publisher
Hale & Iremonger Pty Ltd
PO Box 205, Alexandria, NSW 2015

*National Library of Australia
Cataloguing-in-Publication entry:*

Perrier, John, 1967– .
   Back pain: how to get rid of it forever.

ISBN 0 86806 675 3.

   1. Backache – Popular works. 2. Backache – Treatment.
   I. Title.

617.564

Contents

Acknowledgements   9
Part I: An introduction to back pain

1. Let's get started!   13
2. The structure and function of your spine   15
    - The evolution of the spine   15
    - The design of the spine   18
3. What goes wrong?   24
    - Trauma   25
    - Wear and tear   26
    - Other causes of lower back pain   28
4. Intervertebral disc injuries   32
    - Disc bulging due to weakness   32
    - A prolapsed disc   33
    - Spondylosis   34
5. Facet and sacro-iliac joint injuries   36
    - Ligament sprains   36
    - Coccydynia   37
    - Arthritis   37
6. Injuries to the vertebrae   41
    - Stress fractures (Spondylolisis)   41
    - Displaced vertebra (Spondylolisthesis)   42
    - Crush fractures   44
7. Muscle injuries   45
    - Bruising   45
    - Spasm   46
    - Post-exercise soreness   46
    - Trigger points   46
8. Referred pain   48
    - Normal nerves   48
    - Compressed nerves   51
9. Consequences of nerve compression   56
    - Pain   56
    - Weakness   60
    - Nerve immobility   61
10. The *real* cause of lower back pain   65
    - Joint stiffness and instability   66
    - The behaviour of your pain   68

Part II: How to analyse your back pain

11	What's your problem?	73
	Self-assessment quiz to determine your back pain type	75

Part III: How to get rid of your back pain forever

12	Muscle imbalances	97
13	Designing a personalised exercise program	108
	Stretch your mobilising muscles	108
	Loosen your tight nerves	109
	Mobilise your stiff joints	110
	Strengthen your deep stability muscles	110
14	Exercises to correct muscle imbalances, joint stiffness and neural tension	113
	Which exercises are best for your spine?	113
	The exercises	116
15	Safer sitting	139
	Advice on sitting for all back pain types	140
	Two simple rules for more efficient sitting	141
	A few other points about sitting posture	147
	Further sitting advice for back types B and D only	151
16	How to lift and bend more efficiently	155
	Stabilise your spine	156
	Use a correct lifting technique	158
	Avoid lifting where possible	164
	Summary of safe lifting	164
17	Ways to walk and stand without straining your spine	165
	Bad posture number one—sway back	165
	Bad posture number two—dropped hip	167
	A few more notes on standing posture	168
	Footwear	169
	Other ways to rest your back when standing	170
	Summary of standing and walking posture control	172
18	Simple tips for lying and sleeping	173
	Sleeping positions	173
	Mattresses and sleeping surfaces	177
	Sex and back pain	178
	How to overcome early morning backache and stiffness	178
	Summary	181
19	Easing activities of daily living	182
	Hints on how to perform daily activities without hurting your spine	184
	Employment	188

20	The effects of stress on your spine	191
	Are you stressed?	192
	The fight-or-flight response	193
	Muscular tension as a cause of back pain	195
	The 'gate theory' of pain	196
21	Your physical tolerance to stress	198
	Increasing your physical tolerance to stress	201
	Decreasing your stress level	202
22	How to decrease stress	205
	Some practical considerations for performing the relaxation exercises	206
	The relaxation exercises	211
23	Attitudes, the placebo effect, and the power of the mind	219
	Getting rid of negative thinking	223
	Techniques for positive thinking	225
24	The effects of drugs	230
	Drugs and back pain	230
	NSAIDs for chronic, ongoing back pain	231
	NSAIDs for acute, severe pain	234
	Topical NSAIDs—creams, gels and liniments	235
	Over-the-counter analgesics	237
	Muscle relaxants and sedatives	237
	Summary	238
25	Diet, nutritional supplements and natural remedies	239
	Your daily diet and its relationship to back pain	239
	Vitamins, minerals, nutritional supplements and natural remedies	242
26	Fitness and exercise	248
	Advantages that regular cardiovascular exercise confers upon your spine	248
	Guidelines and frequently asked questions about exercise	251
	Other sports and activities	258
	Summary of how to organise your exercise program	260
27	X-rays and scans	261
	X-rays	261
	CT scans	262
	MRI	263
	Bone scans	264
	How effective is radiology in diagnosing the source of back pain?	265
28	Pregnant women and children	269
	Pregnancy	269
	Children and adolescents with lower back pain	272

29	A few other things that had nowhere else to go	274
	Orthotics	274
	Supports and braces	274
	Taping	275
	Traction	278
	Electrotherapy	279
	Trigger point therapy	281
30	Heat or ice?	282
	Frequently asked questions about heat and ice application	284
31	Myth busting	287
	What *doesn't* cause low back pain	287
	What *won't* cure low back pain	291
32	What to do if you are in acute, severe pain	294
33	Choosing a spinal health practitioner	297
	What makes a good spinal health practitioner?	297
	Is manipulation good for your spine?	303
	Summary	305
34	Which spinal health practitioner is best for you?	306
	Physiotherapy	307
	Chiropractic	308
	Osteopathy	309
	Medical doctors—General practitioners	309
	Acupuncture	311
	Massage	313
	Reflexology	313
	Natural medicine: Naturopathy and homeopathy	314
	Other techniques: Pilates, Feldenkrais, Alexander, Yoga	315
	Surgery	318
	Spinal injections	320
	Summary	322
35	Putting it all together	323

Epilogue	334
Appendices	
Preventing osteoporosis	335
Some common anti-inflammatory medications	336

Acknowledgements

I've occasionally glanced at the 'acknowledgements' at the start of other books. They always commence with well-used phrases such as: 'This book would not have been possible without the generous and dedicated support of many people ... etc.' Usually, I simply skim over this phrase, largely ignoring it as a hackneyed cliché. Well, guess what? It's true!

In my case, this book would not have been possible without the generous and dedicated support of many people. Most of them are busy medical professionals, and all gave freely and generously of their time. To each of these people, I offer my sincere gratitude.

First, to my physiotherapy colleagues, Debbie Creamer, John Miller, Jenny Lawson and Andrew Waldie, for telling me how awful my first drafts were. Thank you very much to spinal surgeon Dr Bill Ryan, doctors David Speed and Andrew Grimes, chiropractor Dr Keith Charlton, and osteopath Mr Graham Sanders, for your technical reviews and comments on the entire text. You are all very clever people.

I would also like to thank Dr Fred Schubert for his help with the radiology section, dietician Lisa O'Brien for reviewing the diet and nutrition segment, and Ian McKenzie for helping with the relaxation and positive thinking chapters. My gratitude also goes to pharmacist Scherelle Waldie for her considerable help with the drugs chapter. Another pharmacist also reviewed this section for me, but she did not want to be identified. Her name, were it a cryptic crossword clue, would read something like 'gets a herb for Mrs Free Horny Ace'. So thanks for your help. Thanks also to Chris Fechner for helping me with my ever-troublesome computer, and to my colleague and co-worker Steven Schamburg for his help not only with the quiz, but for physio in general.

My gratitude also goes out to the secretaries, presidents and committee members of various professional associations, including the Australian Chiropractic Association, the Australian Osteopathic Association, the Australian Natural Medicine Association, the Australian Acupuncture and Chinese Medicine Association, and the Australian Natural Therapists Association, for the information on your various professions. Thanks also to the Australian College of Natural Medicine, the Australian Feldenkrais Guild, the Queensland School of Reflexology and the Arthritis Foundation of Queensland for the advice and material on your specialties. Thanks also to Wendy Lockett for your help on reflexology, and for the foot massage.

I also acknowledge the work of Bert Weir, whose lectures at the Relaxation Centre of Brisbane have already helped thousands of people. Thanks also to Cathy Nash, Clare Stevens, Johnny Godwin and Andrew King for their input. Of course, many thanks to my supermodels Greg Everding and Debbie Creamer, and to Henri Van Nordenberg for his advice on the photographs.

I am also indebted to those patients who completed a back pain questionnaire to help me with my research. Chapter 11, and in fact this whole book, would not have been possible without your co-operation. I hope your backs are still feeling better, by the way.

I am most grateful to Bert, Heather and the rest of the team at my publishers, Hale & Iremonger.

See what I mean about a lot of dedicated people. By the way, if you're reading this and thinking 'Gee, I gave John a lot of help with his manuscript, and he hasn't even thanked me,' then I apologise profusely. I'm terrified that I've left someone out, and, if that includes you, then I thank you from the bottom of my heart.

Last but not least, thank you to my beautiful wife Kath, for putting up with me, and for putting up with the absence of me, while I wrote this book.

Dedicated to Mum and Dad.

Part I

An introduction to back pain

1
Let's get started!

The title of this section, 'An introduction to back pain', is a bit misleading. I'm sure that you already know back pain very well. Whether your particular version is aching, burning, jabbing or gnawing, I'd like to bet that you need no further introduction. I hope that by the end of this book you'll have the knowledge and techniques to say *goodbye* to your back pain forever.

About five *billion* people around the planet are currently suffering, or will soon suffer from, spinal pain of some sort. No, I didn't take a survey. However, medical statistics tell us that about 85% of people will have back problems at some stage during their lives, so my estimate is probably pretty accurate. Five billion cases of back problems! That's a lot of pain. Yet I'm sure that, for you, one case stands out above the rest: Yours.

This book is all about *your* back pain. And, of course, what you can do to get rid of it.

Back pain is not only very common, it is also very likely to recur. Four out of every five back pain sufferers will have more than one attack. Many of these people develop chronic pain that persists for months, years or even decades. This book is dedicated to preventing these all-too-common repeat or chronic problems. Of course, if you've just suffered from your first case of this dreaded affliction, then the techniques and tips that follow will help ensure that it is your last.

As you'll come to appreciate as you read the next thirty-five chapters, back pain is a very individual problem. Techniques that help one person's pain can cripple someone else. For example, consider these two vastly different cases:

(1) An eighty-year-old retiree, whose back stiffens after he has been sitting in his easy chair for an hour, and
(2) A fifteen-year-old gymnast, whose lower spine catches with a sharp pain each time she does a back flip.

These two types of problems are totally different, and so require separate solutions. Likewise, I'm sure your spine has its own unique characteristics and problems. As we go, we'll explore various types of spinal problems, and then provide specific, tailored advice for your particular case. In this way, you will learn solutions that are likely to help *your* problem, not someone else's.

Like most worthwhile pursuits, the solutions may require some hard work. You may have to make changes to yourself, to your habits, your lifestyle, and even to your way of thinking, if you hope to permanently alleviate your back problems. This book will show you how and why you need to take these important steps.

In doing this we will first take a light-hearted look at the evolution of the spine. You will learn how this remarkable piece of engineering progressed from a stiff band of cartilage to become its current complex series of interlocking bits. Then, we'll take a closer look at these interlocking bits to discover how and why the spine works. Finally, to complete Part I, you will learn what can go wrong with your spine.

After that, we'll move onto a self-assessment section. In this part, you'll learn about the nature and behaviour of your problem. You'll complete a very important quiz, which will classify your spinal problem into one of four types. The results of this quiz, along with your gradually accruing knowledge, will enable you during the remainder of the book to identify the advice that most relates to your specific problem.

From this point onwards, the advice flows thick and fast. You will learn how to simplify common tasks such as sitting, lifting and standing. Through this discussion we will interweave advice on things like chairs, work stations and beds, and offer tips to simplify household and work tasks. Importantly, you will learn vital exercises that will help to cure the underlying cause of your problem.

You will also discover many other ways of helping your spine through fitness programs, diet, nutritional supplements and medication. We'll have a thorough look at relaxation and positive thinking, and the role that your mind plays in the rehabilitation process. Not only that, but we'll be debunking a few myths and unproven treatments along the way.

Towards the end, we'll look at how to choose a good spinal health practitioner, and examine the various types of therapies and treatment options that are available to help you.

Finally, the last chapter will show you how to systematically design your own rehabilitation program. Once you have completed this chapter, you will have a blueprint for a program that will help you to get rid of your back pain forever.

Let's get started!

2
The structure and function of your spine
Why a mutant fish is responsible for your sore back

If you asked an inventor or an overpaid corporate engineer to design a gadget, the first thing that they would want to know is what it was supposed to do. No sensible person would design an object, and then assign it a use when they had finished. Usually, the design of something depends upon its purpose. Function dictates structure.

Your spine is no different. Its myriad of strange shapes and complex joints serve very worthwhile purposes. Those funny little pointy bits on the bones did not appear by accident. If you understand the function of your back, and how those demands evolved, then you will find it far easier to appreciate its bizarre structure. Later, armed with this knowledge, you can confidently tackle topics such as diagnosing and preventing back pain.

The evolution of the spine

Mother Nature designed our spinal column over a very long period. Helped by her design team of *natural selection* and *evolution*, she gradually fashioned the extremely complex systems that form the human spine.

The process began about half a billion years ago, when an otherwise inconspicuous ocean-dwelling animal called an Elasmobranch developed a spine. The Elasmobranch's spine was a flimsy affair: its chief function was to provide protection for the bundle of nerve fibres that ran down the creature's back. Despite this inauspicious beginning, the vertebral column had arrived.

Over the next lazy 100 million years or so, other sea life, such as primitive fish, slowly evolved spines. These spines were also very simple, and made from soft cartilage rather than bone. They gradually assumed another job besides protecting the nerves: to provide an attachment for the fish's muscles. This extra control allowed them to swim, and thus survive, more efficiently.

Then, about 400 million years ago, the fish did something that had a huge effect on our spinal development: they migrated to land. With this audacious move came a new problem for the spine. Gravity.

Helped along by the very small changes that are evident from one generation to the next, these early amphibians gradually developed newer, different models of the spine. The quality-control manager, natural selection, tested each new design. Those animals with more efficient spines had a better survival rate, meaning that their descendants, the reptiles, inherited better backs.

By the time mammals arrived about 250 million years ago, the vertebral column had developed many desirable characteristics:

- The individual building blocks of the spine were now constructed from dense bone rather than cartilage. This change allowed them to bear more weight.
- The vertebrae—the back bones—developed joint structures that allowed extra movement.
- Shock-absorbing mechanisms evolved that helped to protect the bones from fracturing in the rough-and-tumble of prehistoric Earth.
- Strange lumps and bumps of bone developed on the vertebrae. These protuberances provided leverage for muscle attachments, allowing more precise movement control.

For a time, everything was going smoothly in Mother Nature's spinal design department. She had an efficient, working model that allowed good movement, offered a firm attachment point for both muscles and ribs, while offering vital protection to essential nerve structures.

Then about fifteen million years ago, probably on an otherwise ordinary Tuesday or Wednesday afternoon, all that contentment dramatically changed. Something happened that would alter the requirements of the spine, and therefore its structure, forever—an apelike creature began to walk on two legs.

Why did the ape do this? Well, nobody knows for sure. However, scientists and anthropologists suspect that the motivation was so that the creature could use its front legs—its arms—for tasks such as using crude tools, or brandishing weapons for self-defence. The two-legged stance also liberated the front legs for the useful purpose of carrying objects, like food. Or beer cans.

Mother Nature and her design team now had to enable the spine to cope with a new functional requirement: to support the trunk in the upright position. Suddenly, the architecture of the lower back needed a drastic overhaul.

Undoubtedly, the first versions were poor. Any decent spinal health practitioner would have made a fortune had they been around during these early reformative millennia. However, as the centuries ticked by, evolution again provided gradual improvements. The pelvis and hips gradually changed their alignment so that the legs were roughly in line

THE STRUCTURE AND FUNCTION OF YOUR SPINE

with the trunk, rather than jutting out at right angles like a quadruped's limbs. The abdominal muscles also changed their function so that they supported the spine in an upright position, rather than simply being a sling for the stomach and intestines.

As we developed, tree climbing became an occasional diversion rather than a semi-permanent home. Our tails, which were no longer necessary, steadily disappeared ... which I, for one, think is a bit of a shame. Imagine how much fun you could have at a party with a fully functioning tail.

Recently, only a mere two or three million years ago, we human beings emerged from the developing gene pool. We now walked upright most of the time. In response, the spine made one further adaptation: it developed some inward and outward curves. Besides providing some extra leverage for the postural muscles, the curves had a springlike effect that helped the spine to absorb shock. Finally, after a 500 million-year journey that started with a mutant fish, the spine arrived at the current model.

Despite the miracle of design, I award Mother Nature only nine out of ten for her efforts in spinal architecture. Why the deducted mark? The lower back is probably the weakest mechanical link in the entire human body. It is responsible for more musculoskeletal pain than any other area. Compared with other masterpieces like the brain and the hand, the lower back looks decidedly amateurish. Paradoxically, the probable reason for this weakness also lies in the mechanism of evolution.

In our earliest caveman days, health problems of all kinds beset the average human being. Even a simple cut or abrasion was often fatal, while the most common form of death was infection from tooth decay! Because of these appalling health problems, most human beings died at a very young age, usually less than thirty. Of course, most reproduction and parenting had to be completed by the early twenties to squeeze into this limited lifespan. Due to the early parenting age, the natural selection process had no chance to attack the residual problems in the lower part of the spine. Most people had already produced their offspring and/or were dead before they had even begun to develop a bad back, which, as we will see later, usually occurs first in early middle age.

So we passed this weak genetic link from one generation to the next, while it patiently waited to make its presence felt when the human lifespan elongated. Now, as the average length of life approaches eighty years, we are, as a race, suffering from far more back pain than our early ancestors could have imagined.

Yet for all its problems, our spine is an amazing and complex piece of machinery. Try to envisage any other design that not only protects the nerves that carry signals from the brain to the limbs, but provides efficient attachment for both ribs and muscles. Of course, this design would also have to allow plenty of movement without being unstable or floppy, protect itself with shock absorption, and stay upright while being supported on only two legs.

As you can see, we place many demands on our spines. Now, we will look at the design that Mother Nature developed to cope with all these requirements.

The design of the spine

Let's now take a closer look at all the knobbly bits and strange twists in your spine. First, we will consider the spine as a whole. Then, we'll examine it piece by piece to see how it achieves its remarkable diversity of roles.

Most of the lumps and bumps have long scientific names, which I'll try to avoid where possible. There's nothing worse than technical jargon to ruin a good story, is there? However, in some circumstances, the anatomical name is actually easier. For example, writing the word 'ligament' is far easier than 'the tough strands of fibre that hold two bones together'. Likewise, I'm sure you'd find it irritating if I repeatedly wrote 'the tough, elastic fibre that joins a muscle to a bone' instead of simply using the word 'tendon'. So I'll use a few anatomical terms, but there won't be many, I promise.

Your whole spine is known as either your vertebral or spinal column. It consists of twenty-six bones, which are individually known as *vertebra*, stacked on top of each other. Two or more of these bones are known by the plural term *vertebrae*.

The spine has four main areas, which have common and scientific names. The upper part, the neck, consists of seven verbebrae and is called the *cervical* spine. The next part, the *thoracic* spine, is distinguished by a pair of ribs that attaches to each of the twelve vertebra. While this book is primarily directed at lower back pain, most of the principles and techniques can also be applied to problems that arise in the thoracic spine.

Below the thorax is our main area of interest, the lower back, or *lumbar* spine. This area has five vertebrae, whose main task is to provide movement. If you have ever experienced lower back pain, I'll bet you sometimes wished that this part didn't exist.

The lumbar spine sits atop a large triangular bone called the *sacrum*, which connects the lower back to the pelvis. The sacrum is an interesting bone, consisting of five vertebrae that fused during the evolutionary process.

THE STRUCTURE AND FUNCTION OF YOUR SPINE

The point at which the sacrum meets the pelvis is known as the *sacro-iliac joint* (say-cro-ill-ee-ack). Known as the SIJ to its mates, this joint does not bend or move very far, as it is fixed in place by many strong ligaments. However, it still contributes to your overall spinal movement by a sliding and gliding motion of the adjacent joint surfaces. These small positional changes at the sacro-iliac joint help to absorb shock, and allow the pelvis to adjust when the lower back moves. Like all joints in the lower back, the sacro-iliac joint can be injured, and can cause pain.

If you have been counting, you will notice that we have now covered twenty-five vertebrae, not twenty-six. The missing bone is the *coccyx* (cox-six) which is a tiny triangular bone that attaches to the bottom of your sacrum. This bone is the remnants of what was once your tail, tens of millions of years ago. The coccyx now sadly lacks any major functional use, and is about as useful to you as is your appendix. Does this mean that the coccyx never hurts? Unfortunately, no. The coccyx still finds a way to be involved in a few different pain syndromes, which we will investigate later.

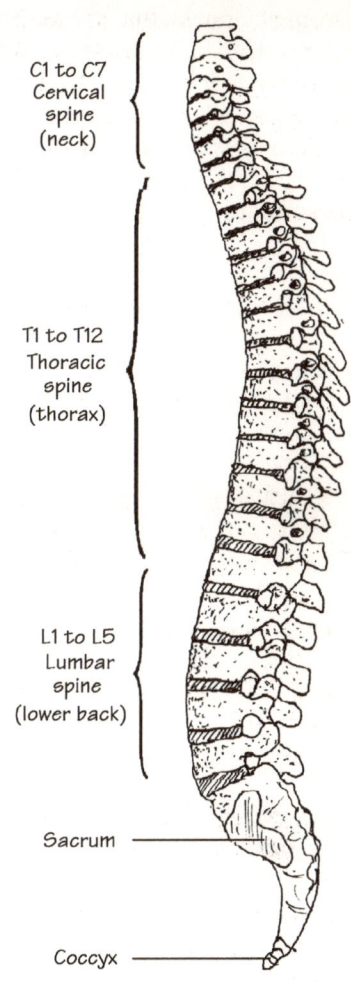

A side view of the whole spine, showing the cervical, thoracic and lumbar areas, as well as the sacrum and the coccyx.

Some textbooks report that the spine has thirty-three bones, not twenty-six as stated above. This difference arises because some health practitioners count the vertebrae that fused to form the sacrum and coccyx as individual bones. Personally, I think that this counting method is a bit outdated. The vertebrae melded together in the evolutionary process a couple of hundred million years ago!

A simple code is used to name each individual vertebra. A letter represents the area—either a 'C', a 'T' an 'L' or an 'S'. You can probably guess that these letters represent the four main areas of the spine: Cervical, Thoracic, Lumbar and Sacral. The coccyx, I guess because the cervical spine already took the letter 'C', does not score an abbreviated nickname. The poor coccyx, doomed not only to a useless existence, but to a complicated, unabbreviated name as well.

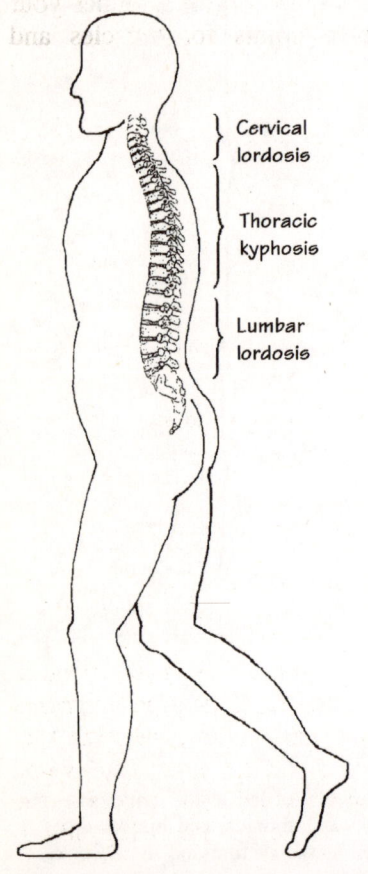

The big names for the curves of your spine.

A number is then added that signifies to which bone you are referring. For example, the first bone in the neck is known as C1, the ninth vertebra in the thorax is T9, while the last bone in the lumbar spine is called L5. (You should also be aware that the Bananas in Pyjamas are known as B1 and B2, and that little robot from *Star Wars* was called R2D2, although I admit this has nothing to do with back pain whatsoever.)

Viewed from the side, your spine resembles an elongated 'S' shape. Some areas curve inwards in a concave fashion, while some curve outwards. In what was probably a move designed simply to confuse ordinary people like you and me, these curves have complicated names. An inward curve in your spine is called a *lordosis*, while a convex curve is known as a *kyphosis*. So, in a normal standing posture, your lower back and neck have a lordosis, while your thoracic spine has a kyphosis. Later, we will see how maintaining the balance of these curves is vital to protecting your spine.

The building blocks of your spine, the vertebrae, have fascinating shapes. The main part of a vertebra, the body, is an oval-shaped cylinder of bone. Actually, it's not really oval shaped—that's just how anatomy textbooks describe it. For me, the vertebral body looks more like a kidney bean.

Projecting off this kidney-bean-shaped body is an arch of bone. When all your vertebrae are stacked on top of each other, this arch forms

THE STRUCTURE AND FUNCTION OF YOUR SPINE

a tunnel through which your spinal cord traverses from your brain to your limbs. Thus, a very hard, stable tunnel of bone protects these vital nerve fibres.

The bony arch has bumps of bone that protrude from it at various angles. If you look at a vertebra from the top, you will see two arms of bone that extend sideways, and one, the *spinous process*, that juts straight backwards. You can feel the spinous process under your skin. These three arms act as anchorage points for muscles and ligaments.

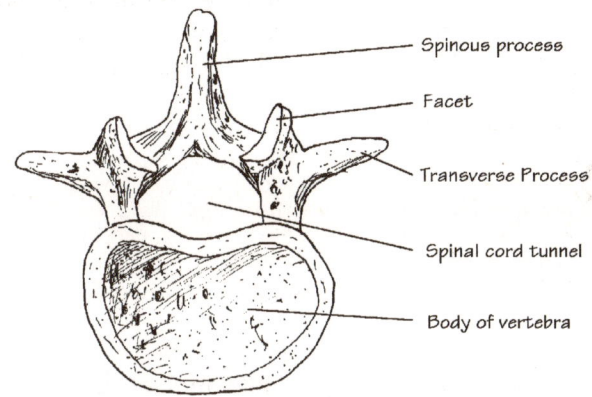

A standard lumbar vertebra, when viewed from the top. See what I mean about the kidney bean? Note also the pointy bits—the processes—and the hole that forms a tunnel for the spinal cord.

The leverage provided by these three arms makes the spine far more efficient. If your vertebrae did not have these bumps, then the ligaments and muscles would have to be far stronger and thicker, meaning that your spine would lose much of its flexibility. It's a great idea when you think about it—using little pointy bits of bone to increase the strength of your spine, without sacrificing its flexibility. A big tick to whoever thought of that one.

Each vertebral arch has four other protrusions on its arch called *facets*. One pair of these facets point up, the other pair points down. When the bones are arranged on top of each other as in a normal spine, each pair of facets connects snugly with the corresponding pair of facets from the next vertebra. Held together by the obligatory ligaments, these articulations are called—wait for it—the *zygapophyseal* joints.

As this word has far too many syllables to be used without sounding pretentious, we'll just call them the *facet joints*. These small joints help to guide and control the movement of your spine. Without them, your torso would be very unstable and floppy. Problems that can affect other

BACK PAIN

joints—such as ligament sprains, swelling, or arthritis—can also affect your facet joints.

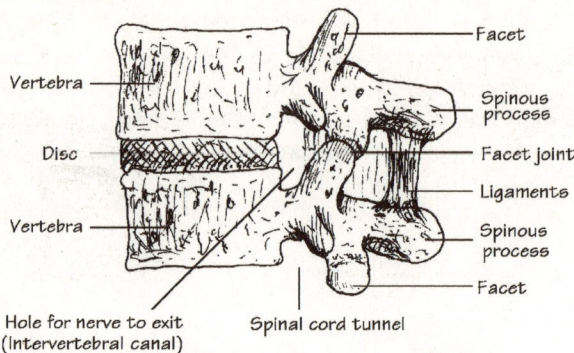

Two vertebrae mating ... er, sorry ... joined together. Note how the facets fit snugly upon each other, forming a facet joint. I've also shown a few ligaments, although normally there's a lot more. Originally I tried to include them all, but the picture looked like a ball of steel wool.

Each vertebra has one other very important connection with its neighbouring bones: a tough, sponge-like structure known as an *intervertebral disc*, or just plain old 'disc' for short. The discs help to absorb pressure and cushion shock, while also allowing some movement between the bones. To help them achieve these aims, they have a very clever structure, comprising a series of leathery rings around a soft centre. (See diagram on the next page.)

The soft centre, or nucleus, of the disc gradually dries and hardens as we age. When we are young, the nucleus of the disc is very liquid. 'Vanilla pudding' and 'jelly' are two terms often used to describe its consistency, although to me these sound more like my favourite desserts.

By the time we are twenty, the nucleus has already started to dehydrate, and by our late forties it is like thick toothpaste. When we are in our sixties, the once nubile nucleus is said to resemble, and I quote, 'crab meat'. Those anatomy experts really have a thing about food, don't they?

To hold the nucleus in place, the disc uses concentric rings of tough fibre known as the *annulus*. These sinewy layers are aligned with a criss-crossed pattern, with one layer slanting diagonally down from left to right, with the next layer tilting in the other direction. This arrangement is sensible, as it ensures that the disc can withstand twisting forces in both directions. If one layer of fibre loosens, the fibres on the opposite slant become more taut. In this way the annulus

THE STRUCTURE AND FUNCTION OF YOUR SPINE

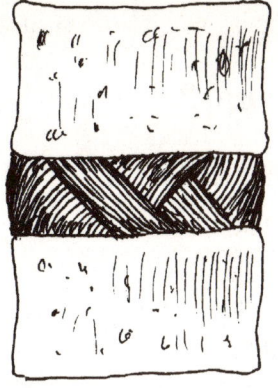 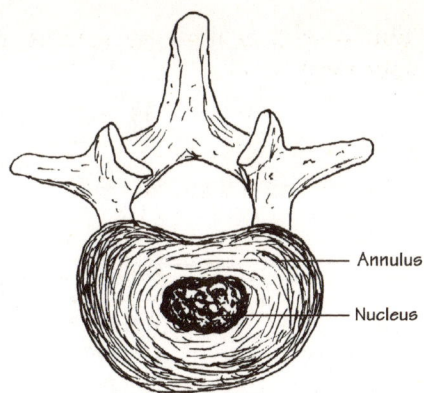

A simplified front view of two vertebrae, showing the criss-crossed orientation of the fibres of the annulus.

A top view of a standard lumbar vertebra, showing the disc. The nucleus is the dark blob in the middle.

retains a firm hold over the nucleus no matter which way you turn.

Finally, many nerves exit the spine to travel to the limbs and trunk, while groups of muscles support and move the spine. As we will be discussing muscles and nerves later in the book, I'm going to ignore them for now. You've already had enough big words for one chapter.

In summary, evolution has designed for us a system of twenty-six strangely shaped vertebrae that form our spinal columns. By using the bony bumps to increase its efficiency, and facet joints and discs to guide the movement, the spine can bend in almost any direction without losing stability. An ingenious tunnel of bone protects the spinal cord, just as it did with those early elasmobranches. Somehow, the whole thing manages to stay upright for two-legged gait.

The spine has come a long way in just 500 million years, hasn't it?

3
What goes wrong?

How to reduce 129 million problems to just three

Back pain is never simple. The spine has potential for an almost infinite variety of problems, which can arise from *any* of its anatomical structures; pain can emanate from not only the discs, joints and ligaments, but the muscles and nerves as well.

To cloud any attempt at an accurate diagnosis even further, the problem may not be isolated to just one type of structure, but spread across a range of interrelated anatomical bits and pieces. For example, an injured disc can push on a nerve, which then causes a muscle to spasm in another part of the back.

Not only that, but injuries can affect each of these structures in many different ways. Consider a facet joint, which can sprain, degenerate, or sometimes even fracture.

To illustrate how difficult arriving at a perfect diagnosis can be, pretend for a moment that the lumbar spine consists only of the bones and joints, and ignore the muscles, nerves, tendons and everything else. Your lower back has five discs, ten facet joints and two sacroiliac joints, making a combined total of seventeen joints. Also, pretend that you can only injure them in two different ways: stiff or unstable, for example. Some simple mathematics will tell you that the total number of potential problems from these seventeen joints is a staggering 129,140,163!

If you are like me, then you consider the term 'simple mathematics' to be an oxymoron. Nevertheless, some readers may be wondering how I derived the seemingly unbelievable number of 129 million different types of back pain from such a simplified situation. This figure represents 3^{17}, i.e. three multiplied by itself seventeen times. This calculation assumes that any combination of joints, from a single joint through to all seventeen joints simultaneously, may be causing the pain. OK, I admit this is highly theoretical argument, but at least it illustrates how difficult it can be to precisely diagnose back pain.

Does this huge number of potential problems mean that no one will ever properly diagnose your back injury? Should you simply concede that your back pain is too complex, and that it will never be cured? Perhaps you should just quit your job, ignore the housework, let the garden overgrow, and retire to a deck chair to sip on a cool drink for

WHAT GOES WRONG?

the rest of your days. Well, as tempting as that may sound . . . no.

Your spine has weak links that are often the first places to break down. So while your spine may have problem number 129,140,162, chances are that you are suffering from a well-defined condition. Moreover, many spinal health practitioners are adept at diagnosing such problems, and sometimes even know how to fix them!

Let's now look at the three basic categories of lower back problems. After that, we'll look at about a dozen specific common conditions in detail. There are three broad groups of spinal problems:

1. Trauma
2. Wear and tear

and, that wonderful group that covers everything else that is too complicated to neatly fit into any other category:

3. Other.

Let's now look briefly at the characteristics of these three main groups.

Trauma

Trauma, as defined by my dictionary, is: **trauma** /ˈtrɔmə/, *n.*, *pl.* **-mata** / -mətə/, **-mas**. 1. Pathol. a . . .

Oh, who cares what the dictionary says. I could never understand what all those little upside-down letters mean anyway. Put simply, trauma is an injury sustained by a *violent force*.

By violent, I mean *violent*. A sneeze does not count as violent, nor does picking up a box. Moreover, I don't consider that sexual activity is violent, not even very acrobatic sex . . . none that I have ever been involved in, at any rate.

Usually a traumatic injury will involve high speed, such as a car crash or sporting accident, or a great force, such as a collapsing wall. In other words, traumatic back pain is readily distinguishable by its *history*. Humpty Dumpty was a classic example.

The symptoms of physical trauma are very recognisable: bruising, swelling, and severe and/or unusual pain. The location and extent of the injury will not follow any typical pattern, as these signs depend on other factors, such as the shape of the bumper bar that hit you, or how much alcohol you consumed before attempting to walk home past the seaside cliffs.

If you are unlucky enough to suffer from a traumatic injury to your vertebral column, then you will probably require specialist help. By all means try the principles outlined in this book, but be aware that your injury might respond differently to 'normal' back pain.

Wear and tear

The vast majority of people who complain of back problems, which probably includes you, suffer from wear and tear of some description. The main characteristic of these injuries is that the pain resulted from a nonviolent incident. It includes those people who first felt their symptoms after undertaking an activity that was unusual, or after attempting a job that was heavy, prolonged or repetitive. This group also includes people whose pain simply starts for no apparent reason.

Some typical histories associated with wear-and-tear injuries include:

- I was just trying to move the piano a few metres . . .
- It was match point, and as I lunged for the winning volley I felt a twinge . . .
- I must have slept on it strangely . . .
- We drove back from the country last weekend . . .
- My boss has been annoying me at work, so I'm feeling really stressed . . .
- I just bent over to tie my shoelaces and felt something go . . .

As you can see from this list, our natural human reaction is to look for a cause—someone or something to blame—for our back pain. Most people implicate the activity that immediately preceded their pain, like tying their shoelaces, for example. They heap all the blame for their lower back problem upon this single unfortunate incident, and respond by buying a pair of Velcro sandals, vowing never to tie another set of shoelaces again.

But wait! Before you spend your hard-earned dollars on footwear that will cast your wardrobe back to the 'seventies, think about the situation more carefully. You've tied your shoelaces thousands of times before without any problems. Why did the pain start this time?

The reason that your pain began suddenly is that your spine had already developed considerable wear and tear. You may have felt a few warning signs, such as a few twinges here and there, a bit of stiffness in the mornings, perhaps some backache 'like everybody gets'. Or you may not have felt any warning signs at all. Either way, your back would not have broken down in such a simple situation had it been strong and healthy. Almost certainly, your spine had already degenerated, and this incident was simply letting you know that your spine had reached its breaking point.

The shoelace-tying incident was, to use a badly chosen metaphor, the straw that broke the camel's back.

A spine that is one hundred per cent healthy can withstand amazingly high pressure. Consider the gruelling force that some athletes exert on their spines—a Rugby prop forward, for example. Or think of the punishment absorbed by the lower back of a builder's labourer who lifts a hundred railway sleepers before he's even downed his first meat pie for the day.

The reason that your back pain arrived so suddenly after tying your shoelaces, with so little provocation, is best understood if you think of your spine as being similar to a light bulb.

Every night, you walk into, say, your bedroom, and switch on the light. You repeat this process hundreds of times, night after night after night. Then one evening, without warning or fanfare, the light flickers, emits a mild hiss, and dies. Usually, of course, this happens when your wife is already in the car, honking the horn with increasing regularity, while you search frantically in the dark for your bow tie ... but I digress.

What happened to the light bulb? Simply, the wear and tear in the filament had progressed to the point where it could no longer manage. So it collapsed.

No sensible person would assume that the light bulb expired because of the way that they flicked the switch. Your lower back is the same. The daily grind to which you subject your spine gradually wears it away. Slowly but steadily, the years take their toll, sometimes without any warning signs at all. Then, one day, for no apparent reason, your spine 'goes'. Just like a light bulb.

If a qualified light technician had carefully examined the light bulb's filament a week or so before it blew, he or she could probably have told you that it was deteriorating. In the same way, if a competent spinal health practitioner examined your back just before the onset of your pain, then the damage would already have been evident. However, no one ever checks their light bulbs in advance. Unfortunately, most people take the same attitude with their spines. We prefer, for some reason, to find out the hard way.

The term for this process of gradual deterioration is *repetitive microtrauma*. Understanding this concept is important, as it underlies almost every non-traumatic spinal injury. Microtrauma refers to tiny injuries; injuries that are so small that you cannot feel them. Yet when the damage accumulates over many years it can reach a devastating level.

To explain further how accumulated microtrauma relates to lower back pain, we should also consider how the body attempts to heal these insidious injuries.

When performing your usual daily activities, many normal stresses and strains are placed upon the discs, ligaments and bones. These stresses cause microscopic damage that is quite normal, and is usually so insignificant that you don't realise that it has occurred. Usually the body heals these injuries quickly, so that the tissues have repaired themselves by the next day.

However, if the activity that caused the microtrauma was too stressful, or is repeated too frequently, then your body cannot fully repair the microscopic tears in time. When you again stress the now slightly injured tissues, further microtrauma is the result. As this cycle continues, the inflammation and scar tissue steadily accumulate. Of course, these changes further weaken your spine, rendering it even more vulnerable to injury. A vicious cycle develops. After days, weeks or even years, you suddenly notice pain or stiffness. An injury!

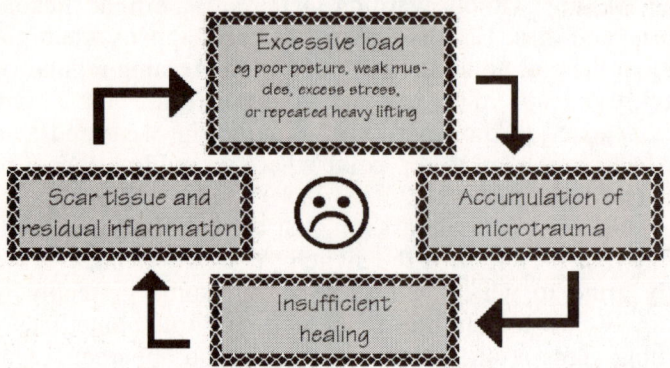

The vicious cycle of microtrauma, from which it can sometimes be very difficult to escape. Hence the sad face.

Often during my years of clinical practice I have explained to patients that their sudden or recent back pain was due to the gradual degeneration associated with repetitive microtrauma. Most patients naturally then ask what caused the degeneration. This very simple question has a very complex answer!

My usual time-limited response was to cite a few straightforward examples such as poor posture, stress and bad habits, while muttering that some day I'd write a book to explain it properly. Well, here it is! Most of the chapters in this book are dedicated to unravelling the complex answer to the question of why our backs degenerate with such alarming frequency.

Suffice to say at this stage that most back pain, probably including yours, is due to repetitive microtrauma.

Other causes of lower back pain

This broad band of spinal problems covers all those pesky conditions that won't fit neatly into one of the previous categories. They range from common conditions such as an achey flu, to the downright serious,

WHAT GOES WRONG?

such as spinal cancer. Luckily, most of the nasty conditions are rare. I've listed some other causes of back pain here, not to alarm you, but so that you are aware that they exist:

- cancer and other tumours
- viral conditions, such as the flu, Ross River Fever, etc.
- shingles
- kidney problems
- inflammatory conditions, such as ankylosing spondylitis
- stomach ulcers
- tuberculosis
- meningitis
- infected bones
- lung problems
- gall bladder problems
- an aortic aneurism (a weakened blood vessel in your tummy).

Below is a list of warning signs that may suggest that your problem is serious. Spinal health practitioners call these signs 'red flags'. *Please read them carefully*. If you have any of these warning signs then don't be brave or overly fearful: make an immediate appointment with your doctor.

- Constant pain that never varies in intensity.
- Pins and needles or numbness that does not vary in intensity.
- Pins and needles in both feet or hands that are in a 'sock' or 'glove' distribution.
- Back pain that began with another illness.
- Recent unexplained weight loss.
- Problems elsewhere, such as unexplained vomiting, fever or shortness of breath.
- Severe headaches and neck stiffness that are associated with your back pain.
- Family or personal history of cancer or other serious pathology.
- Persistent morning pain and stiffness that takes more than two hours to warm up.
- Unusual skin rashes that occur with your spinal pain.
- Weakness or severe clumsiness in the legs.
- Pins and needles or numbness in the genital region, particularly if it is combined with incontinence or bowel disturbances.
- Pain that is worse with rest, particularly persistent night pain.
- Back pain that began following a urinary tract infection.
- Night sweats.

Do you have any of these signs? If so, put this book down, go to the telephone, and make an appointment with your doctor. Go on, do it now.

Let's look at three simple cases to further illustrate the difference between trauma, wear and tear, and unusual spinal pathology:

Graham, a 22-year-old salesman, went out on the town to celebrate his football team's win. After stumbling out of a taxi at three in the morning, he somehow negotiated the nine steps that lead up to his front door. Fearing his wife's rebuke for his late homecoming, he leaned over the railing to pick a flower as a peace offering. In his drunken state he overbalanced and plummeted downwards, landing awkwardly on his back atop a box full of garden tools. He felt something crack in his spine, and experienced considerable discomfort as he crawled back up the stairs. The next morning he felt very stiff, and experienced a stabbing pain in his spine with every step. His back sported a large bruise shaped suspiciously like a garden trowel.

Deirdre, a 35-year-old manager, had experienced very little previous back pain. A couple of times her thoracic spine had ached during stressful periods at work, but apart from those minor incidents her back had remained healthy. During the first game of the new netball season, Deirdre felt her back twinge as she lunged for a goal-saving intercept. The next morning she felt very stiff as she dressed for work. The pain continued to increase during her first sales meeting. By mid afternoon her symptoms were unbearable, and she was unable to sit for even five minutes without agonising pain. At this point Deirdre's secretary drove her home and she retired to bed.

Paul is a 45-year-old engineering consultant. He is unfit and a heavy smoker. About two months ago he noticed a gnawing ache in his lower back, but as he was very busy at work he declined to see a spinal health practitioner. Two weeks later he felt some pins and needles in his left calf, but again ignored this sign as he was now even busier. Although mild, the symptoms were very persistent, and Paul could not find a position that relieved his pain. Nevertheless, by rubbing his spine with liniment and taking regular doses of aspirin, Paul could continue working. The pain gradually progressed until Paul felt it continuously, with almost no variation except after taking the pain-relieving drugs. The pins and needles often kept him awake at night. His wife Grace had been nagging him to seek treatment, so he finally decided that he would make an appointment—when he had time, of course.

Can you deduce the type of injury with which each person is afflicted?

Graham, silly fellow, suffered a spinal trauma, while Deirdre has degeneration caused by repetitive microtrauma. Paul is the unluckiest of all—he has spinal cancer. Notice that the intensity of the symptoms does not necessarily show the severity of the underlying condition.

I hope that you can now see the difference between the three main causes of spinal pain. For the rest of this book, we'll concentrate on the second category, wear and tear, which constitutes a vast majority of all back pain cases.

Wear and tear can affect your spine in many different ways and places. Spinal health practitioners use many different terms to diagnose these problems. You may be told that you are suffering from a low back sprain, lumbago, soft tissue damage, a slipped disc, a touch of arthritis, spondylosis, degenerative joint disease, sciatica, a pinched nerve, or any one of a thousand other labels. What do these terms all mean?

Over the next few chapters, we will look at the spine piece by piece. By examining each structure individually, you will see how wear and tear usually affects the lower back. You will see, in an uncluttered, straightforward way, the problems that commonly afflict the spine.

The purpose of this discussion is *not* to help you diagnose your own problem—that task is best left to a qualified spinal health practitioner. However, you will at least develop a clearer understanding of the most often-quoted causes of spinal pain.

4
Intervertebral disc injuries
Middle-aged mayhem

The intervertebral discs are one of the most common causes of lower back pain. Their awkward tilted position at the bottom of the back (a legacy from our ancestral four-legged days) means that the stresses and strains of everyday life take a very destructive toll on the disc tissue.

Yet despite this anatomical vulnerability, I believe that disc injuries are frequently overdiagnosed or misdiagnosed. Unfortunately, some spinal health practitioners use 'lower disc injury' as their one and only diagnosis of back pain. Certainly, the discs in the lower back are responsible for many problems—most good research suggests about forty per cent. They are not, however, the only cause of back pain, as some practitioners would have you believe.

Furthermore, saying that you have 'done a disc' does not give you very much useful information. Imagine how you would feel if you went to a practitioner with a sore foot, only to be told that you had 'done your foot'. Yet, because of the widespread ignorance of lower back pain, the diagnosis of 'done a disc' seems to be generally acceptable. Not good enough!

We will now discuss three common ways in which the disc can be injured:

- disc bulging due to weakness
- a prolapsed disc
- spondylosis.

We will also briefly discuss what effect these injuries have on the function of your spine.

Disc bulging due to weakness

Recall that the disc is composed of two main parts: a series of leathery fibrous rings called the annulus, which surround a jelly-like nucleus. During your normal day-to-day activities, the nucleus exerts enormous pressure on those fibrous rings. Researchers have performed experiments in which they inserted tiny pressure gauges into the discs of

INTERVERTEBRAL DISC INJURIES

living subjects, and found that even while resting in bed, the nucleus created a force of about 25 mmHg inside the disc. This pressure rose to 50 while standing, 70 during normal sitting, and a staggering 200 mmHg during forward bending.

Although these forces are high, they are usually comfortably within the holding capability of the annulus—if it is healthy and strong. However, if the annulus's fibres weaken through wear and tear, then they may have difficulty in firmly containing the nucleus. The whole segment becomes unstable. Here, the pressure of the nucleus causes the annulus to bulge outwards, which can sometimes cause pain and stiffness.

Not only that, but the bulge can then impact on other structures such as nerves or ligaments, causing even further pain. We will talk more about nerve injuries in Chapters 8 and 9. The symptoms of a clinically evident weakened disc range from mild aches to agonising pain.

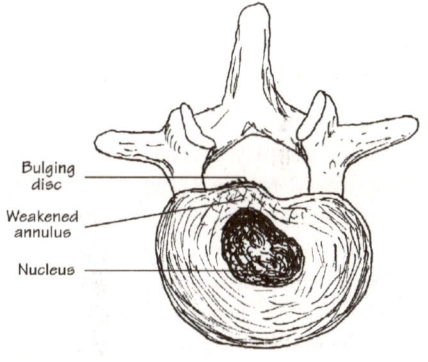

A weakened annulus can allow the nucleus to bulge.

A prolapsed disc

Sometimes, particularly in cases of severe degeneration or trauma, the annulus can completely tear. This creates a channel from the nucleus to the outside of the disc. Any further strain can completely squeeze the nucleus from the centre of the disc, literally like toothpaste from a tube. This severe condition is known as a *prolapsed disc*, or is sometimes called a *disc herniation*.

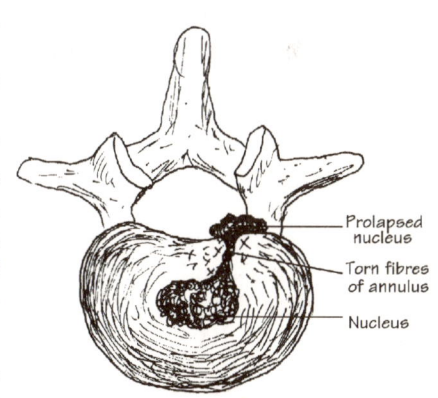

The squeezed-out nucleus then causes a violent inflammatory reaction, which, no doubt, feels like a red-hot branding iron pressing into your back. This nasty response occurs because the infection-fighting cells in your blood do not recognise the nucleus, and attack it as though it were a foreign body.

In the case of a herniated disc, some of the nucleus is completely squeezed out from the centre of the disc.

This may sound like a stupid thing for your cells to do. However, it

BACK PAIN

makes a bit more sense if you realise that your blood stream is never supposed to have contact with the nucleus. In a healthy spine, the nucleus is wholly contained by the annulus from conception until death. However, this situation does not hold for anyone unfortunate enough to suffer a prolapsed disc, resulting in the immune system attacking the nucleus as though it were an unwelcome intruder, such as a germ, or even a splinter.

The symptoms of a true prolapsed disc can be very unpleasant: excruciating pain that accompanies every movement, severe muscle spasms, and even shock-type reactions, such as profuse sweating and clammy hands.

Luckily nature gave us a defence mechanism against these debilitating injuries: the gradual hardening of the nucleus as we age. Thankfully, the outer fibres of the disc are still healthy enough to contain the nucleus when we are young. By the time we are seniors, our disc has dehydrated to the 'crab meat' stage. Obviously, crab meat cannot possibly herniate, so our senior citizens are also safe from the agony of a true disc prolapse.

However, those people aged 30 to 50 years have a problem: the nucleus is still reasonably mobile, but the outer annulus fibres have often started to deteriorate. It will come as no surprise to you that this age group has the peak incidence of disc-related back pain.

Does this mean that older people do not suffer from disc-related lower back pain? Unfortunately, no. The outer fibres of the disc can still tear, become inflamed, and so cause pain. Translated into medical-speak, a stiff and inflamed disc is known as spondylosis, which we will now discuss.

Spondylosis

Spondylosis is a frequent cause of backache. Literally meaning 'stiff vertebrae', this condition is found frequently among those of us who are more than thirty years old.

Spondylosis develops when the annulus suffers from repetitive microtrauma. Like most injuries, the annulus heals these tiny tears with scar tissue. Unfortunately, this scar tissue does not stretch as elastically as do the normal annulus fibres, meaning that the disc becomes stiffer than normal. This tightness renders the disc even more vulnerable to further microtrauma, which produces even more scarring.

Can you see how quickly a vicious circle develops? A tear leads to scar tissue that causes stiffness, which leads to further tearing and scar tissue, which begets even more stiffness.

After this cycle has revolved many times, the disc becomes so tight that it blocks the vertebrae above and below from moving properly. The lower back joints seize up like a rusty hinge. Subsequently, your back becomes inflamed, painful and generally feels stiff to move.

The entire degenerative process can take months, years, or even decades to reach the painful stage. Like most wear and tear type injuries, spondylosis builds silently and painlessly, until one day an unusual activity—a heavy lift, a long drive, or an unaccustomed sporting activity, for example—provokes a more sizeable tear of the annulus. Spinal health practitioners call this situation an acute-on-chronic injury, meaning that an old injury has suffered from a new tear.

As you can deduce from the above three conditions, disc injuries sometimes become chronic, long-lasting conditions. The vulnerability of the disc tissue, combined with the ongoing stress that we heap upon our lower backs, often produce a vicious cycle of microtrauma. Both factors have to be addressed to effectively control disc-related pain.

Later, you will learn both prevention techniques and rehabilitation exercises. We will now turn our attention to other frequent pain-producing structures of the lumbar spine.

5
Facet and sacro-iliac joint injuries
Sprains, strains and rusty bones

Recall that the facet joints form a connection from each vertebra to those above and below, while the two sacro-iliac joints connect the sacrum to the pelvis. Problems that can affect other joints, such as ligament sprains and arthritis, can also affect these joints.

Ligament sprains

Like all joints in the body, the facet and sacro-iliac joints are held together by tough fibrous ligaments. If these ligaments are subject to traumatic force, or if they are repeatedly stressed, then they can tear or weaken.

The simplest way to classify ligament tears is as a grade one, two or three. A grade one tear means that although the fibres have been injured, they are all still intact, while a grade two sprain implies that some fibres have snapped. A grade three sprain is the worst, as it means that the ligament has totally ruptured.

Paradoxically, a grade two sprain is often more painful than a grade three tear. This unexpected effect occurs because a second-degree tear heals with scar tissue, which can be very painful when moved or stretched. However, a ligament with a third-degree rupture does not usually reattach or repair itself, and so cannot produce pain as it theoretically no longer exists!

Spraining a healthy back ligament is no easy task. This injury would require a violent traumatic force, probably with an unusual direction or twist as well. However, a ligament with prior degeneration is far more vulnerable. Here, a simple action such as an incorrect lift might sprain a facet joint. Likewise, an everyday activity such as jumping off a low bench might strain the sacro-iliac joint, which normally absorbs the shearing strains and jarring forces of such an action.

What happens to your back if you sprain a ligament? The response of the back ligaments is identical to ligaments in other parts of your body: the underlying joint becomes inflamed, is painful to move, and swells (although the puffiness from sprained spinal joints is not usually visible from the surface of the skin). Think of a sprained ankle and you'll get the general picture.

When the sprain settles, two possible outcomes can lead to ongoing back pain. First, the thickening and tightness of the scar tissue make the whole joint stiff and immobile. Conversely, the ligament may not knit tightly enough, meaning that the joint becomes loose and unstable.

If your back joints become either stiff or unstable, then the potential for future wear-and-tear is increased. Naturally, each type of injury requires a different approach to achieve its best resolution. We will discuss the subjects of joint stiffness and instability in detail later in the book, as they are very important concepts to your understanding of back pain.

Coccydynia

This condition, with the wonderful sounding name of cox-ee-din-ee-ah, is the common term for a sprain of the ligaments that hold the coccyx to the sacrum.

As the coccyx no longer has a real function and does not bear any weight, it rarely suffers from degenerative injuries. Due to its sheltered position, there is only one way that you can sprain it: by falling onto a hard surface and landing on your bottom. Ouch!

Many years ago, surgeons decided that as the coccyx was a rather useless piece of bone, they might as well just remove it from anyone suffering with pain in this area. Coccygectomy, I believe, was the medical term for this procedure. However, they soon noticed an unexpected result: about three-quarters of their patients were experiencing just as much pain in their coccyx, even though the bone was in a jar on their mantelpiece. How could this be? The answer will be revealed in Chapter 9. Hint: It has something to do with the nerves.

Arthritis

Arthritis is common in the sacro-iliac joint and facet joints in the spine. The discs and vertebrae are also frequently diagnosed with arthritis, which is another way of saying advanced spondylosis.

Very few concepts in medicine are misunderstood as frequently as is arthritis. Mountains of misinformation, half-baked opinions and bad advice have confused the truth about what is really a remarkably simple condition.

I'll be straightforward. Arthritis is simply wear and tear of a joint.

Pretty boring, heh? Just plain old wear and tear, not the lifelong agonising condition that the word 'arthritis' conjures up in most people's minds. Sure, some people have a genetic predisposition to developing arthritis. But for most people, arthritis is simply wear and tear that was left unchecked.

To further understand the meaning of arthritis, let's do what medical people do, and break the word into its Latin (or was it Greek?) roots. The first part, *arth*, means 'joint'. For example, an *arth*roscopy means 'to look into a joint'. The second part of the word, *itis*, means 'inflamed'. An inflamed appendix is therefore known as appendic*itis*, an inflamed pharynx as pharyng*itis* while inflamed tonsils are called ... I'll let you guess.

Put these two bits, *arth* and *itis* together, and they mean simply 'inflamed joint'. So how does the joint become inflamed? Through wear and tear, of course.

I hope that you now understand that arthritis is simply joint wear and tear resulting from years of accumulated microtrauma. Got it? Good. Now, I'm going to confuse you a bit.

In this discussion, I am referring to the common condition of *osteo-arthritis*. This type of arthritis commonly affects the spine, hips and knees. However, there are about 150 other sorts of arthritis that fall into a completely separate category. Some of their complicated names include *ankylosing spondylitis*, *juvenile chronic arthritis* and *rheumatoid arthritis*. In contrast to normal osteo-arthritis, these conditions *are* diseases, and can usually be detected by means of a blood test.

The symptoms of these other arthritic diseases vary. Some of them are associated with skin rashes, lumps and bumps, while others cause generalised aching and stiffness. The pain associated with these diseases ranges from boring aches to a complete severe crippling of all the joints. But don't fret: most of these diseases are rare, and many, such as rheumatoid arthritis, do not usually affect the lower back.

If you have one of these conditions, then you should still uphold the principles of back care described in this book, but be aware that your condition probably requires specialist management.

Whenever I diagnose someone as suffering from spinal wear and tear, I avoid using the word 'arthritis', as it is too easily confused with the above conditions. Why use an ambiguous term when 'degeneration' or 'wear and tear' are less confusing and more descriptive? So for the rest of this book, the word 'arthritis' will refer to normal, common osteoarthritis, not its more sinister namesakes. Let's now take a closer look at other aspects of this much-misunderstood condition.

Osteoarthritis is *not* caused by age. Sure, it's far more common in the elderly population, but it is definitely not a direct consequence of age.

FACET AND SACRO-ILIAC JOINT INJURIES

For example, some people have arthritis in one knee, while the other is fine. Yet both their knees are the same age, aren't they?

A characteristic of arthritic joints is that they sometimes make creaking, scraping noises as they are moved. The medical term for this noise is *crepitus*. Feeling or hearing coarse crepitus can make your neck hairs stand on end, just like when someone scrapes their fingernails down a blackboard, or rubs two pieces of styrofoam together. Just the thought makes me shiver.

The crepitus sound originates from the lining of cartilage that covers each joint surface. Normally, this cartilage is silky-smooth, which facilitates the gliding of the joint surfaces over each other. However, the wear and tear associated with arthritis makes the cartilage rough and ragged, which can produce a sandpaper-like crunching sensation when the joint is moved. In short, the joint surface gets rusty.

If the wear and tear continues unchecked, the two joint surfaces begin to grind each other away. Small flakes of bone and cartilage crumble off, and generally float around the joint cavity making a nuisance of themselves. Eventually the arthritis can completely denude the joint surfaces of cartilage, meaning that the bones must glide on each other's rough, chalky surface. At this point the joint becomes extremely stiff and painful, and will possibly swell.

Please, for the sake of your spinal health practitioner's sanity, seek treatment *before* your joints deteriorate to this point.

Previous joint injuries, particularly those that heal too loosely or stiffly, can predispose you to 'arthritis' later in life. This susceptibility can also occur following disc-related injuries, as the nucleus is less effective at absorbing and dissipating shock, meaning that the facet and sacro-iliac joints have an extra burden to bear.

Furthermore, a previously injured disc sometimes loses height, particularly if the nucleus herniated. If the disc is too low then the vertebral bodies sometimes rub together. Just as a builder's thumb develops a callous to protect it from the constant friction of work tools, the vertebral body responds to this frequent rubbing by developing extra layers of calcium.

Eventually, the extra calcium forms small lumps that resemble a series of small parrot beaks. These outgrowths, known as *osteophytes*, are not intrinsically painful. However, they can cause plenty of trouble if they impact on other pain-sensitive structures, such as nerves.

Once the degeneration has progressed to this stage, it is usually visible on X-ray pictures. Despite this fact, it is very misleading to diagnose arthritis using X-rays alone. Consider a typical case, in which the patient has been experiencing pain for, say, two weeks. Upon sighting the degeneration on the X-ray, the patient is told that they have the dreaded affliction of arthritis, and are often informed that they will 'just have to learn to live with it'. This bad advice is often reinforced with fallacies such as 'you're just getting old', and 'treated' with handfuls of pain-killing tablets. This diagnosis and treatment are, most often, inadequate.

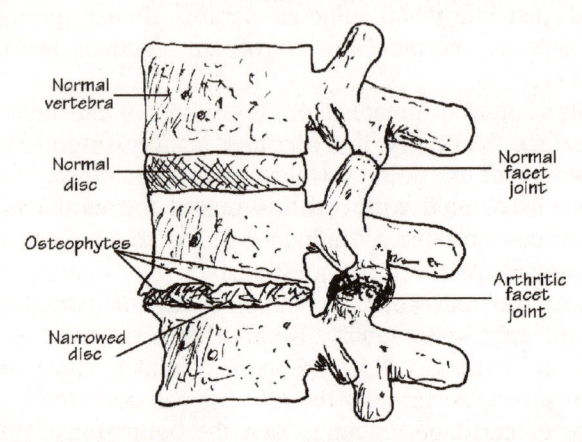

In this picture, the upper level is normal. However, the lower level has a degenerated disc and facet joint. Note the little bony outgrowths—the osteophytes—which can push on other structures, such as nerves, causing pain and stiffness.

Consider this: the facet joints and discs take years, even decades, to degenerate. Yet the X-ray would have looked practically identical had it been taken a month previously, despite the pain only being present for about two weeks. It follows that if the joints and discs could be returned to their condition of a month previously, then the pain should disappear, although 'arthritis' still shows on the X-ray.

The joint wear and tear associated with arthritis can be likened to a surgical incision in the skin: the scar may be present many years later, but it does not necessarily cause any pain or stiffness. Likewise, arthritis is not necessarily permanent. If the joint movement can be returned to normal, then the pain, inflammation and stiffness should disappear, even though the degeneration is present in the spine.

In short, please don't treat arthritis as an incurable condition. It is simply advanced wear and tear of a joint or disc. Osteo-arthritis is not a disease of the whole body, and as such there will never be a magic cure. Trying to develop an arthritis pill is as silly as producing a 'sprained ankle pill'. However, with sensible management, exercise, treatment and prevention, the symptoms of arthritis can usually be eliminated.

6
Injuries to the vertebrae
My bones are broken?

The vertebrae themselves rarely cause lower back pain. These sturdy bones are well cushioned by the discs, and held firmly in place by many ligaments that stretch between their bony arms. However, occasionally things can go astray with the structure of the bones themselves, leading to various painful conditions.

For example, the entire vertebral body can suffer with a crush fracture, which we'll talk about later in the chapter. For now, we'll talk about another pair of related conditions that can affect the bones: *stress fractures* and *displaced vertebrae*.

These two disorders have the most confusing official names in all of physical medicine. They are respectively named *spondylolisis* and *spondylolisthesis*. As you can imagine, these terms sit confusingly beside 'spondylosis', which we discussed earlier. If you're not yet confused then throw in *spondylitis*, which refers to inflamed vertebrae.

Spondylosis, spondylitis, spondylolisis, spondylolisthesis ... sorry, I needed months of study at university to remember these names, so I was determined to use them at least one more time before we pack most of them away for the remainder of this book.

Just for fun, why not try to remember those terms to throw at the next person who gives you unwelcome advice about your sore back.

Stress fractures (Spondylolisis)

Some patients are horrified when they are diagnosed with a vertebral stress fracture. Judging from their aghast expressions, visions of life in a wheelchair flood instantly to mind. If you have a spinal stress fracture, then do not fear, for the chance of paraplegia is negligible and need not concern you. In a fracture of this type, the ligaments, discs and muscles remain intact, and provide ample support to prevent any such catastrophe.

A stress fracture, by definition, is a break in the bone that occurred *without trauma*. It is a classic example of the devastating effects of accumulated microtrauma. Of course, vertebral fractures can occur in accidents as well, in which case they are likely to have consequences that are more serious. As traumatic spinal fractures usually require specialist help, we won't be discussing them in detail.

The most common site for spinal stress fractures to develop is in the vertebral arch of the bottom two vertebrae. In particular, the point between the upper and lower facet joints is the most vulnerable area.

As stress fractures usually develop gradually, most victims do not realise that they are occurring. The back may issue some warning signs that the fracture is increasing—such as morning stiffness, pain following activity, or dull aches—while sometimes the pain can start seemingly out of the blue.

Two main factors predispose your spine to stress fractures. First, the movement of lumbar extension: i.e. bending backwards. This effect is multiplied if the extension is combined with twisting or sideways tilting. The second major cause of stress fractures is jarring, jolting or heavy-impact forces.

When these causes occur together—a jarring force while the spine is positioned in extension—massive tension is created on the vertebral arch. If the extension and jarring are repeated many times, the bone starts to weaken, and can ultimately break.

Stress fractures are more common in sports people than in the general population. Think of the demand that certain sports place on your lumbar spine and you'll see why this is so. Activities such as gymnastics demand a high degree of lumbar extension combined with jarring. Try to envisage the huge spinal stress when those young girls do that backward flip-flop thing.

Many top-class cricketers, especially the fast bowlers, break down with lumbar stress fractures every year. In particular, those bowlers whose delivery action is neither fully front-on nor fully side-on have the most trouble. This type of activity—spinal extension, combined with a half twist, superimposed with a heavy jarring force and repeated often—is a sure recipe for a stress fracture. Kicking a football, weight-lifting, surfing, serving a tennis ball and diving also place similar high-risk demands on your lower back.

Displaced vertebra (Spondylolisthesis)

You might have heard the term 'slipped disc' being used to describe back pain. This term has no medical meaning, and is simply a common expression for a bulging or prolapsing disc. When talking here about a 'displaced vertebra' I am referring to an entirely different condition.

A displaced vertebra occurs when a bone, usually one of the lowest two lumbar vertebrae, slides forward over the bone below. Please note that these slips are almost never sudden events, and are not accompanied by pain, clicking, clunking, or any other sensation.

INJURIES TO THE VERTEBRAE

Is a displaced vertebra painful? Well, funnily enough, no. The bones themselves don't cause much pain. Many people with a displaced vertebra go about their business—playing sport, dancing in nightclubs, drinking beer on the hill at the cricket, whatever—blissfully unaware that their bones are not aligned with each other.

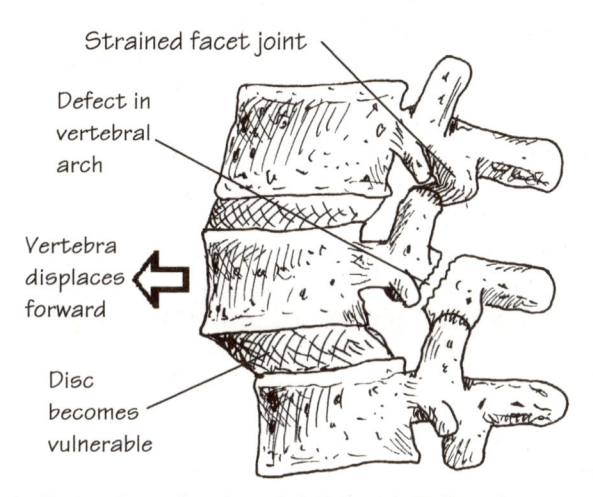

Strained facet joint

Defect in vertebral arch

Vertebra displaces forward

Disc becomes vulnerable

A displaced vertebra (spondylolisthesis). Believe it or not, but this injury is usually painless.

The displaced vertebra may possibly cause pain by pressing on other sensitive structures, such as nerves or ligaments. It also causes problems because the adjacent discs and facet joints degenerate more rapidly than usual. Without the support of each other, these structures quickly become overworked. Lucky they don't belong to a union! Once the overburdened discs and joints degenerate, they display the 'normal' signs of injury.

Displaced bones occur for three main reasons: either a breakdown of the vertebral arch, a natural birth defect, or severe degeneration.

(1) A BREAKDOWN OF THE VERTEBRAL ARCH

If the vertebral arch breaks down on both sides, half of it becomes separated from the main body of the vertebra.

Influenced by the inward curve of the lumbar spine, gravity gradually pushes the vertebral body forward, leading to the 'displaced bone' effect. This type of slip usually occurs during early childhood, and is often painless. Once growth has ceased, the bones don't go anywhere in a great hurry.

(2) NATURAL BIRTH DEFECT

Some people are simply born with wonky or incomplete vertebrae. This defect allows one bone to move forward on the other, usually in the toddler stage of life. Calling it a birth 'defect' is probably a bit harsh, as a naturally occurring displaced vertebra usually does no harm to its owner at all. As with type one, this type of slip almost never progresses in adult life.

(3) DISC AND LIGAMENT DEGENERATION
If the discs and facet joints have severe degeneration, then they may not be strong enough to withstand the ordinary stresses and strains of gravity. The pressure slowly stretches and elongates the ligaments and discs until they are too loose to effectively stabilise the vertebra. This laxity then allows one bone to gradually slide forward on the next, leading to the 'displaced vertebra'. The slippage usually takes place over several years.

Note in all causes of displaced vertebra, the vertebral arch, which shields the all-important spinal cord, maintains a relatively high level of stability.

Crush fractures

The term 'crush fracture' is wonderfully descriptive, isn't it? Simply, it refers to a condition in which the vertebral body is crushed, so it fractures. Just this once I wish that some whiz-bang medical expert would invent a more complicated name so that we spinal health practitioners could sound more intelligent when diagnosing this condition.

Like all broken bones, vertebral crush fractures are sometimes caused by violent trauma. However, crush fractures are usually associated with *osteoporosis*, a condition in which the bones become very weak and brittle.

The highest risk group for osteoporosis, and thus vertebral crush fractures, is elderly women. Almost one-third of all women over the age of sixty-five have a vertebral crush fracture. This condition varies in severity from a localised dint in the end of one vertebra, to a complete collapse of a whole row of bones.

A series of stress fractures can alter the curve of the spine. A *dowager's hump*, a hunchbacked posture which is associated with osteoporosis, is an extreme example.

A spine with multiple crush fractures will usually be painful and extremely stiff. However, as with spinal stress fractures, many people function perfectly well with one or two minor crush fractures. In the Appendix we will talk more about the risk factors, treatment and prevention of osteoporosis.

7

Muscle injuries

No such thing as a torn back muscle?

If disc injuries are the most over-diagnosed lower back complaint, then muscle tears run a close second. I believe that many people are erroneously diagnosed as having a back muscle problem when they are suffering from a disc or joint injury. Perhaps this mistake occurs because the pain associated with many lower back injuries is often *perceived* as arising from the muscles.

Why are back muscles so rarely injured? There are three simple reasons. First, muscles are, by nature, very adaptable. In contrast to most other back structures, the muscles tend to strengthen, not degenerate, with repeated or heavy use. Second, most back muscles are long and elastic, and are thus able to stretch a considerable distance before they tear. By contrast, the ligament and disc fibres are very short, and tighten long before the muscles reach their limits of extensibility. Third, muscles are very robust. Enormous force is required to tear a muscle, which would no doubt tear many other structures as well.

Also, consider that the signs of a true muscle tear—severe bruising and swelling—rarely, if ever, occur in a non-traumatic lower back injury. If your spinal health practitioner diagnoses you as having a back muscle tear then he or she is probably, in my humble opinion, misdiagnosing another injury.

However, muscles can cause pain in four instances that we'll now examine: bruising, spasm, post-exercise soreness, and 'trigger points'.

Bruising

Back muscles, like all other structures in the body, can suffer from bruises and bumps. Under normal circumstances a bruise will always be traumatic, and will be recognisable from the history of the injury. This type of injury is usually confined to the football field, the late-night pub, or other similarly violent situations.

The medical term for a bruise, *haematoma*, infers that the symptoms of bruising arise from broken blood vessels—the arteries and veins. The amount of bluish discolouration does not always represent the severity of the underlying bruise, but simply reflects how much blood escaped from the tiny blood vessels before they clotted.

Spasm

All muscles in your body can be roughly divided into two groups. The characteristics of these groups vary in many ways, one of which is their response to the injury of a nearby joint: one set of muscles weaken, while the other group tend to spasm in the same situation.

Some lower back muscles, particularly the large, surface muscles, belong to the group that go into spasm. In particular the *paravertebral* muscles, which run down the length of your vertebral column, tend to automatically tighten if you injure your lower back.

Despite being frequently diagnosed, *muscle spasm is not a primary cause of lower back pain*. It is a response to other injury; muscles don't decide to spasm by themselves! To relieve the pain associated with muscle spasms, the joint structures that caused the original pain must be addressed. Working on the muscle in isolation from the underlying problem will have very little lasting benefit.

Post-exercise soreness

Like all muscles in the body, back muscles can become sore and inflamed from overuse. If you play a rugged five-setter of tennis, followed by a session at the gym and then chop enough firewood to last until the end of winter, don't be surprised if your muscles become a tad sore. The peak discomfort from this type of problem is usually about one or two days later. Please remember that although your muscles feel sore, your pain may be arising from another source.

Trigger points

A trigger point is a small, localised thickening in a muscle, which is commonly known as a 'knot'. These knots develop in response to unremitting, long-term overload that can be due to many factors: sitting or standing with a poor posture, for example. Excessive demand can also come from frequent overuse, like a job that requires repetitive bending. Weak muscles are far more prone to being overworked than are muscles with good tone.

The condition of nearby joints also effects muscle knots. As mentioned above, an injury will cause the nearby muscles to react with either spasm or inhibition. If a joint is chronically or repeatedly injured, then the nearby muscles will constantly be irritated into spasm or inhibition. After days, weeks, or even years of this constant irritation, the muscle responds by developing trigger points in its most sensitive areas.

Trigger points tend to develop in the area that the main nerve fibres enter the muscle belly. This point is naturally more excitable than the rest of the muscle, and so is prone to a reaction, such as a localised knot.

Once they have arrived, trigger points behave like a bad guest and overstay their welcome. They can even refer pain to other areas of the spine or legs, and sometimes mimic other conditions.

Some people find that a deep massage helps to relieve their lower back pain. Often the relief is due to the relaxation of spasm, or the release of tension from trigger points. Unfortunately, the massage does not change the reason that the spasm or trigger points initially developed, so the pain returns. When dealing with muscle-related lower back pain, you must correct the underlying factors if you wish to fully cure the problem. As you will learn as this book progresses, massage alone is a poor way to treat lower back problems.

But ignore that last paragraph if you can persuade someone to give you a pleasant relaxing back rub. It's probably not going to do you any harm, and, if it feels good, why not!

8
Referred pain
Is your back problem getting on your nerves?

Nerves injuries and referred pain are the most complicated and confusing areas of lower back pain. However, as you've already survived the spondylosis-spondylitis-spondylolisis-spondylolisthesis bit, I reckon you've got a fair chance of emerging unscathed by the ruthless complexity of nerve injuries.

Don't feel worried if you find this section difficult at first. Even many spinal health practitioners misunderstand the ins-and-outs of nerve injuries, for the simple reason that they are so complicated.

So just try to get a general feel for their nature and behaviour. As the next two chapters unfold you will see how many common conditions, not only in your spine, but in your limbs as well, are caused by nerves. Let's now demystify this complex and rapidly developing area of spinal health care.

Normal nerves

Nerves have two main jobs:

- to carry signals to the muscles to make them contract
- to carry sensory signals up to the brain—these signals include sensations such as touch, warmth, vibration and texture.

Suppose you wish to move your big toe. Your brain sends a signal, which is like a mild electric current, charging down your spinal cord. The spinal cord is protected not only by the vertebrae, but also by a sheath of tough fibrous tissue that looks like an elongated sock. This canvas-like sheath is called the *dura*.

Many non-medical people have never heard of the dura, which is surprising, as it is a frequent cause of back pain and stiffness. If you would like to know what the spinal dura feels like, then find a newborn baby and poke your fingers gently around the top if its head. Eventually you will feel a soft spot, just above its forehead, that has no bony covering. (This hole gradually closes over during the baby's first year of life.) If you push gently into this hole, you will feel a firm, canvas-

REFERRED PAIN

like structure under your fingers. This is the cranial dura, which is continuous with, and very similar to, the spinal dura.

So the dura covers the brain, then extends down over the spinal cord, resembling what I imagine a tadpole's body suit would look like. At the other end, the dura attaches onto the coccyx, that tiny bone at the bottom of your sacrum. Sometimes, if your dura is not moving properly, you feel pain at this attachment point. This syndrome can cause the symptoms that fooled those knife-happy, coccyx-removing surgeons that we mentioned in Chapter 5.

When the electrical signal reaches the appropriate level of your spine, it branches sideways from the spinal cord along a small filament known as a *nerve root*. Next to the nerve root is another similar nerve root, which carries signals in the opposite direction. The two nerve roots function like opposing lanes on a highway, allowing the signals to travel in different directions without colliding.

Just as the two little nerve roots emerge from the protective covering of the dura, they combine. At this point the nerve technically becomes known as a *spinal nerve*.

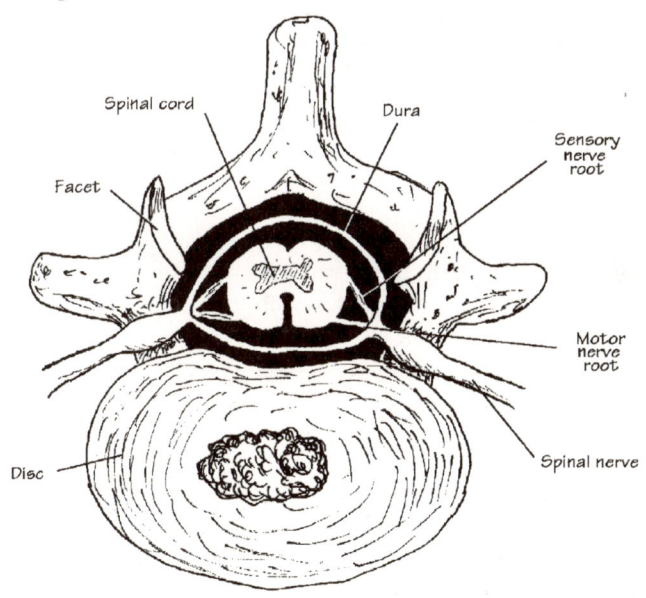

There's a lot to learn in this picture, isn't there? Let's start in the middle. That roundish, lumpy-shaped thing is the spinal cord. Those two stringy bits poking out each side are the nerve roots: the top one transmits the sensory signals, while the lower one delivers outgoing orders to your muscles. Encapsulating this whole area is the canvas-like spinal dura. You can also see the two pairs of nerve roots combining to form the spinal nerves, which exit the vertebral column through small tunnels. Whew! If you understand all of this, then you are halfway to becoming a decent spinal health practitioner.

The spinal nerve then leaves the protected sanctity of the spinal cord tunnel through a hole known as the *intervertebral canal*. These canals are formed on one side by the facet joint, and on the other side by the disc. We'll see later in the chapter how this area is a frequent site for nerve-related injuries.

Once they have passed through these small canals, the spinal nerves form a tangled mishmash of webbing. They emerge on the other side of this fishnet-type structure as *peripheral nerves*, which then travel to the trunk, hips and legs. From now on, we'll refer to 'peripheral nerves' as just good old 'nerves' for simplicity.

Are you keeping up with me? I hope that all of this complicated talk of dura, nerve roots, spinal nerves and peripheral nerves is not getting on your nerves. (Ha ha.)

Each of us has about half a dozen main nerves that travel into the legs. We'll conveniently ignore most of them, although I couldn't sleep properly at night if I didn't at least mention two: the *femoral nerve* and, importantly, the *sciatic nerve*. These two nerves are often accomplices in lower back pain. The femoral nerve travels down the front of your thigh to your knee. In contrast, the sciatic nerve travels through your buttocks and down the back of your thigh.

Many people misunderstand the nature of nerves. Just for fun, try the following one-question quiz.

Q1. The sciatic nerve is as thick as ...
   (a) a delicate strand of a spider's web
   (b) a human hair
   (c) a strand of knitting wool
   (d) a drinking straw
   (e) your little finger.

If you said (e), then congratulations! You have passed this test with the incredible grade of 100 per cent. However, if you answered with one of the first four options, do not fret, for most people are like you, and underestimate the robust nature of the nerves. They are not delicate, fine little things, but are tough, fibrous, rope-like structures, capable of withstanding tremendous forces without complaint.

I hope that you now have a rudimentary understanding of the workings of a normal nervous system. I realise that the subject is complex; you've done very well. Now we'll turn our attention to a more specific topic: nerve injuries.

Compressed nerves

Compressed nerves are a frequent consequence of spinal injuries. A nerve can be compressed when any structure—be it a bulging disc, a swollen joint, even a cancerous tumour—pushes into it anywhere along its path. Spinal health practitioners refer to compressed nerves using a variety of names, including 'pinched nerves' and 'referred pain'. These terms are generalisations that imply roughly the same thing, although you will soon see some subtle differences between them.

One tag that many spinal health practitioners apply to back-related thigh pain is the term 'sciatica'. This diagnosis implies that the sciatic nerve is being compressed by a disc as it exits the lower back. You will soon see that this is a very poor description of what really happens. By the end of the next two chapters, you will see that there are many causes of leg pain.

Not only that, but you will learn how compressed nerves can cause a variety of other unpleasant symptoms in your legs, such as tingling, numbness and weakness. You'll also be surprised to discover that compressed nerves can cause seemingly unrelated signs, such as stiffness, tenderness, and even swelling.

Theoretically, any structure in the lower back can compress a nerve. However, if we follow the path of the nerve from the spinal cord to the limbs, we come across three places that they are particularly vulnerable:

- inside the spinal cord tunnel
- as they pass through the intervertebral canal, and
- where the nerves rub against other structures.

Let's look at the implications of these three common points of nerve compression. Don't worry if you can't remember the exact details of every condition, just try to develop a feel for the general nature and importance of nerve injuries.

(1) INSIDE THE SPINAL CORD TUNNEL

The tunnel through which the spinal cord travels does not have very much spare room, as the spinal cord takes up at least half of the area in most places. If a bulging disc protrudes into this otherwise almost impenetrable area, it quickly encounters the dura—that long, canvas-like sock of tissue.

BACK PAIN

The dura is a bit of a sook when it is pushed around, as it is used to being protected within a very sheltered environment. So the pressure of the disc quickly causes the dura to become inflamed and tender, in much the same way that soft hands develop a blister more quickly than roughened, callused palms. The result is widespread pain, which is worsened by any movement that moves the dura or stresses the disc.

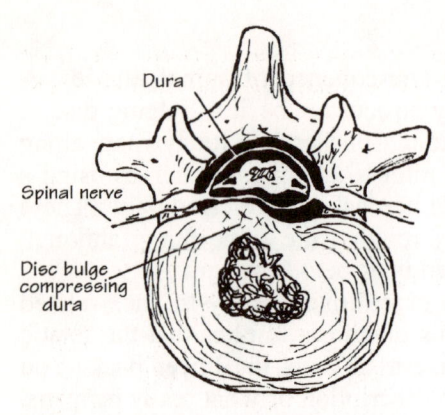

Here a bulging disc is pushing onto the spinal dura, which is likely to cause its owner considerable pain and stiffness.

A severely prolapsing disc can also cause two other nerve-related problems inside the spinal cord tunnel. These conditions are called *central stenosis* and *nerve root compression*.

Central stenosis
'Stenosis' means 'narrowing'. A diagnosis of *central stenosis* means that the tunnel through which the spinal cord travels has become narrowed. This narrowing, especially if it is due to a disc prolapse, can be serious, and should not be dismissed lightly.

The consequences of untreated central stenosis can include severe pain, pins-and-needles, and gross muscle weakness. You may be suffering from central stenosis if you have any of the following three symptoms:

- pins and needles in a 'sock' distribution (a 'glove' distribution may occur if the stenosis is higher in the spine)
- 'saddle paraesthesia' i.e. pins and needles in the genital region, combined with an inability to pass urine or defecate correctly (known as *cauda equine* syndrome)
- uncontrollable spasms in the leg muscles.

This condition requires immediate specialist assessment, so if you have any of these signs, please don't mess around. Make an appointment with your doctor today.

Nerve root compression
The second possible outcome of a severe disc injury occurs when the nucleus pushes onto the nerve roots—the small pair of filaments that emerge from the spinal cord.

The nearest nerve root to the disc is the one that carries signals to the muscles. If something compresses this nerve root, it interrupts the muscle-bound messages, causing weakness in the legs and feet. These symptoms also indicate severe damage, and so you should ensure that any weakness or clumsiness in your legs or feet is thoroughly investigated.

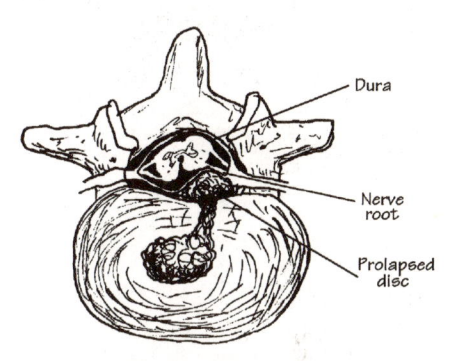

Here the nucleus of the disc has prolapsed so badly that it is pressing not only on the dura, but onto the motor nerve root as well. As you will see in the next chapter, this type of problem can cause not only pain, but weakness in the leg muscles as well.

Luckily, the nerve root that carries the sensory signals up to the brain is a long way forward in the spinal canal. Even severe disc problems do not normally reach the sensory nerve root, so we are spared what would doubtless be extraordinary pain.

Luckily, both central stenosis and nerve root compression are rare. However, compression of the dura is far more common, and is one of the most likely consequences of an unstable disc.

(2) IN THE INTERVERTEBRAL CANAL
The intervertebral canal is a bit like Uganda in the 1970s: it is a very dangerous place through which to travel. These narrow pairs of holes are formed by the discs on one side, the facet joints on the other, with bone on the top and bottom. Injury to any of these structures can therefore press on the spinal nerve.

For example, the inflammation that follows a facet joint sprain can swell into the intervertebral canal, pressuring the spinal nerve. Or a disc can bulge or prolapse into the canal, leading to nerve-related pain.

Chronic problems, such as arthritis, can also create havoc in the intervertebral canal. As the joints or discs degenerate, osteophytes (calcium deposits) can accrue on their edges. As these calcium deposits increase in size, they can encroach so far into the canal that the nerve has very little room through which to pass. Even simple movements like walking cause pain.

When the intervertebral canal is severely narrowed in this way, it is called *intervertebral stenosis*. This condition, in which the bones themselves are effectively squashing the spinal nerve, can be difficult to cure. Note that although this name is similar to 'central stenosis', these two conditions have different ramifications.

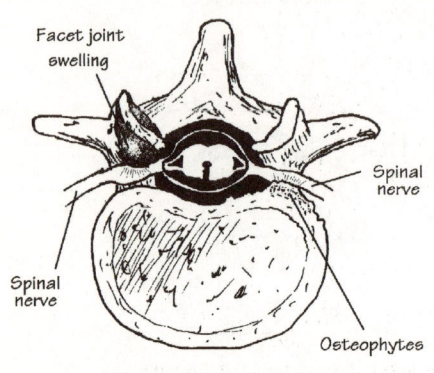

So you can see that many lumbar structures—including not only the discs, but also the joints and even the bones—can compress the spinal nerves in the intervertebral canal.

Two things are wrong with this vertebra. On the left side of the picture, the facet joint is swollen, which encroaches into the intervertebral canal from the top. On the right side, the vertebral body has developed bony spurs—osteophytes—which are also intruding into the intervertebral canal. Either of these two injuries can cause pain and stiffness by itself. However, when they occur together on the same side, the intervertebral canal becomes severely narrowed, and the spinal nerve has very little room to move. This condition is known as 'intervertebral canal stenosis'.

(3) WHERE THE NERVES RUB AGAINST OTHER STRUCTURES

Many structures can compress the nerves as they travel through the hips and limbs. There are many sites at which the nerves are vulnerable, including old injury sites, natural bony attachments, and branches at which the nerves divide. I won't list all the common sites here, as that would involve about a hundred ten-syllable words, that would doubtlessly make excruciatingly boring reading. Instead, I will illustrate this concept using a single example.

You have a small muscle in your buttocks called the *piriformis*. In many people, the sciatic nerve pierces directly through this muscle, rather than running alongside it. Guess what happens if the piriformis muscle gets tight, or if it goes into spasm? That's right—it clamps around the sciatic nerve. This causes pain, tightness, and all of the other symptoms associated with compressed nerves. This set of symptoms occurs commonly enough for it to score a name all of its own: *piriformis syndrome*.

In summary, we have seen three places in which the nerves are frequently compressed: inside the spinal cord tunnel, as they pass through the intervertebral canal, and where the nerves rub against other structures. By combining this knowledge with the earlier discussions about anatomy and joint movement, you should now be starting to get a feel for the myriad of ways in which back pain and referred pain can be generated.

REFERRED PAIN

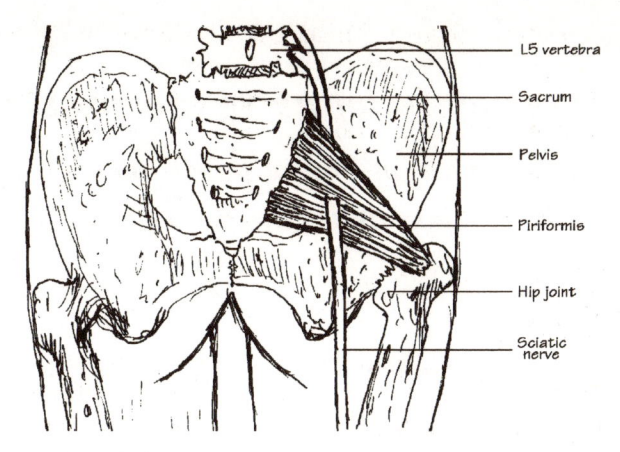

A view of your pelvis from the back. This illustration depicts a case of piriformis syndrome, which can, for reasons that should now be obvious, be a real pain in the butt!

Nerve compression can produce a wide range of symptoms, including pain, weakness, and stiffness. Now we'll look at these symptoms to discover the surprising characteristics and origins of each condition.

9
Consequences of nerve compression

Pain, pain, pain and more pain—oh, and some weakness and stiffness as well

Anyone who has ever suffered from a compressed nerve can attest to the most common symptom: pain. However, nerve-related pain is unusual because it varies wildly in its nature and character. Furthermore, nerve compression pain often appears in seemingly unrelated areas that are far removed from the source, and often trick you into thinking that you are suffering from another injury.

In the first part of this chapter, we are going to explore why nerve injuries have such different presentations, and why the pain refers such a long way from its origin. After that, we'll look at two other consequences of nerve injuries: muscular weakness, and nerve immobility.

Let's now look at the most frequent consequence of nerve compression: pain.

Pain

TYPE OF PAIN
The signs and symptoms of a sprained ligament or torn muscle are readily identifiable and consistent. Yet the symptoms of compressed nerves vary wildly. They range from dull gnawing aches to sharp shooting pains, and even sensations such as pins and needles or numbness. Sometimes they make your legs feel tender, or overly sensitive. Why do nerve injuries provoke such a seemingly unrelated variety of feelings?

The reason that nerves produce such assorted symptoms is that different parts of the nerve can be injured. Each nerve is composed of two parts, in much the same way as an electrical cable is made from a metallic wire with a rubberised coating. In your nervous system, the parts that carry the signals are called the *neurones*. The outer protective covering is called the *connective tissue*. Either part can cause pain if it is compressed. Furthermore, the nerve itself can become inflamed and painful if it is compressed for a long period.

Let's have a brief look at each of these three possibilities. However,

CONSEQUENCES OF NERVE COMPRESSION

please be aware as you read that, like most back pain diagnoses, these conditions are not necessarily clear-cut, isolated situations. They can, and often do, overlap.

Referred pain from the connective tissue
When a structure such as a ligament or muscle is injured, you feel pain because the local nerve endings register a painful stimulus. This message goes along the nerve and into the spinal cord, which forwards it to the brain.

So what happens when the outer, connective tissue part of nerve is compressed or injured? Exactly the same thing, for the nerves have a nerve supply too! The feeling of a connective tissue injury is readily recognisable to most people: a deep, aching, familiar type pain. Often the pain is diffuse, and is sometimes described as 'like a toothache'. In short, an injury to the nerve connective tissue feels very similar in *character* to most other sprains and strains.

However, injury to nerve connective tissue—which, by the way, includes the dura—has one minor difference. Most nerves have a very diffuse, web-like nerve supply, and the brain can not always localise the exact source of the problem. The result is that the brain often misinterprets the painful signals, incorrectly 'guessing' their source. You experience the pain in the 'wrong' area. These misguided symptoms are simply known as *referred pain*.

This inaccuracy on your brain's part is not surprising—no offence intended. The poor thing is being continually bombarded by signals from all over the body, and cannot be expected to monitor every square millimetre with unerring accuracy. Your spinal cord should also shoulder some of the blame, as it too must receive, process and then deliver thousands of similar signals, often all at once.

This does not imply in any way that the symptoms are 'all in your head'. Do not believe anybody that tells you so. The nerve damage is real, and would be apparent if you carefully examined the nerve fibres. However, you would probably find that the damage was on a different part of the nerve to where you expected it to be.

Think of this misinterpretation as similar to the brain trying to place the source of an aroma. Upon first sensing the smell, your brain may be able to roughly tell you what is causing it—say, a freshly baked apple pie. However, you probably would not be able to discern the exact location of the pie, as your sense of smell is too diffuse. In the same way, your brain can tell what type of sensation is coming through the nerve—pain—but cannot always pinpoint its exact location.

Referred pain of this type arises from not only the nerves, but from other parts of the spine as well. For example, a lumbar disc can create referred pain in the buttocks, tummy or groin, as can an inflamed facet joint. This type of referred pain is extremely common in many back pain sufferers.

'Nerve pain' from the neurones

The second major type of nerve pain arises when the neurones are injured. In other words, the signal-carrying part is compressed, torn or somehow strained. This situation produces an entirely different character of pain from connective tissue injuries.

Normal neurones carry their signals using a series of chemically generated electrical impulses. If the neurone is compressed, false electrical signals are created. Your brain cannot distinguish from where, how or why the false signals arose. This results in feeling pain or other sensations that appear in distant areas.

To illustrate this point further, imagine that you are chatting on the telephone to your Aunty Doris, who lives on the other side of the country. Halfway through the call, a linesman working down the street clamps some electrodes onto the telephone lines, and, unbeknownst to you, he uses special equipment to join the conversation. You would find it impossible to discern the location of the linesman. Your brain would simply make its best guess, and assume that the new signal was coming from its usual source: Aunty Doris's bedroom telephone. Gasp! Does she have a new toy boy?

Likewise, an injury to the neurones will create a whole new signal. This strange message will then travel up the rest of the neurone in the normal way, making it impossible for your brain to place its origin, or even to discern its intended meaning.

Neurone-related symptoms are called *dysesthetic pain*, (dis-ess-THET-tick ... try not to lisp) which means 'pain that does not feel normal'. Dysesthetic pain is often a stabbing, burning or electric sensation. Other words sometimes used to describe neurone-related nerve pain include 'searing', 'crawling' or 'jabbing'. These symptoms can be very disturbing, as they are unfamiliar to most people.

Neurone injuries can also give rise to two other symptoms: *para-esthesia*, or pins and needles, and *ana-esthesia*, or numbness. I have added the hyphens to simplify pronunciation. I find it amusing that the term 'anaesthesia', which is difficult to pronounce, hard to spell and poorly understood, has more letters than a good old-fashioned word like 'numbness'.

In short, neurone injuries produce unfamiliar pain. Because the neurone is protected by the connective tissue these symptoms usually represent more severe damage than does ordinary referred pain.

Inflammation of the whole nerve

Normal nerves have two systems that keep them healthy. The first system uses a thick liquid that slowly circulates around the nerve, which delivers the chemicals that allow it to fire its electrical impulses. If the nerve is compressed, then the flow of this fluid is retarded, meaning that the nerve cannot fire properly. This misfiring produces the main symptom of a lack of nerve fluid: pins and needles. To show how easily this occurs, just sit on your hand for twenty minutes or so and see what happens.

The second system that keeps the nerves functioning is a very rich and elaborate blood supply. The nerve system is a real hog for oxygen: it consumes twenty per cent of the available oxygen in your blood, despite only weighing about two per cent of your entire body mass.

If your nerve is severely compressed, then its blood supply dwindles. This creates an imbalance between oxygen supply and waste removal, so your nerve swells. It can sometimes become so tight that even your blood cannot force its way in, and, deprived of oxygen, your nerve starts to die. Despite initially being healthy before it was compressed, your nerve now has its *own* problems.

This process explains why back injuries create seemingly unrelated tenderness, inflammation and sometimes even mild swelling in distant parts of your trunk or limbs. These symptoms are frequently misdiagnosed as tendonitis, RSI (repetitive strain injury) or chronic muscle strains.

AREA OF PAIN
We have seen how nerve injuries can vary in character, from dull aches to localised pins and needles to distant inflammation and tenderness. The other strange aspect of all these types of pains is that they often appear far removed from the injury source. Why do we feel pain in such strange and seemingly unrelated areas? The answer to this question varies according to which section of the nerve was affected.

First, let's consider the *spinal nerves*. They have specific distribution areas known as dermatomes. Pictured on the following page, the sites of referred pain or other symptoms correspond to which segment of your back is injured.

You can see from the diagram on the next page that an injury that compresses a thoracic spinal nerve is likely to cause pain in the chest that resembles a lung or rib problem. The L1 spinal nerve refers lower abdominal pain, mimicking appendicitis or a hernia, while an L2 injury can appear as a hip joint strain or groin muscle tear. The L3 and L4 refer respectively to the front and back of the thigh, tricking the unwary into believing that they have a quadriceps or hamstring muscle strain. Note that L5 sometimes produces no pain in the back or thigh, only in the calf and foot region. This tricks many people with an L5 injury into thinking that they have a leg problem. Finally, the first two sacral nerve roots create pain down the back of the legs. Can you see how easily a spinal problem can fool you into believing that you have another injury?

BACK PAIN

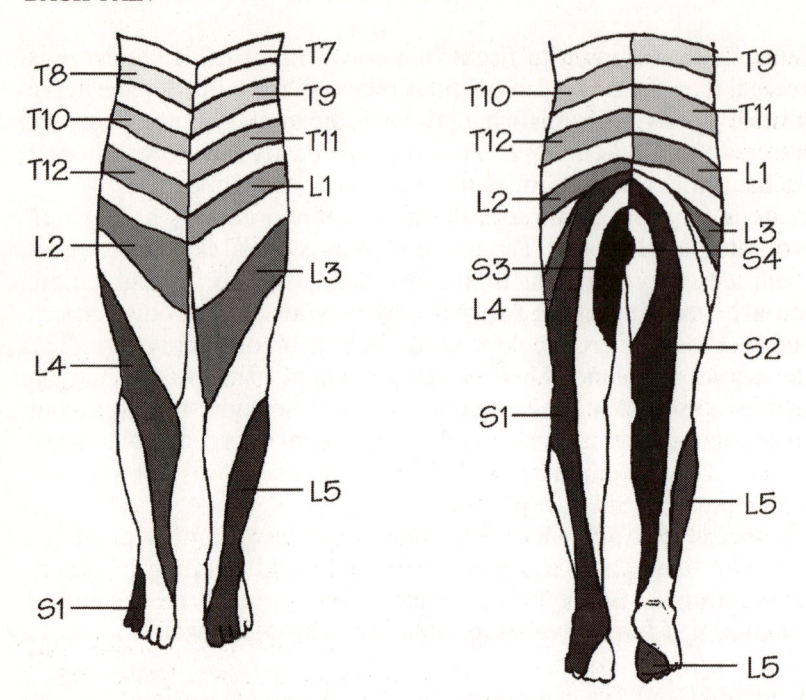

This picture shows the areas to which each spinal nerve normally refers. The left diagram shows the front view, while the right side shows the back of your trunk and legs. These areas, known as 'dermatomes', can be very handy in helping to localise the source of your problem. For example, can you see that if you had pain or pins and needles in your big toe that the L5 spinal nerve would be the most likely culprit?

An injury to the *dura* produces a different type of pain. While roughly corresponding to the dermatomes above, the pain tends to be more diffuse. Any generalised or unexplained pains in the back, buttocks or legs can often be attributed to a dural injury (see diagram on the next page).

Finally, a *nerve* injury will produce pain in the region supplied by that nerve. For example, a compressed femoral nerve will refer pain to the front of the thigh, while the sciatic nerve will send pain over the hamstring muscles.

Enough talk of pain! Let's now look at the two other main consequences of nerve compression: weakness and nerve immobility.

Weakness

Recall that the nerve root nearest the disc carries the signals to the muscles to make them contract. Compression of this nerve root will cause weakness in the leg and foot muscles, rather than pain. (Unfortunately, this type of injury is still usually painful, as whatever is pushing on the nerve root will also undoubtedly be compressing the dura.)

If the nerve root is squashed, then the strength loss will be specific to a few muscles. Muscles, like the surface of your skin, are supplied by different nerve levels. As a rough guide, compression of the upper lumbar segments will cause weakness in your hip and knee muscles. Problems in the lower lumbar nerve roots create weakness in your ankles and toes, while the sacral nerve roots supply the calf muscles.

As mentioned earlier, muscular weakness is usually a sign of a severe problem. If you have any apparent muscular weakness associated with your back pain, please see a spinal health practitioner immediately.

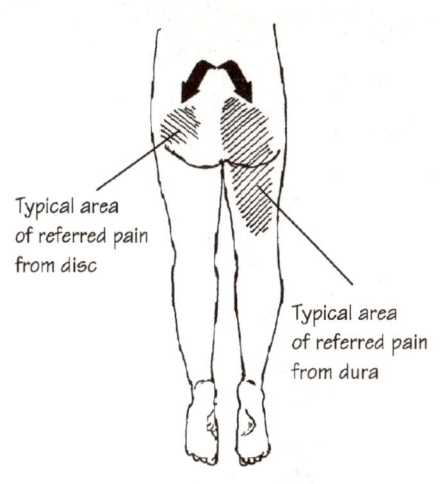

Typical area of referred pain from disc

Typical area of referred pain from dura

On the right is a typical pain pattern that would arise if your dura were compressed at a low spinal level—say at the L5–S1 area. If the dura were compressed higher in your lumbar spine, then you would be more likely to feel pain in the front of your thigh. In general, the pain distribution is similar to the dermatomes shown in the preceding diagrams, but it feels deeper, more vague, and rarely travels below your knee.

The shading on the left side of the picture shows a typical area of referred pain from a lower lumbar disc. Note that this type of pain has nothing to do with compressed nerves, but is simply your brain misinterpreting the source of the trouble.

Nerve immobility

Nerve immobility is a common and painful consequence of compression. Stuck nerves not only create pain and stiffness in other parts of the hips and legs, but can also exaggerate the original back pain.

Many people are surprised to hear that nerve movement can be restricted, or that nerves need to be regularly moved and stretched. This confusion probably occurs because most people picture nerves as delicate, fine structures that have to be mollycoddled along inside the body. Nothing could be further from the truth. As mentioned in the last chapter, nerves are robust structures, with some being as thick as your finger and as strong as rope.

Your nerves must glide and stretch when you move your legs and trunk, far further than do muscles. This flexibility requirement is so large because nerve cells are very long. They travel vast distances in the body, sometimes even more than a metre, despite the nucleus of the cell being smaller than a pinhead.

To give some further appreciation of the scale of distance, pretend that the head of the nerve is the size of a basketball. In the same scale of measurement, the tail-like neurone would measure a staggering 2.5 kilometres! This long cell length means that a nerve might have to cross many joints on its journey through the limbs. So compared to most muscles, which only cross one or two joints, the movement requirements of nerves are huge.

Luckily, the nerves are well adapted to cope with this movement demand. They have a mechanism in which they slide along inside a tunnel formed by the other bodily tissues. This effect can be likened to a brake cable, in which the central wire slides happily inside its outside casing.

Usually, this sliding mechanism works extremely well. However, if a nerve is compressed then its movement will be impeded. To use our previous analogy, suppose that you compress the outside of the brake cable—clamping it with pliers, for example. The inside wire will not slide properly, and any attempt to move it will simply increase its tension. Your nerves are the same: compression along their path will greatly inhibit their movement, leading to a rapid escalation of tension when you move your limbs or trunk.

The most obvious symptom of neural tension is stiffness. That pulling feeling behind your knees when you bend forward is almost certainly due to immobile nerves, and is not, as many people believe, due to muscle tightness. Neural tension can also occur in the dura, which causes back stiffness, as well as deep, tight, achey feelings in your whole spine.

Furthermore, neural tension can create problems further along the nerve's path. For example, a back injury can create tension in the sciatic nerve, which can irritate its attachment point on the outside of the knee. If this irritation is repeated enough times, the knee itself can develop pain and tenderness. A whole new injury! This interplay between tension points helps to explain why some people have 'pain everywhere', from headaches and neck pain to a stiff back, and down to aching legs and feet.

One area that deserves special mention here is the thoracic spine: the bit between your neck and your lower back. Thoracic injuries such as spondylosis or bulging discs can readily push on the dura. This pressure hinders the sliding and gliding movements of the dura, which causes it to become, in essence, tight.

This tension in the dura can then cause symptoms in other parts of

CONSEQUENCES OF NERVE COMPRESSION

the body such as headaches, lower back pain, and even leg pain. The thoracic spine can also cause pain in the coccyx, by virtue of the dura's attachment to this otherwise insignificant bone. While this range of symptoms seems remarkable, clinical experience has shown that it is not only possible, but also common.

The easiest way to think of the nervous system is to consider it as one big, tangled nerve, like a rope with fraying ends, rather than dozens of smaller, independent nerves. The thoracic area, by virtue of its position in the approximate middle of this frayed rope, has a strong effect on the movement of the other fibres.

Let's look at some cases to help clarify these difficult neural tension concepts. Please remember that these histories are examples only, and by no means exhaustive. Nerve immobility is very complex, and can rear its head in a surprising number of areas:

Gillian, a forty-year-old economics professor, had tenderness and pain around her tailbone, her coccyx. The pain had been worsening for months, and she now had to sit on a doughnut-shaped cushion for relief. When questioned by her spinal health practitioner, Gillian could not recall any trauma; the pain had simply started by itself. During the examination, the spinal health practitioner noticed that Gillian's dura was very immobile, and so checked the rest of her spine. This examination revealed that a bulging thoracic disc was pushing onto the dura, hindering its movement. When combined with Gillian's poor sitting posture, the tension in the dura eventually created pain at its attachment point on the coccyx.

Jock, a twenty-five-year-old elite footballer, felt a rip in the back of his thigh when kicking a football. Assuming he had torn his hamstring muscle, he iced the injury for a few days before strengthening it at the gym. Jock resumed training, and after three weeks of dedicated exercise he rejoined his team in time for the finals. However, twenty minutes into the next game he again felt a tear, and left the field a shattered man. When he sought treatment, the practitioner noticed that Jock's sciatic nerve did not glide properly, and elicited pain when stretched. His piriformis muscle was also tight. The diagnosis: Jock's piriformis muscle was hindering the sliding motion of his sciatic nerve, which was why it tore when he kicked the football. It was not a hamstring muscle tear after all.

I hope that you are beginning to see the breadth of complaints that can have nerve immobility as a component. Torn muscles, tendonitis, non-responsive injuries, fibrositis, even headaches, can be caused by neural tension. Tight nerves not only cause lower back pain, but are a consequence of it as well.

SUMMARY OF NERVE-RELATED INJURIES
OK, that just about brings us to the end of nerve-related injuries. Don't worry if you can't remember exact details of each condition. However, I hope that you can see that the usual practice of simply diagnosing any back-related leg pain as 'sciatica' is close to useless.

You should now understand that leg or buttock pain can come from many sources. Referred pain can arise from the connective tissue of the spinal nerve or dura, or simply from misinterpreted signals from injured spinal structures. Other strange symptoms or shooting pain can occur if the neuron is compressed. A pinched nerve can also develop tenderness and inflammation, as well as becoming tight due to hindered mobility.

When you multiply the many types of referred pain by the variety of spinal injuries, such as disc bulging, stenosis or facet joint sprains, you will appreciate just how complex nerve-related pain can be. This intricacy can be very deceiving, and many people with nerve-related injuries think that they are suffering from another condition. Nevertheless, by performing a thorough assessment, a good spinal health practitioner can accurately diagnose the source of your nerve-related symptoms.

10

The real cause of lower back pain

Why your spine is like a door that was fitted by an incompetent handyman

You learned, in Chapters 4 to 7, of some frequently quoted causes of low back pain. We've discussed details on many different conditions, from disc problems to arthritis, and bone injuries to muscular trigger points. You'll be pleased to know that most of the big words are now out of the way.

Does this newfound knowledge fix your back pain? Well, sorry, but no.

Unfortunately, the anatomical source of your pain doesn't tell you much about the real cause of your problem. Sorry to say this, but all of that seemingly vital information you absorbed from those four chapters is not really as important as I made out at the time.

There are three reasons for this:

1. Many of these problems are normal occurrences in an otherwise pain-free spine. For example, about two-thirds of people with no history of back pain whatsoever have a bulging disc. Furthermore, almost everyone over the age of sixty has arthritic changes in their spine, whether or not they are experiencing any symptoms.
2. Some people with severe low back pain do not have any identifiable condition at all. Even highly detailed scans and tests show that their spine is 'normal', despite long-term, crippling pain.
3. The same injury can create entirely different symptoms from one person to the next. To illustrate this point, suppose that two people have an identical L4-5 disc bulge. Both people are the same sex, height, weight, age and occupation. Yet despite all these similarities, one person might experience a dull aching pain while sitting, the other a sharp catching pain when hanging out the washing.

So can you see that investigating the anatomical source of your pain will not really tell you what is wrong with your spine? Nor does it tell you how to treat it. Of course, having a basic working knowledge of common low back complaints is useful, but it is far from a complete answer.

So what is the *real* cause of back pain?

Pay attention very closely now, because I'm going to tell you the secret to the true origin of all back pain. It's not bulging discs, it's not sprained ligaments and it's not degenerated joints. The *real* cause of back pain is this:

Voodoo.

That's right, voodoo. The ancient mystical art of placing a painful curse on someone else by sticking pins into a miniature doll of their likeness. I know this for a fact, because I saw it once on 'Gilligan's Island'.

OK, OK, I'm only kidding. (You *knew* that, didn't you.)

What I really meant to say was that when we look at specific, localised reasons for long-standing or repeated back pain, one major cause leaps out at us: *your back segments do not move properly*. More specifically, your back joints might be *stiff* or they may be *unstable*.

In short, a stiff or unstable joint underlies virtually every case of chronic lower back pain.

The big words for these conditions are *hypomobile* and *hypermobile*. However, as I thoroughly confused myself for the first three months of my university study by frequently getting them back-to-front, I will spare you this problem by using the everyday terms. Let's look in more detail at these vital concepts.

Joint stiffness and instability

Normally, your back uses a series of small slides and glides to create an overall movement. For example, when you extend your spine backward, each facet joint slides a tiny distance over its lower neighbour, and your discs compress and stretch by a similarly minuscule amount. These tiny individual vertebral movements combine to create an obvious bend in your spine. Think of a limbo dancer, and you'll see how effectively these tiny glides and slides add together to create a large overall movement.

Sometimes, however, these small gliding movements do not occur normally. The joint surfaces may not glide over each other as freely as they should, meaning that the joint is *stiff*. Conversely, the bones may not be held together firmly enough, making the joint *unstable*.

The unbalanced gliding and sliding makes the joint move with an abnormal movement pattern. The alteration in joint movement may be only a few millimetres, or a fraction of a degree, but that is all that is required to place enormous extra stress on one side of the joint.

To picture this effect, suppose an incompetent handyman changes the hinges on the door, but accidentally aligns one of them with a twist of just a few degrees. (Not that I ever did that, of course.) Here, the entire action of the door will be faulty. It probably won't close properly, and

THE REAL CAUSE OF LOWER BACK PAIN

the wood will probably warp or split. Although the errant hinge position was barely detectable to the naked eye, the effect of the misalignment on the motion of the door was dramatic.

Your joints are the same. Like a door hinge, even a minor difference in their alignment or position is enough to cause major stress during movement. This stress, when repeated thousands of time during normal everyday movements, causes an accumulation of microtrauma that ultimately causes inflammation and injury.

Can you see how stiffness and instability have such an important influence on the condition of your spine? A well-balanced joint will last for years. However, a joint that is either stiff or unstable will quickly degenerate, causing pain.

Joint stiffness and instability occur for many reasons. Chapters 15 to 19 discuss lifestyle factors, such as poor postures or movement habits, that can cause or amplify the problems of stiff or unstable joints. Later in this chapter, we'll take a brief introductory look at the *behaviour* of your back pain, which will outline some principles that will help you to analyse these lifestyle factors.

On a local spinal level, two specific factors are usually responsible for abnormal joint movement. Let's take a brief look at them.

The major cause of **instability** is *that the muscles do not control and support the joints properly*. Weak, lazy muscles allow the joints to move too far. These same muscles are responsible for maintaining the joints in the correct position during prolonged postures. Weakness in the muscles can lead to excessive gravitational stretching of the defenceless joint, leading to laxity and subsequent instability.

The role of the muscles in controlling your joints is very important. It is so important, in fact, that all of Chapter 12 is devoted to this interesting and vital area.

Spinal joints can also become stiff, just as can other joints such as your hip, knee or shoulder. The most common cause for joint **stiffness** is the *minor imperfections in your body's healing process*. In other words, scar tissue.

If you injure yourself, either through trauma or wear and tear, your body makes its best effort to restore everything to its original form. A mighty job it does, too. However, tiny variations in the shape, elasticity and position of the new tissue can alter the flexibility of the healed joint. Sometimes, the new tissues will be too tight, meaning that the joint becomes stiff. Excess scar tissue, or even extra bone, can accumulate around the edges of a joint, impeding its movement.

Of course, the same effect can apply in reverse, in which the scar tissue may not form tightly enough, meaning that the joint becomes unstable.

Despite appearing to be opposites, joint stiffness and instability are closely related. Paradoxically, unstable joints sometimes create feelings of stiffness during movement. I realise that this statement sounds absurd, as stiffness and instability are diametrically opposing conditions. However, if we look at a simplified example using the shoulder joint, you will see that this contradiction makes perfect sense.

Imagine, if you can, that you've just dislocated your shoulder—popped the arm bone right out of its socket. I'm sure that you can envisage the pain and stiffness as you try to move your inflamed and injured arm. Can you feel the stiffness?

But wait! A dislocated shoulder is an example of a very unstable joint—in fact, dislocation is the most extreme form of instability. Yet your movement after such an injury feels very tight and restricted. In short, the instability has caused your joint to feel stiff. The same process can occur within your spine, whereby a joint that is too lax and loose can actually make your overall movements feel tight and restricted.

Now imagine that you didn't move your arm around properly while your shoulder healed itself—you silly person! Then three months later, you attempted to lift your arm overhead, only to discover that your shoulder joint had lost much of its normal range of movement. This type of injury is now a true stiffness, rather than an apparent one. So, instability can sometimes lead to genuine joint stiffness as well.

Of course, your body's healing process is continually trying to repair and realign the joints to their normal state. However, nature is often not strong enough to overcome the laws of physics, which tell us that a force will follow the path of least resistance. In other words, when you move your spine, the loose, unstable joints bend first, while the stiff joints remain locked in position.

Because the loose, unstable joints are being moved most often, they steadily become even looser. Conversely, the stiff joints do not move very often, and so become even stiffer.

If you have chronic, long-lasting back pain, then my guess is that at least one of your spinal joints has entered into this difficult-to-escape cycle, in which the stiff joints get tighter and the unstable joints become even more lax.

But never fear! Later, you will learn exercises to help you reverse this process. Not only that, but we will investigate ways to prevent these imbalances occurring in the first place.

The behaviour of your pain

In your daily life, you probably find that certain postures and activities cause more pain than others. Alternatively, you may notice that your back feels 'stirred up' after certain tasks, rendering it liable to further injury. Or do you avoid certain activities because they will worsen your back pain? All of these instances are *aggravating factors*.

Furthermore, some postures or activities probably relieve your back pain. Or, if you have an extremely sore and irritable back, you may have found some activities that you can perform without worsening your pain, giving *relative* relief. These are the *relieving factors*.

By analysing these aggravating and relieving factors, you can learn more about the behaviour of your problem.

For simplicity, we will divide all activities into two groups: those that involve flexion, and those that involve extension. I realise that many injuries also respond to twisting, sideways bending, compression, distraction and a host of other biomechanical forces. However, were we to include every type of force, this book would be useful for no other purpose than a doorstop.

By 'flexion activities' I mean those that involve the loss of the normal lumbar *lordosis*. (Do you remember this word from Chapter 2?) Here, the lower back is held in a position in which it curves outwards, not inwards.

Bending forwards is the most straightforward example. Sitting with a slumped back is another. Other examples include putting a golf ball, tying up your shoelaces, and bending forward to weed the garden. You can probably think of dozens of other postures or tasks that classify as flexion activities.

'Extension activities' are just the opposite. Here, the lumbar lordosis is held in its normal inward-curving posture, or is even increased.

Bending backwards is the most obvious example of an extension activity, while reaching high is another. Standing in a queue also falls into this category, as does walking, serving a tennis ball and shooting a basketball. Any posture where your lumbar spine is held with an inward, lordotic curve counts as an 'extension activity'.

The first part of the quiz that follows in Part II will tell you whether your problem is most likely to be due to underlying joint stiffness or instability. The second part will help you to decide which postures aggravate or relieve your pain. Let's get to it.

Part II

How to analyse your back pain

11

What's your problem?

Why some spinal health practitioners are like bad car mechanics

I hope that you now understand that a diagnosis—such as a disc bulge, arthritis or a joint sprain—does not tell you much about how to treat your injury. Unfortunately, this difficulty is often reflected in the advice that people receive from their spinal health practitioner. The back care advice is either roughly aligned with the anatomical structure that is causing the problem, or, more usually, is the same for every case regardless of the problem. Some have a handout, booklet or advice sheet that they distribute to every back pain patient, while others have a standard spiel of verbal advice.

A spinal health practitioner who gives the same advice for every back injury is like a mechanic that changes the same part on every car, no matter what the problem. Sometimes, the advice will be fine. However, most times it will not help, and occasionally will be downright harmful.

These simple hypothetical conversations may help illustrate this point:

CASE 1
High & Mighty Spinal Health Practitioner: Well, Mr Cypher, we've just received the results from your very expensive series of tests, scans, X-rays and blood tests for your back pain.
Mr Cypher: What do they say?
H&MSHP: Well, it looks like you have a bulging disc at the L4-5 level.
Mr C: Really? What should I do about it?
H&MSHP: Well, you should rest in bed until the pain goes away, lose some weight, keep your back straight when sitting and don't lift any heavy boxes.

CASE 2
High & Mighty Spinal Health Practitioner: Well, Mrs Fechner, we've just received the results from your very expensive series of tests, scans, X-rays and blood tests for your back pain.
Mrs Fechner: What do they say?

H&MSHP: Well, it looks like you have arthritis in your right L3-4 facet joint.
Mrs F: Really? What should I do about it?
H&MSHP: Well, you should rest in bed until the pain goes away, lose some weight, keep your back straight when sitting and don't lift any heavy boxes.

Get the picture? In short, the most accurate diagnosis in the world does not necessarily tell you how your back is going to behave. Sure, some diagnoses will give you a big hint. However, trying to give advice or exercises without considering the nature and behaviour of the problem is doomed to failure.

The hypothetical situation above is unfortunately common. Although simplified, it represents the actions of many spinal health practitioners. How would you feel if you went to an optometrist for an eye check, only to receive a standard set of lenses from the shelf? Pretty annoyed, I would think. Yet many people often receive the standard set of back care exercises and advice, regardless of their problem. Can you see how silly this is?

Well-meaning friends often fall into a similar trap. Often they will smother you with advice about how to get rid of your pain, what exercises to do, and what activities to avoid. If I were you I would politely thank your well-meaning friends for their advice, then disregard it. Unfortunately, they are simply telling you what helped *their* lower back pain, not *your* lower back pain.

So what do we do?

The answer is to listen to our backs, and analyse what they are saying. Instead of *us* telling our backs how they *should* behave, we let *them* tell us how they are *going* to behave.

An old truism in medical practice says that if you listen to a patient for long enough then they will tell you what is wrong with them. And if you listen a bit harder, they'll probably tell you how to fix it! This approach illustrates how we have to attack back pain prevention.

I'm sure that you will agree that this approach makes a lot of sense ... in theory. But now we have another problem. In Chapter 3, we saw how, even in a highly simplified situation, there were 129,140,163 different combinations of back pain. With so many different causes of lower back pain, how are we going to cram separate advice for each type into one modest book?

Luckily, we don't have to. For as it turns out, most back pain falls into one of four categories of behaviour. If you can determine which category your back pain falls under, then you have a far better chance of garnering the right advice to suit your particular situation.

To correctly analyse your back pain behaviour, you must consider two areas. First, you must evaluate whether the major part of your problem is due to stiffness or instability—its *nature*. Then, you must evaluate what types of activity cause and ease the pain—its *behaviour*.

By combining these two factors, we arrive at one of four descriptions of your back pain. This description—which we will label as either 'A', 'B', 'C' or 'D'—will guide the advice and exercises that are most appropriate for your back pain.

Not my back pain, not your neighbour's, and not some 'textbook' case.

Your pain.

Self-assessment quiz to determine your back pain type

Do not skip this section. It is very important, so please ensure that you carefully complete the following quiz before continuing with the rest of this book. If you do not complete this section with care, then you may misdiagnose yourself, meaning that the benefit of the tailored advice in the rest of this book will be wasted.

I ask that you take the time to do this analysis slowly and properly. Sure, it will take a while—probably 30 to 45 minutes. But what a tiny price to pay for a lifetime of relief! Furthermore, you should be alert, preferably sitting at a desk, with a pen in your hand. Lying rugged up in bed on a cold winter's night is not very conducive to hard-edged analysis of your spinal pain.

So now I'll pause for a minute while you grab a pen and paper, brew a coffee if you like, then seat yourself comfortably at a desk.

Go on, do it . . . .

I'm waiting . . . .

Good.

Now, just a few housekeeping notes before we start. First, in developing the following quiz, I have assumed that you are currently suffering from lower back pain of some description. If not, then you will have to use your memory of previous incidents as best you can.

Second, for simplicity, I have used the term 'hurt' and 'pain' to represent all symptoms. Obviously, some people have other problems, such as stiffness, weakness, pins and needles, pulling, tightness, whatever. In this case you should mentally substitute your symptoms wherever the terms 'hurt' or 'pain' are used. In short, you should lump all of your related problems together under the one banner of 'back pain'.

Third, when observing the reaction of your back pain to a certain posture or activity, you will find it useful to note the behaviour of any referred or nerve-related pain in your legs. These symptoms are a sensitive indicator of the behaviour of the underlying spinal injury.

In particular, any activity that makes the referred pain travel further down your leg is probably worsening your underlying problem. For example, if your pain is normally in your lower back, but refers to your thigh during a particular activity, then I would consider that this activity is aggravating your problem. This premise holds true even if the severity of the pain has not worsened.

Conversely, if a position or activity makes your referred pain *centralise* (not travel as far down your limbs) then it is probably helping your problem. For example, you should consider that a pain in your upper thigh is not as severe as a pain that extends to your calf muscle, even if both pains have the same intensity. Generally, you should count any activity that leads to centralisation of pain as a relieving factor.

Fourth, you'll need a few simple household items. First, a large bath towel. Second, a firm surface—preferably a table that is strong enough to bear your weight. In some sections it will help if you can find someone you trust to serve as an assistant observer.

Sometimes a direct classification of your back pain might be very difficult. For example, your back may have two or more problems. If you have two or more *areas* of pain, then I suggest that you mentally separate them. Begin with the area of pain that causes you most problems on a day-to-day basis. Ignore any occasional or uncommon pains.

Similarly, if you have different *types* of pain—a continuous dull ache, with occasional jabbing pain, for example—then try to tackle them one at a time. Begin with the problem that limits you most, focusing your initial analysis on it. Then, when you have controlled that problem, you can work on your other pains.

You should also try to ignore your previous symptoms, and focus on the problems that have been hurting you during the last, say, one week. Back pain can change with time, so concentrate on your present, ongoing pain, rather than your initial or previous problems.

In short, you should concentrate on the *one* aspect of your *worst* area that has bothered you *recently*.

Without further ado, you can now start on the very important task of self-analysing your spinal pain. In the first part of the following analysis, you will discover whether your back is painful because it is stiff and restricted, or because it is unstable and weak. In the second part, you will discover whether your back pain is worse during flexion activities (when your back is bent forward) or during extension activities (when your back is held straight). Then, in the third section, you will perform some quick movement tests to discern if immobile nerves are a component of your problem.

Take a pen, and divide a sheet of paper into two columns. Or, if you are a new-aged techno-freak, boot up your computer, open a spreadsheet or database software package, and create a table with two columns, each with a simple addition function. But hurry. We old-fashioned people can't sit around and wait for you forever.

Mark the first column with the heading 'STIFF' and the second with the heading 'UNSTABLE'. Now just simply read the following quiz, and make an appropriate tally in each column.

Please, make sure that you remember to:

- concentrate on the *one* aspect of your *worst* area that has bothered you *recently*
- regard any activity that makes your pain spread further as an exacerbating factor
- regard any activity that makes your pain centralise as a relieving factor
- mentally insert other symptoms such as leg pain, stiffness or pins and needles, if appropriate.

BACK PAIN

Back Pain Quiz

PART ONE: THE BEHAVIOUR OF YOUR INJURY

Type of pain
Add one point to the STIFF column for each of the following words that describe your main area of pain:

- tight
- pulling
- stiff
- inflexible
- tense
- unbending
- rigid

- taut
- consistent
- seized
- restrained
- rusty
- like a lead pipe
- jammed.

Add one point to the UNSTABLE column for each of the following words that describes your main area of pain:

- catching
- collapsing
- lacks strength
- weak
- unsupportive
- gives way
- fragile

- floppy
- spasmodic
- unstable
- unexpected
- grabbing
- insecure
- unpredictable.

Aggravating and relieving factors
Add one point to the STIFF column for each of the following statements that are true.

1. My back often feels tight in the morning.
2. My back takes a few minutes to loosen after prolonged rest or inactivity.
3. Stretching my back usually relieves my pain.
4. When my spine hurts, my range of movement is usually very restricted.
5. Wearing a back brace or corset only helps to relieve my pain a minor amount, or does not help at all.
6. My back rarely causes pain during subtle movements, such as small positional changes on a chair.
7. I am familiar with the normal daily tasks that cause me back pain—it rarely causes pain unexpectedly.
8. General exercises, such as walking or swimming, usually make my back feel considerably looser.
9. I am over the age of sixty.
10. Manipulation from a spinal health practitioner usually helps my pain significantly.

WHAT'S YOUR PROBLEM?

11. A daily stretching program helps to relieve my back pain considerably.
12. Heat helps to relieve my pain and stiffness considerably.
13. My back pain is almost always in the same area of my spine—it never moves from side to side.
14. Even though my back might be painful, I am confident that it will not give way when I move.
15. My back joints never click or clunk in response to simple movements, such as gentle twisting, bending or extending.
16. Many of my other joints, such as my knees, hips and shoulders, are stiff and immobile.
17. Even though my back might be painful, it still feels reasonably strong.
18. My back never catches during simple movements, such as leaning across a desk, or reaching up toward a high shelf.
19. Even when my back is painless, it still feels stiff to bend and move.

Add one point to the UNSTABLE column for each of the following statements that are true.

1. My back feels no worse in the morning than at other times.
2. My back usually feels no stiffer after a prolonged rest or inactivity.
3. Stretching my back does not relieve my pain, or helps only a minor amount.
4. Even though my spine hurts, I can still move through a full range of motions.
5. Wearing a back brace or corset helps my pain significantly.
6. My back sometimes grabs when I make subtle movements, like small positional changes on a chair.
7. My back sometimes unexpectedly gives way when I perform normal daily tasks.
8. General exercises, such as walking and swimming, do not relieve my back pain very much.
9. I am under the age of twenty.
10. Manipulation from a spinal health practitioner does not seem to help my pain very much, makes it worse, or provides only transient (maximum 1-2 days') relief.
11. I have tried stretching my joints every day, but it provides no long-term relief.
12. Heat does not seem to help my pain very much, or provides relief for less than one hour.
13. My back pain sometimes moves from one side of my spine to the other without much provocation.
14. I am not very confident when my back is painful, as I fear that it may give way if I move it in the wrong direction.

BACK PAIN

15. My back joints sometimes click or clunk in response to simple movements, such as gentle twisting, bending or extending.
16. Many of my other joints, such as my shoulders and ankles, are loose and floppy.
17. My back feels very weak when it is painful.
18. My back sometimes catches during simple movements, such as leaning across a desk, or reaching up toward a high shelf.
19. When my spine is pain-free, I can bend and move it without obvious stiffness.

The above two sets of nineteen questions are usually complementary. In other words, if for you Question one is true in the first section, then it is unlikely that Question one in the second section is also true. If you have ticked the same question in both Section 1 and Section 2, then you may wish to re-examine your answers.

Special questions
Answer Yes or No to the following five questions.

1. Have you ever suffered from urinary stress incontinence? (i.e. leaking urine in response to physical activity).
2. Have you ever had lower abdominal surgery? (Ignore this question if you specifically retrained your lower abdominal muscles following the surgery.)
3. Does your spine sometimes catch with pain when you roll over in bed?
4. Does your spine sometimes catch with pain when you stand up from a chair?
5. Does your spine sometimes catch with pain when you cough or sneeze?

Examine your responses to the above five questions, if you entered No to *all* of them, then add 5 points to the STIFF column.

If you answered Yes to *any* questions, find your score below and add this score to the UNSTABLE column:

    1 yes = 1 point   4 yes = 7 points
    2 yes = 3 points   5 yes = 10 points
    3 yes = 5 points

For women only
1. Are you currently pregnant? If so, then add five points to the UNSTABLE column.
2. If you have ever been pregnant before, or are currently pregnant:
   • If your back pain was worse during pregnancy, add two points to the UNSTABLE column.

WHAT'S YOUR PROBLEM?

- If any longstanding back pain seemed less severe when you were pregnant, add four points to the STIFF column.

Spinal movement tests

Please use commonsense when performing the following two movement tests. Although they are very simple, they may aggravate your spine if it is very irritable. Discontinue the tests as soon as you feel that they are hurting your spine.

Ideally, have someone else observe you perform these movements. They can then assist you to answer the following seven questions. If you have no-one available, then I suggest that you perform each movement a few times BEFORE you read the questions. You and/or your assistant must carefully observe how you *naturally* perform these movements.

Movement test one: Flexion

Bend forward toward your toes as far as you can. Remain in this flexed position for about three seconds. Carefully note any feelings of stiffness, insecurity or pain. Slowly return to an upright position.

Once you and/or your assistant are satisfied that you have naturally performed this movement a few times, read and answer the following four questions. You will have to observe very carefully, as the responses may be quite subtle.

1. Did you feel any short catches of pain at the beginning or middle of the movement? Please ignore any pain that you felt when you were fully flexed. If so, add two points to the UNSTABLE column.
2. Did your knees *automatically* buckle or slightly bend as you *returned* from the flexed position? If so, add two points to the UNSTABLE column.
3. Did you instinctively brace your hands on your legs for support? If so, add three points to the UNSTABLE column.
4. When returning to the upright

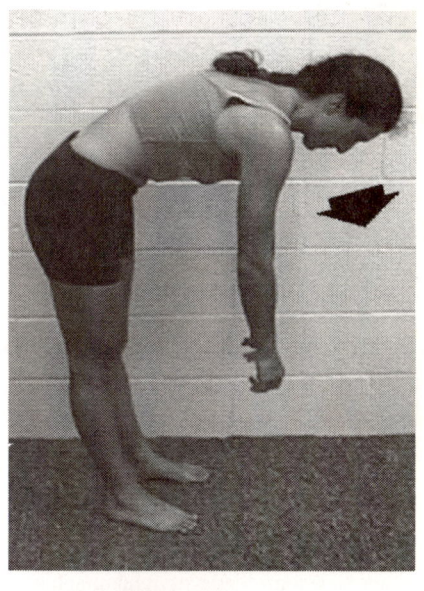

Let me introduce my friend and co-worker, Debbie. She is not only a great physiotherapist, but plays a mean classical guitar. Here, she is mid-way through the movement of lumbar flexion.

81

position, did you use your hands to 'walk' up your legs? If so, add four points to the UNSTABLE column.

Movement test two: Extension
Stand with your feet comfortably apart. Keep your knees straight, lean backwards as far as you can, so that your back arches. Stay in this position for about three seconds, carefully noting any feelings of pain, stiffness or insecurity. Then return slowly to the upright position (see opposite page).

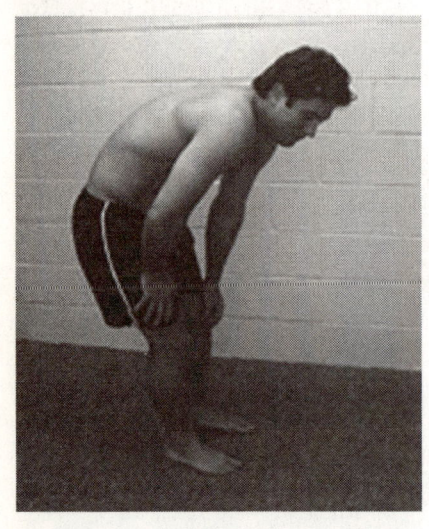

This is another friend of mine, Greg. Besides being a good drinking buddy, he is a fantastic architect, and will hopefully design my next house for me on the cheap. In this picture, he is demonstrating a typical movement pattern for an unstable lumbar spine during flexion. Note how he is subconsciously bracing his hands on his knees for support, and is buckling his knees slightly as he tries to return to the upright position. If his spine were *very* unstable, then he might even instinctively 'walk' his hands up his legs, rather than confidently straightening his spine. Compare this action with the preceding photograph of Debbie and you will see a clear difference.

Once you and/or your assistant are satisfied that you have naturally performed this movement a few times, read and answer the following three questions. You will have to observe very carefully, as the responses may be quite subtle.

5. Did you feel any short catches of pain at the beginning or middle of the movement? Please ignore any pain that you felt when you were fully extended. If so, add two points to the UNSTABLE column.

6. Did you *instinctively* brace your hands into your lower back for support as you moved? If so, add two points to the UNSTABLE column.

7. Did your lower back develop a crease (a horizontal skin fold) when you were fully extended? (Use a mirror to check if necessary.) If so, add two points to the UNSTABLE column.

Now examine your responses to the above seven questions. If you scored points in *any* of these seven questions, then please skip the next question and move on to the next section, entitled 'Analysis'.

If you scored *no* points in *every* one of the preceding seven questions, then consider this question.

WHAT'S YOUR PROBLEM?

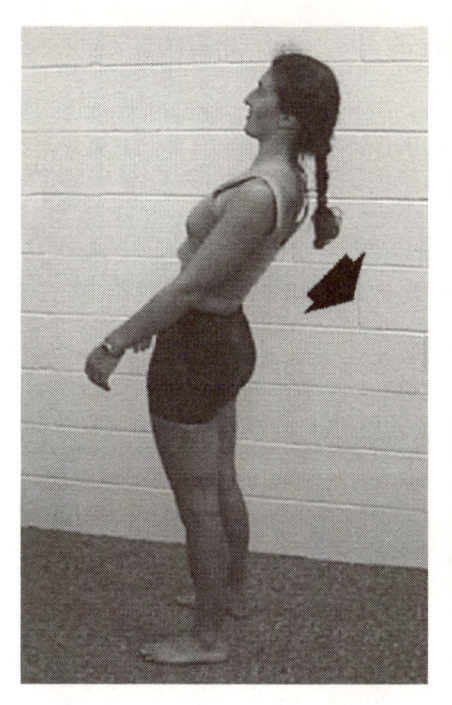

The movement of lumbar extension

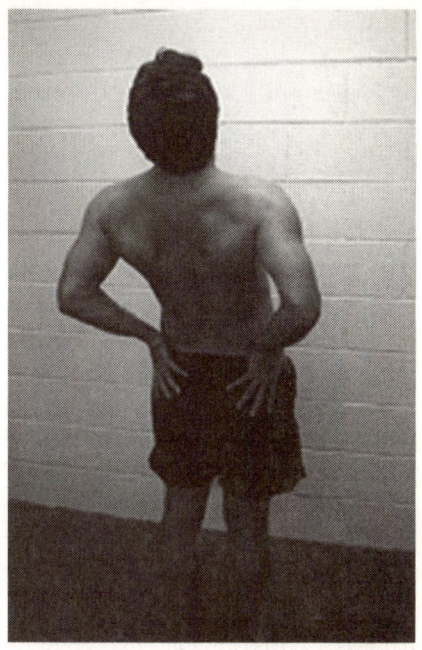

Here Greg is bracing his spine with his hands while extending his lower back. Although you may feel that this is a normal, natural thing to do, your spinal joints may be unstable if you subconsciously use this confidence-boosting movement pattern.

Did either movement (i.e. bending forward and arching backward) cause feelings of stiffness, tightness or pulling in your spine? Please ignore any tension in your legs.

- If so, then add five points to the STIFF column.
- If not, then do not change your score.

Analysis
Tally up the points in each column. Now we are going to perform some simple math. Don't panic at this thought, because the equation is very easy. Just add thirty points to your STIFF points, then subtract your UNSTABLE points. We'll call this your S-U score.

So your S-U score = 30 + STIFF points − UNSTABLE points.

You should end up with a number that is probably between zero and sixty. For example, suppose your STIFF points were four, and your

BACK PAIN

UNSTABLE points were sixteen. Your S-U score would be eighteen (30 + 4 − 16 = 18).

Please add carefully. I urge you to double check your answer, as it is amazing how easily simple but important errors can appear in your results. Write down your S-U score, as we will come back to it soon, then please move on to the second part of the test.

PART TWO: THE NATURE OF YOUR INJURY
Create another two columns on your page, computer screen, or whatever. This time, label them 'FLEXION' and 'EXTENSION'. As before, please concentrate on the *one* aspect of your *worst* area that has bothered you *recently*. Remember to consider whether the activity in question makes your pain travel further (down your leg, for example) or whether it makes the pain move closer to your spine. Please also remember to mentally insert other symptoms, such as leg pain, stiffness or pins and needles, if appropriate, Away we go again.

General questions
Add one point to the FLEXION column for each of the following statements that are true about your main area of pain.

- I sometimes feel pain when I sit.
- Sitting in a soft padded chair hurts me more than if I sit in a hard chair.
- Leaning forward, such as working over a low bench, sometimes makes my back hurt.
- My back sometimes hurts when I'm in the car.
- Tasks that require lifting make my back hurt.
- Repeated bending, such as when stacking a low shelf, makes my back hurt.
- Lying on my back on a soft bed, couch or hammock sometimes makes my back ache.
- I find that a hard mattress is better for my back pain than a soft mattress.
- If I sit for more than one hour, then I sometimes find it difficult to straighten up.
- I am able to stand for at least four hours without worsening my back pain.
- I can walk for at least one hour without worsening my back pain.
- I can repetitively reach up, such as putting things away in high cupboards for one hour, without any back pain.
- Lying on my tummy or flat on my back does not hurt my back.

WHAT'S YOUR PROBLEM?

Add one point to the EXTENSION column for each of the following statements that are true about your main area of pain.

- My back sometimes hurts if I have to stand for long periods, like in a queue.
- The longer I stand, the worse my back hurts.
- Walking sometimes hurts my back.
- My back hurts more if I walk downhill rather than uphill.
- My back sometimes hurts if I have to reach up, as when putting something in a high cupboard.
- I can drive for at least four hours without any pain.
- Lying on my tummy makes my back uncomfortable.
- Despite the advice I have been given, a hard mattress does not seem much better for my back pain than a soft mattress.
- If I lie on my tummy or flat on my back for more than an hour then I sometimes find it difficult to arise from the bed.
- I can sit for at least four hours without my back pain increasing.
- I can perform repetitive bending, such as light weeding in the garden, for at least an hour without worsening my back pain.
- I can bend forward, such as when tying my shoelaces, without any pain or stiffness.
- Lying on my back on a hard surface sometimes hurts my back.

Employment and activities of daily living

Add one point to the FLEXION column for any of the following activities that tend to make your back hurt.

- sweeping
- vacuuming
- raking
- picking up objects from the ground
- leaning/working over a low bench
- driving
- lawn bowls
- putting a golf ball.

Add one point to the EXTENSION column for any of the following activities that tend to make your back hurt.

- reaching up to peg clothes on the line
- putting away objects in high cupboards
- walking around the shops
- prolonged standing
- jarring, vibrating or pounding forces
- lying flat on your tummy or back
- serving a tennis ball
- surfing, diving or bowling a cricket ball.

BACK PAIN

Factors that ease your pain
Add one point to the FLEXION column if any of the following activities ease *your pain.*

- standing
- walking
- lying on your tummy
- supporting your back with a small roll when you sit
- gently arching backward when standing.

Add one point to the EXTENSION column if any of the following activities ease *your pain.*

- sitting
- curling up into a ball
- lying on your back with your knees bent up
- standing with your hands supported on your knees
- leaning forward onto a bench when working.

Rate your pain
The following four scenarios describe simple activities. You must estimate how much pain you would experience after each activity, and rate it on a scale of zero to five. When rating your pain, a score of zero means that you would not experience any pain at all. A score of five represents the worst spinal pain that you have ever experienced.

Scenario 1: You have to sit in a soft chair for two hours. On a scale of zero to five, how much pain would you experience? *Add this score to the FLEXION column.*

Scenario 2: You have to weed the garden for half an hour, repetitively bending to ground level. On a scale of zero to five, how much pain would you experience? *Add this score to the FLEXION column.*

Scenario 3: You have to stand in a very long bank queue for two hours. On a scale of zero to five, how much pain would you experience? *Add this score to the EXTENSION column.*

Scenario 4: You have to walk for half an hour—say about three kilometers (two miles)—at a steady pace along flat ground. On a scale of zero to five, how much pain would you experience? *Add this score to the EXTENSION column.*

Movement tests
Now, you are going to perform some more movement tests that are similar to those that you performed in Section 1. As before, please use

WHAT'S YOUR PROBLEM?

commonsense when performing these tests, and cease them if they are exacerbating your pain.

Movement test one: Flexion
Bend forward toward your toes as far as you can, with your fingers lightly touching your legs as you do. Remain in this flexed position for about three seconds. Carefully note any feelings of pain, stiffness or insecurity. Slowly return to a standing position.

Choose one of the following four responses that best matches what you experienced.

- If you felt pain, stiffness or insecurity before your fingertips got to your knees, add three points to the FLEXION column.
- If you felt pain, stiffness or insecurity when your fingertips were at shin level, add two points to the FLEXION column.
- If you could stretch all the way forward to your toes, but felt pain, stiffness or insecurity at the end of range, then add one point to the FLEXION column.
- If you did not feel any pain or stiffness, then do not change your score.

Movement test two: Extension
Stand with your feet comfortably apart, with your hands loosely touching your bottom. Keeping your knees straight, lean backwards as far as you can, lightly sliding your hands down the back of your thighs as you do. Stay in this position for about three seconds, carefully noting any feelings of pain, stiffness or insecurity. Then return slowly to the upright position.

Choose one of the following four responses that best matches what you experienced.

- If you felt pain, stiffness or insecurity as soon as you attempted to move, add three points to the EXTENSION column.
- If you felt pain, stiffness or insecurity when your fingertips were level with the upper part of your thigh, add two points to the EXTENSION column.
- If you felt pain, stiffness or insecurity when your fingertips were level with the lower part of your thigh, then add one point to the EXTENSION column.
- If you could fully arch your spine so that you could reach the back of your knees without feeling any pain, stiffness or insecurity, then do not change your score.

BACK PAIN

Movement Comparison
Compare how your back felt during the second test with how it felt during the first test. Choose one of the following five responses that best matches what you experienced.

- If leaning backward hurt much more than bending forward, then add four points to the EXTENSION column.
- If leaning backward hurt a bit more than bending forward, then add two points to the EXTENSION column.
- If neither movement hurt, or if they hurt about the same amount, then do not change your scores.
- If bending forward hurt a bit more than leaning backward, then add two points to the FLEXION column.
- If bending forward hurt much more than leaning backward, then add four points to the FLEXION column.

Analysis
Now, tally the marks in each column. Again, we are going to perform some easy arithmetic. Just add thirty points to your FLEXION points, then subtract your EXTENSION points.

This will give you a score that is probably between zero and sixty. We will call this your F-E score. To put it another way: Your F-E score = 30 + FLEXION points − EXTENSION points.

For example, if you had a tally of ten in the FLEXION column, and eighteen in the EXTENSION column, your F-E score is 30 + 10 − 18 = 22. If you tallied five in the FLEXION column, and two in the EXTENSION column, then your F-E SCORE is 30 + 5 − 2 = 33.

ANALYSIS OF F-E AND S-U SCORES
You should now have two scores: your F-E score and your S-U score. These scores tell us a lot about the behaviour and nature of your pain.

You may have already guessed that your F-E score indicates what type of activity causes the most aggravation to your back. Scores greater than thirty are aggravated by flexion activities, while scores less than thirty are aggravated by extension activities.

Similarly, a high S-U score indicates a lot of stiffness and rigidity in your joints, while scores lower than thirty indicate that instability and weakness are your major problems.

To simplify our classification system, we're now going to combine the two scores to give your back pain a label, either A, B, C or D. Look at the table on the next page. The top line shows the F-E score, from zero to sixty, while the vertical axis shows the S-U score. *Mark your two scores on their respective lines.* Note that I have deliberately omitted the score of 30, for if you scored exactly 30 then you are 'on the line'.

Now by intersecting the two scores, you will land in one of the four

WHAT'S YOUR PROBLEM?

quadrants of the table. These quadrants, labelled from 'A' to 'D', show your *back pain type*.

		F-E SCORE											
		0	5	10	15	20	25	35	40	45	50	55	60
S	0	A						B					
U	5												
	15												
S	25												
C	35	C						D					
O	45												
R	55												
E	60												

We are going to refer to your 'back pain type' many times during the rest of this book, so please remember it.

I hope that now you can see that your back pain type provides a concise description for the nature and behaviour of your problem. Let's look at a few examples, and discuss a few of the possibilities.

Let's suppose that your F-E score was 42 points, and your S-U score was 41 points. These scores would land you firmly in the lower right quadrant, clearly making you a type 'D'.

However, what if your F-E score was 42, but your S-U score was 'on the line' at 30 points. These scores would land you between the 'B' and the 'D' quadrants. Here you should assign yourself a dual category, in this case 'BD'. A coupled rating like this indicates that

89

BACK PAIN

although your back tends to become sore with flexion activities, it is not clearly definable as either stiff or unstable.

Similarly, say your F-E score was close to the line at 29 or 31, while your S-U score was, say, only 8 points. This would indicate that your back was very unstable in both directions—not an unlikely scenario. Here you would assign a rating 'AB'.

Commonsense will tell you that each back pain type has the following characteristics:

Type A: Tends to be painful during EXTENSION activities, and is generally UNSTABLE. A good example of a Type A spine is a young sportsperson, such as a gymnast or cricketer, who has developed a stress fracture (see Chapter 6). If you are a Type A, your spine will sometimes catch with pain when you perform an extension movement, and may ache after the activity. It can sometimes be difficult to find a relieving posture until the injury has settled, but sitting or lying curled up on your side sometimes helps a little. Even though your spine is obviously painful, you still have a fairly good range of movement.

Type B: Tends to be painful during FLEXION activities, and is generally UNSTABLE. A weak, unstable disc (see Chapter 4) which bulges during sitting, and grabs when you try to arise from the chair, is a classic type B injury. This type of problem will also sometimes cause a sharp catching pain during forward bending, and may ache following activities such as housework or gardening.

Type C: Tends to be painful during EXTENSION activities, and is generally STIFF. Intervertebral canal stenosis (see Chapter 8) is a typical—and often difficult—case. Facet joint arthritis (see Chapter 5) is also frequently a Type C injury. This type of problem will usually present as a deep vague ache, with loss of movement. Prolonged standing is sometimes difficult. Walking and lying flat can temporarily exacerbate your symptoms, which can usually be relieved by sitting or bending. You will never win a limbo competition, as your flexibility is very limited.

Type D: Tends to be painful during FLEXION activities, and is generally STIFF. Those people with disc spondylosis (see Chapter 4) may fall into this category. Usually, type D spines ache during prolonged sitting, or after a few hours of housework or gardening. The pain is usually relieved by going for a walk or a swim, or lying flat on your tummy or back. You sometimes feel one hundred years old when attempting to bend, such as when putting on your shoes, or dressing in the morning.

Please realise that I have developed this method of classifying back

WHAT'S YOUR PROBLEM?

pain for this book. It is not presently a generally accepted classification system, so please don't show up to your spinal health practitioner next week asking for advice regarding a Type D back with a very high S-U score. They'll probably refer you to a psychiatrist if you do!

Now, you have one more job: to measure the length and mobility of your nerves, to check whether you have any signs of neural tension.

PART THREE: NERVE IMMOBILITY TESTS

The following three tests provide a rough indication of whether you have any immobile nerves. As you learned in Chapters 8 and 9, nerve injuries cause a lot of spinal pain, so it is important that we include them in our analysis. In all three tests, an assistant may be useful to help you to estimate your range of movement.

Nerve test one: The 'Straight Leg Raise' Test

You will need an ordinary bath towel for this test. Lie on the floor, flat on your back. While keeping your left leg on the floor, use the towel around your right foot to lift your leg into the air. Keep your knee perfectly straight. Keep raising your leg until you feel pain, tightness or stiffness in either your back or your leg. Note the approximate angle of lift, then steadily return to the starting position.

Now repeat the same test on your left leg, again noting the angle at which you *first felt* pain or stiffness. If your legs felt different, then use the lesser angle (i.e. the reading from your stiffest or most painful leg) to answer the following question.

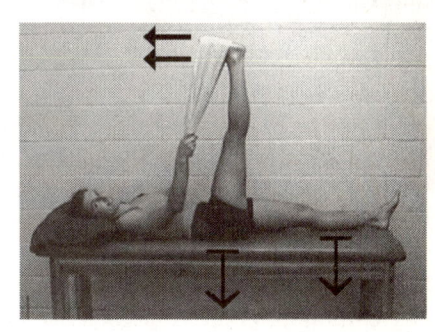

Debbie shows that her sciatic nerve has full extensibility. Note that her left leg is still on the bed, and that her right knee is perfectly straight. Also, her pelvis is flat and relaxed.

How far could you lift your leg before you first felt pulling, tightness or pain in your back or your leg?

- If you could lift your leg less than 30 degrees, then you score three points for this test.
- If you could lift your leg between 30 and 60 degrees, then you score two points for this test.
- If you could lift your leg between 60 and 90 degrees, then you score one point for this test.
- If you could lift your leg more than 90 degrees without any stiffness or pulling in your legs, then you do not score anything.

BACK PAIN

Nerve test two: The 'Slump' Test
Sit on a table, or other firm surface, with your bottom fully supported. Preferably, the surface should be high enough so that your feet are clear of the floor. Perform the following three stages, stopping the test when you first feel any pain, stiffness or pulling in either your back or your leg.

Stage One: Allow your back to fully slump into a 'C' shape. Let your neck bend forward, so that your chin is on your chest.

Stage Two: Straighten one knee so that your leg becomes horizontal. If you cannot fully straighten your knee, then stop the test at this point.

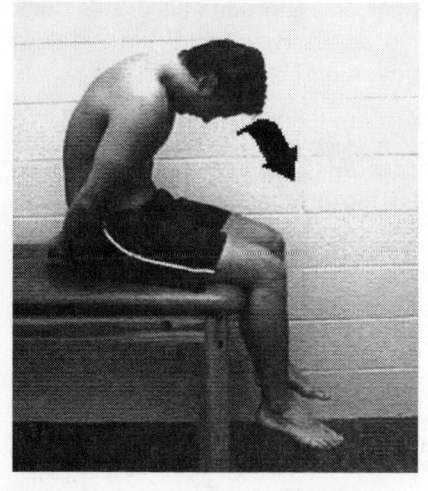

The 'Slump' Test, Stage One. Note that although Greg's spine is slumped, he is not bending forward or backward.

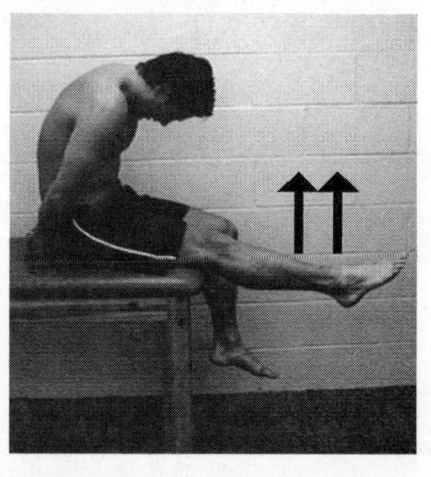

'Slump' Test, Stage Two—straightening your knee.

Stage Three: While keeping your leg extended, bend your toes back toward you as far as possible.

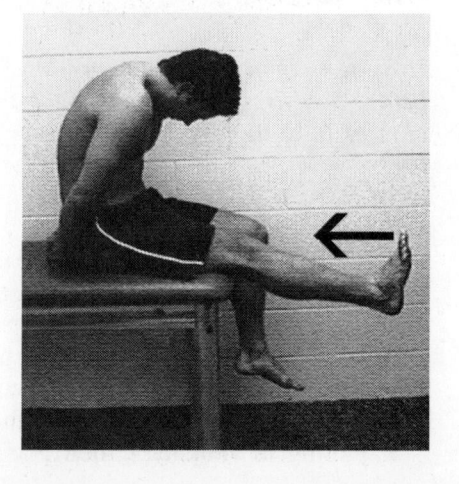

'Slump' Test, Stage Three—bending your foot back.

WHAT'S YOUR PROBLEM?

Now repeat the same test on your other leg, noting the stage at which you *first felt* pain or stiffness. If your legs responded differently, then use the lesser angle (i.e. the reading from your stiffest or most painful leg) to find your score.

- If you first felt pain or tightness during Stage One, then you score three points for this test.
- If you first felt pain or tightness during Stage Two, then you score two points for this test.
- If you first felt pain or tightness during Stage Three, then you score one point for this test.
- If you could perform all stages without feeling any pain or stiffness, then you do not score anything.

Nerve test three: The 'Prone Knee Bend' Test

If you have arthritic or injured knees, you may find that the range of movement in your knee limits this test.

Lie on your tummy on a firm surface, and slowly bend one knee. If possible, have an assistant gently push your heel further toward your bottom. If you do not have anyone to assist you, then reach back and try to grab your foot to continue the stretch. Alternatively, you can try to use the towel around your ankle for assistance. In all cases, keep your spine as flat and relaxed as possible, and keep your hip bones on the floor.

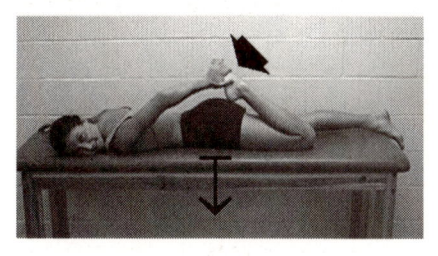

The 'Prone Knee Bend' Test at end range. Note that Debbie's hips are still comfortably on the bed, and that she is not arching or moving her spine.

Note the angle of your leg at which you first felt any stretching in the front of your thigh, or any back pain. Slowly return. Repeat the test on the other leg, and remember the response from your stiffest or most painful side.

How far could you bend your leg before you first felt pulling, tightness or pain in your back or your thigh?

- If you felt pain or tightness when your leg was bent less than 90 degrees, then you score three points for this test.
- If you felt pain or tightness when your knee was bent more than 90 degrees, but not quite touching your bottom, then you score two points for this test.
- If you felt pain or tightness when your foot was touching your bottom, then you score one point for this test.
- If you could bend your knee so that your foot was touching your

bottom and you did not feel any pain or stiffness in either your back or your thigh, then you do not score anything.

Please write down your scores for these three tests. You will use them occasionally throughout the rest of this book to help tailor the advice and exercises to your problem.

I hope that you now have a clear idea of your spinal pain, and to which category it belongs. Well done, and well diagnosed. You have the makings of a fine spinal health practitioner.

You can now use your newfound knowledge—of both anatomy and the behaviour and nature of your problem—to discover how to get rid of *your* back pain.

This quiz is displayed on the author's web page (address on p. 334).

Part III

How to get rid of your back pain forever

Now you're really getting somewhere. You have read the background information, and completed the assessment. Now you are going to learn some causes and cures of back pain. We will discuss not only aspects of your everyday life, such as postures, habits and work-related tasks, but also factors that arise from within yourself, such as muscle imbalances, stress and diet.

If you are like most people, then you probably feel that you already have enough problems, such as money, relationships, bad hair days and political correctness. 'Why,' you are probably asking yourself, 'is this guy telling me to try to identify even more problems?'

Never fear! For whenever I indicate a potential problem area, I'll provide a simple, workable solution as well. For example, if we discuss weak muscles, I'll tell you exactly how and why to perform appropriate strengthening exercises. If your sitting posture is suspect, I'll give you some practical hints on how to make it more efficient. Of course, all of the advice will be linked to your back pain type, *so the hints will be tailored to your particular problem.*

Naturally, all of this advice will be useless if you do not do one thing.

Change.

Yes, that's right, change.

Who, me?

Yes, you.

You'll have to change, because if you've had chronic or recurrent back pain in the past, then something that you are doing, or not *doing, is creating problems. Otherwise, your body would have naturally healed your injury long ago. Your behaviour is only the sum of your habits, and you must decipher which of them are causing the micro-trauma that doubtless underlies your problem.*

As you read the next twenty-three chapters, you'll come across many recommendations for the rehabilitation of your lower back. I suggest that you read every chapter, even if you feel that the topic is irrelevant. You may be surprised to discover an aspect of your problem that you hadn't really considered.

After each chapter, make some mental or physical notes about which aspects of back pain are most relevant to you. This information will be useful later, as in the final chapter you will learn how to combine your newfound knowledge to create a personalised rehabilitation program. This program will integrate all the information, tips, hints and tricks that you've learned, and will constitute your strategy to get rid of your back pain forever.

12

Muscle imbalances

Are you too strong for your own good?

Muscle imbalances are one of the most common causes of wear and tear in the body. They create all sorts of injuries, including arthritis, tendonitis, worn ligaments and headaches. And, importantly for you, muscle imbalances cause an enormous amount of back pain. Let's answer some basic questions about muscle imbalances, starting with the most simple.

What is a muscle imbalance?
Every joint in your body has at least two muscles that control it. These muscles are designed to work in harmony with each other, with each contributing a certain amount of pull when you perform a movement. In this way, a joint will move evenly and smoothly along its normal axis.

However, this symmetry of force does not always occur. Sometimes, the muscles around a joint pull it with an unequal force. This situation is known as a muscle imbalance.

At a basic level, muscle imbalances occur due to one of two reasons. First, one muscle might be stronger or tighter than the others. Second, one muscle might be weaker or more lax than the others. As you will soon learn, the differing strengths of opposing muscles have great implications for the health and wellbeing of your joints.

Do I have a muscle imbalance?
You might be a big, ugly, two-metre tall giant who plays professional football, or you might be a tiny, sweet, little old lady who crochets for a living. Although I've never even met you, I'm reasonably sure that the answer to the above question is 'yes, you probably *do* have a muscle imbalance'. How can I make this far-reaching assumption? Simply, most adult humans have developed a muscle imbalance of some sort, even if just a single tight or weak muscle.

The odds are swayed further in my favour if you've ever suffered from back pain. In one study, some researchers examined a large group of people, half of whom had experienced previous back pain, while the other half had always been symptom-free. The researchers were able to discern, with ninety per cent accuracy, to which group each subject belonged, simply by studying the muscle balance of each subject. They had no other information to go by whatsoever. In short, if you have back pain, then I am almost certain that you have a muscle imbalance that is contributing to your problem.

My guess is that you will find the following information extremely useful. Balancing your muscle tone is a front-line, A1 strategy in your fight against back pain.

Which muscles are usually affected by a muscle imbalance?
All of the muscles in the body can be roughly divided into two groups: *mobilising* muscles, and *stabilising* muscles.

Mobilising muscles are, as the name suggests, the muscles that normally move a joint. Your biceps muscle in your upper arm is an example: when you contract your biceps, your elbow bends.

The mobilising muscles score all of the exciting jobs that the human body has to do, like serving a tennis ball, drinking from a can of beer, dancing a foxtrot, or pedalling a bicycle. In general, they function when we consciously call upon them, then act in one quick burst, then rest and restore their energy. They tend to be long and large, and are often located just under your skin, where they have good leverage over the joints that lie deep below.

The names of many of the mobilising muscles are familiar to most people. This group includes well-known members like the *hamstrings*, the *quadriceps*, the *deltoids* and the *triceps*. When any of these muscles contract, the adjacent joint moves.

Conversely, the stabilising muscles have the job of holding your body together, which they do in two related ways. First, they routinely maintain your body's posture or position, such as sitting or standing. Second, the stabilising muscles counter the force of your mobilising muscles during joint movement. Without the stabilising muscles, your mobilising muscles would probably pull your joints out of place!

Your mind *subconsciously* recruits your stability muscles for all the tedious, boring jobs, such as posture maintenance, joint stability, and holding your organs in place. Because of this requirement, your stability muscles function with a continuous, low-intensity contraction, and you are usually barely aware that they are working. They tend to be short muscles that are situated deep within your body, alongside the joints that they protect.

Unfortunately, the stabilising muscles are not as well known to the general community, and most strengthening programs pay scant attention to this vital group. Who, apart from medically trained practitioners, has ever heard of the *lower trapezius*, the *subscapularis*, or the *vastus medialis oblique*?

What does all this have to do with muscle imbalances? Well, in the human body, the mobilising muscles tend to become overactive and tight,

MUSCLE IMBALANCES

while the stabilising muscles tend to become weak and lax. This is such an important point, that I'll risk boring you by repeating myself. The mobilising muscles tend to tighten, and the stability muscles tend to weaken.

Keep this point in mind as you read the rest of this chapter—no, the rest of the book as well.

How does a muscle imbalance cause joint wear and tear?
In normal movement, the mobilising muscles move the bones, while the local stability muscles dutifully hold the joint in place. However, if you have a spinal muscle imbalance, the stability muscles will be relatively weak, and will be unable to counteract the force of the mobilising muscles.

In this situation, your spinal joints slide and glide in a slightly faulty movement pattern. This eventually creates joint instability and/or stiffness, which, as you know, leads to excessive microtrauma. Repeat for ten years or so and hey *presto!*, you've got a sore back.

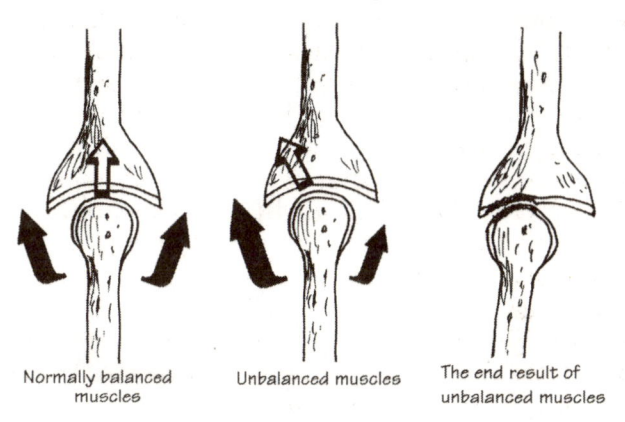

Normally balanced muscles   Unbalanced muscles   The end result of unbalanced muscles

The left picture shows the movement pattern of a normally balanced joint. The dark arrows show the equal pull of the muscles, and the clear arrow shows the resultant straight movement.

The centre picture shows how this situation changes if the muscles are imbalanced. Note the different sizes of the black arrows: the left one is probably an overactive mobility muscle, while the right side is most likely a weakened, inhibited stability muscle. The clear arrow shows that the resultant movement of the joint is slightly crooked.

The third picture shows the end result of a long-term muscle imbalance. Note the degeneration to the joint surface. Of course, this diagram is a highly simplified version of what happens in your spine, but the principle remains the same.

The effect of the muscle imbalance on your joints can be likened to what happens over time to your car tyres. If your car's wheels are properly balanced and aligned, then the tyres will wear evenly across their surfaces, and will last for years. However, if your wheels are badly aligned or unbalanced, one side of the tyres will wear out far more quickly.

A joint with a muscle imbalance is like a misaligned tyre: its abnormal movement pattern makes one part of the joint surface wear out more quickly than it should.

Weak stability muscles not only cause problems during movement, but also during stationary postures, such as sitting or standing. Here, the weak stability muscles cannot counter the effect of gravity, meaning that your vertebra must rely on the ligaments and discs to keep them in place. This extra pressure places a great burden on your lower back, which deteriorates far more quickly than normal.

Which stability muscles are important to the balance of your spine?
The muscular system around the spine is very complex. However, research has shown that two stability muscles are particularly important for the control, balance and stability of your spine.

These two structures are so important to many aspects of back pain control that you would be well served to make their acquaintance now. Without further ado, I would like to introduce you to these two vital players in the management of your back pain: your *transverse abdominal* muscle and your *multifidus* (mul-**tif**-ee-dus) muscle.

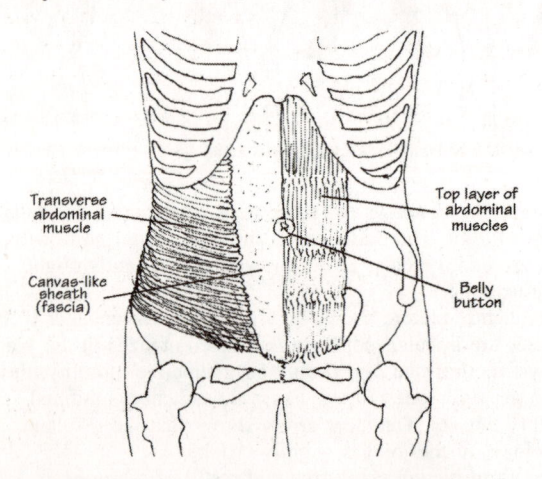

The left side of this picture shows the *transverse abdominal* muscle. Can you see that it wraps around your trunk, forming a natural corset to protect your spine?

The right side of the picture also shows your uppermost tummy muscle (called *rectus abdominus*, if you're interested) which is not so adept at protecting your spine.

MUSCLE IMBALANCES

Your transverse abdominal is the deepest of your four separate tummy muscles. This underused muscle wraps around your tummy like a wide belt, and forms a natural corset for your spine.

By contrast, your multifidus is a collection of small muscles that run down the centre of your back, directly next to the pointy spinous process at the back of each vertebra.

These two muscles, by virtue of their positions and well-leveraged attachments, are the most efficient providers of spinal protection and stability. Like Batman and Robin, the Lone Ranger and Tonto, or that pair of flair-wearing '70s cops Starsky and Hutch, these muscles work best in tandem with each other. When they contract at the same time, they firmly stabilise your spine both front and back, providing a platform for controlled, safe spinal and limb movement.

If these two muscles weaken, your spine loses stability, and must use other stomach and back muscles to substitute. However, the only other muscles available are the local mobilising muscles. This recruitment creates poor muscle balance, which almost inevitably causes pain.

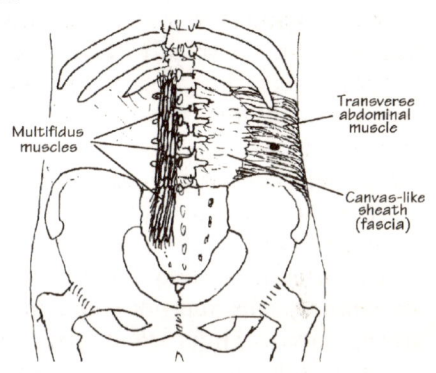

On the left side of this picture, which shows your trunk from the back, is the *multifidus* muscle (pronounced mul-TIF-ee-dus). The multifidus is really a collection of many tiny muscles. Can you see that their close association with the vertebrae makes them ideally positioned to protect your spine?

These theories sound alright, but have they been proven?
Previously, the actions of the stability muscles was very poorly understood, resulting in strengthening programs that were ineffective at best. Luckily for us, many researchers have recently investigated the causes and effects of weakened spinal stability muscles. Although I won't directly quote much research in this book, this stuff is important, so I'd like to share it with you. (Also, much of it was conducted at my old *alma mater*, the University of Queensland, so it is a good opportunity to give them a plug.)

The research team used whiz-bang modern technology such as electromyography, biofeedback and ultrasound scanners. These machines not only had pretty lights, and emitted lots of important-sounding beeping noises, but they also allowed the examiners to see what role the transverse abdominal and multifidus muscles play in preventing back pain.

In one project, the researchers studied two groups of people. The

BACK PAIN

subjects in the first group had healthy, pain-free spines, while the members of the second group had, like you, lots of lower back pain. The researchers found that those people with back pain had much smaller, weaker stability muscles than the other group.

Furthermore, the back pain subjects could not actively, consciously contract their stability muscles, no matter how hard they tried. Conversely, the members of the pain-free group could consciously tighten their stability muscles without difficulty.

Subsequent studies provided additional insights. For example, they demonstrated that the multifidus muscle tended to be smaller and weaker on the painful side than on the good side. Not only that, but the muscle next to the affected vertebra was smaller than the muscles at other non-affected levels. This finding showed a clear relationship between the strength of the multifidus muscle and lower back pain.

The researchers also showed that after an injured spinal joint heals, the stability muscles did not spontaneously recover their strength. In other words, once you injure your spine, the stability muscles remain weak until you retrain them. This finding helps to explain why many people suffer from repeated or chronic spinal injuries. Does that sound familiar?

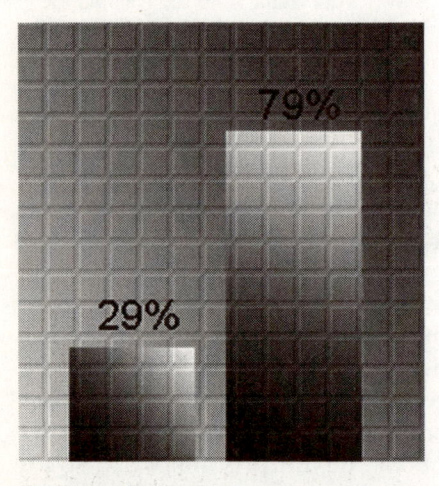

In order to observe how these muscles protect the lower back, the team also investigated the automatic, subconscious reactions of the transverse abdominal and multifidus muscles. The experimental subjects were asked to rapidly lift and lower their arm, while the researchers monitored their deep stability muscles. They found that the muscles contracted *automatically* in people with healthy spines, thus protecting the lumbar joints. However, the muscles of those people with back pain did nothing to help protect their spines. They just sat quietly bludging, as if nothing were happening. The spinal discs and joints had to fend for themselves. It is no wonder that this group had back pain!

The left column shows your expected rate of back pain recurrence if your stability muscles are awake and toned.

The right column shows your likelihood of recurrence if, like most people, your brain has forgotten that your stability muscles exist. Which side would you rather be on?

To seal the case that these muscles are vital for preventing lower back pain, the researchers divided forty back pain suffers into two halves. They placed the first group on a traditional back pain prevention program, which included

MUSCLE IMBALANCES

anti-inflammatory medication and regular swimming. They showed the second group how to strengthen their deep stability muscles. A year later, the researchers reviewed both groups.

The results were conclusive. The first group had a 79 per cent recurrence rate of lower back pain. However, the second group, who had strengthened their deep stability muscles, had only a 29 per cent recurrence rate. Which group would you rather be in?

These, and many other studies show that the function of the stability muscles is extremely important—possibly the *most* important factor—in preventing back pain. The research strongly suggests that you include strengthening of the transverse abdominal and multifidus muscles in your back care program.

By the sound of it, weak stability muscles cause lots of problems. But what about tight mobility muscles?
Tight mobilising muscles create pain because they lead to poor postures and movement habits, which inevitably stresses the spinal joints. For example, say that your hamstring muscles, which stretch over the back

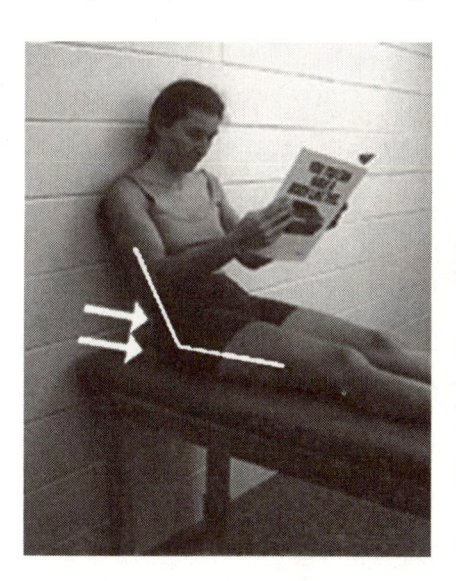

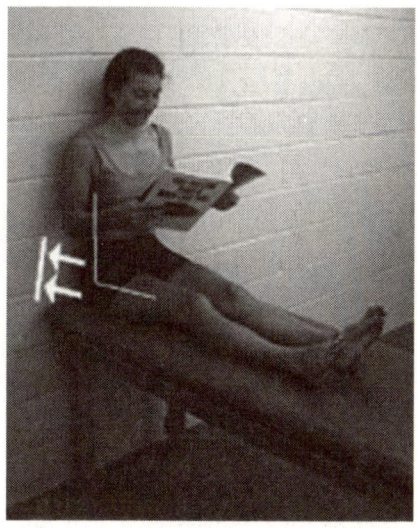

In the left photo, Debbie's tight hamstrings are preventing her from fully bending her hips, as indicated by the lines. As a result, her bottom must slide away from the wall, so her lower back loses support.

However, in the right photograph, Debbie's hamstrings have miraculously loosened. She can now bend her hips to a greater angle. Her bottom can stay against the wall, and thus maintain support for her lower back. By the way, a tight sciatic nerve has the same effect. We'll talk more about sitting posture in Chapter 15.

of your hips and knees, are tight and inflexible. When you adopt certain postures—for example, sitting with your legs stretched out in front of you—your spinal joints must bend further than usual to compensate for your hamstring tightness. This extra pressure generates strain on your back joints, ultimately causing premature breakdown.

Another example is the muscle at the front of your hip called the *iliopsoas* (pronounced ill-ee-oh-SO-ass; ignore the 'P' and you'll get it right). In a normal standing position, your iliopsoas is stretched between your back and your hips. If this muscle is tight, it pulls your spine further inward, increasing your lordosis until its curve is excessive. This poor posture, which is compounded by weak abdominal muscles, leads to problems such as pain during prolonged standing.

Why do muscle imbalances occur in the first place?
Muscle imbalances occur for many reasons. The most common reason that muscle imbalances occur is very simple: they just happen. The big word for this is *idiopathic*.

Simply, the nature of the mobilising muscles—their cellular formation, nerve supply, fibre type, and a million other factors that are too complex to enter into here—encourages them to become stronger and tighter. Conversely, the same factors work to weaken and loosen the stability muscles.

Furthermore, evolution was not kind to many of our stability muscles. For example, the abdominal muscles once had the cushy job of simply holding our intestines in place as we meandered around on all fours munching grass. However, as we progressed to two legs, the hapless abdominals were forced to include 'spinal support' in their job descriptions. This change did not happen overnight, and unfortunately, it did not happen with complete effectiveness.

Unfortunately, these two factors—muscle type, and the evolutionary boo-boo—are common to all of us, and cannot be changed. So forget about them. However, five other situations will magnify the difference between the two groups of muscles.

(1) Repetitive, high speed or heavy movements
When you perform any movement repetitively, quickly or with great force, your body sensibly recruits its mobility muscles, which are designed for these types of tasks. This gives the mobilising muscles a work-out, meaning that they become stronger. However, the stabilising muscles do not receive an equivalent input to improve their holding capacity. This difference in recruitment results in asymmetric muscle development, which, if regularly repeated, ultimately leads to a muscle imbalance. Many sports people fall into this category.

(2) Mental tension

The mobilising muscles are more readily activated than the stability muscles. If we again look at human evolution, this makes perfect sense, for if you need to move quickly to avoid danger, the mobilising muscles are obviously the group of choice. Your postural muscles are not much use in this situation.

In modern society, the stress of physical survival has been replaced by many other anxieties. When these stresses build up, our body places the mobilising muscles on full alert, ready to fight or flee. Of course, this response is rarely necessary, so the tension simply accumulates in the mobility muscles.

After being held in a tensed state for a long period, the mobility muscles become naturally tighter, stronger, and even more responsive. Meanwhile, the stability muscles are receiving less input, and are relatively weakening. Guess what happens after a while? A muscle imbalance.

We'll be talking in detail about mental tension and its effects on back pain in Chapter 20.

(3) Lack of consistent exercise and stretching

A muscle that is not regularly stretched throughout its full range quickly tightens, and may undergo permanent shortening if the lack of use continues. When tight, muscles tend to become overactive, heightening the potential for a muscle imbalance to develop.

Weakness develops at a similarly alarming rate. Consider space astronauts, who, after only a few weeks in zero gravity, become so weak that they cannot support their own body weight. Therefore, immobility due to injury, or a sedentary, couch-potato lifestyle, will rapidly lead to development of a muscle imbalance.

(4) Injury to a nearby joint

As we briefly mentioned in Chapter 7, nature has provided each group of muscles with a different response to injury. The mobilising muscles tend to spasm or tighten if a nearby joint is injured. Conversely, the stability muscles become inhibited in the same situation.

Can you see how a joint injury has the potential to create an instant muscle imbalance? When you suffer an injury, the local mobilising muscles become tight, while the nearby stability muscles weaken. These opposite reactions create an instant imbalance.

A nagging, chronic injury can have a potentially devastating effect on the balance of nearby muscle groups. The injury encourages the adjacent mobilising muscles to spasm, while simultaneously inhibiting the stability muscles. Unfortunately, this imbalance can worsen the injury, which then exacerbates the muscle imbalance, and so on. This vicious cycle can be very difficult to break—unless you know how, of course!

(5) Poor posture
A poor posture is generally one which relies on your joints to hold you upright, rather than using the muscles for stability. Many people subconsciously adopt a poor posture to avoid using fatigued or weak postural muscles. This not only heightens the muscle imbalance, but causes degeneration in your overstrained ligaments and discs.

Will going to the gym or doing weight-lifting exercises help me to strengthen my stability muscles?
No.

Note this point clearly: general strengthening exercises, such as sit-ups, back extensions and a whole host of other 'normal' exercises, will not strengthen your stability muscles. These types of exercises call upon the mobilising muscles, and so may even worsen your imbalance.

Many athletes are under the impression that they can prevent imbalance problems simply by working the major muscles either side of a joint: the hamstrings and the quadriceps in the thigh, for example, or the biceps and triceps in the arm. This theory has two drawbacks. First, almost all weight-lifting exercises concentrate on the mobilising muscles, not stability muscles. The fact that these mobilising muscles are on opposite sides of the joint is of little consequence. Second, the exercises encourage the mobility function of the muscles, not the stabilising, postural function that is necessary to prevent injury.

In short, strength alone will not protect you from injuries: even extremely strong weightlifters suffer from pain, stiffness and other injuries. The key to protecting yourself from injury and degeneration is *balance*.

Does this mean that you should quit all sports, and avoid gym programs like the plague? No, it doesn't! Not at all. You probably have many other perfectly good reasons to go to the gym. If you are feeling stronger, keeping fitter or looking better as a result of your gym program, then fine. Keep at it. However, if you are doing a weight-lifting program in the hope that extra strength will cure your spinal pain, then you may wish to reassess your motives.

Similarly, I am not advocating that general aerobic exercise is bad for your spine. In fact, as you will see later, the opposite is true. However, the type of exercise, how you perform it, and which muscles you target, will decide if your program will be successful in increasing your spinal stability.

I hope that you can now see the vital role that muscle balance plays in preventing your lower back pain. The evidence is very strong. If you have chronic or frequent bouts of back pain, then the exercise routines in the following two chapters will be one of the most useful strategies to help you cure your problem.

13
Designing a personalised exercise program

You may be wondering: 'So I have spinal muscle imbalances, stiff joints, and neural tension. But how do I fix them?'

What a good question! I'm glad you asked. In simple terms, you must address four areas to properly rehabilitate your spine. You must:

1. Stretch your mobilising muscles.
2. Loosen your tight nerves.
3. Mobilise your stiff joints.
4. Strengthen your stability muscles.

In this way, balance and flexibility will be restored to your entire lower spine, and your joints will again sit and move with a normal alignment. From there, it's only a short metaphorical hop to a permanently pain-free back.

Let's look at techniques to perform these four very important functions. Then, in the next chapter, we will detail the individual exercises step by step.

Stretch your mobilising muscles

When you stretch muscles, your body subconsciously derives devious ways to avoid the unpleasant pulling sensation. As if they had a mind of their own, your limbs cannily shift into a position where the tension is minimised. Of course, this sneakiness lessens the uncomfortable feelings, but also ruins the effectiveness of the stretch. So when stretching, you must use careful positioning so prevent your limbs from tricking you.

Once you have achieved the desired position, you must *relax*. Any extra tension will simply flow through into the muscles, causing them to tighten, thus reducing the effectiveness of the exercises. In most cases the stretching positions have been designed to allow gravity to do a lot of work, so an easy method to increase the intensity of your stretch is to relax even further.

Do not bounce, jerk or tense the muscle. You should steadily maintain each stretch position for at least ten seconds. This technique allows

DESIGNING A PERSONALISED EXERCISE PROGRAM

time for the muscle fibres to elongate, producing a more effective result. You can hold the stretch for even longer, up to one minute, if your concentration allows.

Another useful method for stretching tight muscles is to use a technique known as contract–relax–stretch. The contract–relax–stretch technique was popularised many years ago by researchers who derived it from a theory known as *proprioceptive neuromuscular facilitation*.

Even though they are effective, simplicity dictates that I won't be describing propriomuscle neurothingamijig stretches in this book. However I was dying to use that big phrase somewhere in this book to show how clever I was (it's got fifteen syllables, you know) and this was the most obvious place.

Loosen your tight nerves

Recall from Chapter 8 that nerves are not delicate structures, but are as thick and robust as a piece of rope. You may well feel that it would be pretty difficult to stretch a piece of rope. Guess what ... you're absolutely right. However, this does not mean that you should ignore the *mobility* of your nerves.

Recall from our earlier brief discussion in Chapter 9 that as the nerves traverse through your spine and limbs, they move inside a tunnel formed by the other tissues, just like a brake cable. When you perform the nerve-loosening exercises in the following chapter, you will be encouraging the nerve to regain its normal sliding and gliding movements inside this tunnel. In short, you will be stretching the things that are stopping the nerve from moving. Please do not underestimate the value of this practice, as many cases of back pain are caused or worsened by immobile nerves.

Two techniques can help you to loosen your nerves. First you can 'floss' the nerve, in much the same way that you floss your teeth. By holding your nerve in an elongated position and then performing a gentle oscillation, your nerve will slide and glide across whatever is blocking it. As you repeat this technique, your nerve will hopefully unstick itself.

The second technique is to simply stretch your nerve. With some luck, the nerve will gradually pull away from whatever is causing its movement to be blocked. When loosening your nerves in this fashion, you should aim for the same principles of careful positioning and relaxed, prolonged holds as you do with muscles.

Unfortunately, nerve stretching is even more unpleasant than muscle stretching, so you must monitor your limb position very carefully to ensure that they aren't cheating on you.

Mobilise your stiff joints

Spinal joint stretching, known as joint *mobilisation*, can be difficult to accurately perform on yourself. This predicament is because, as mentioned previously, the laws of physics demand that the body will always take the path of least resistance. Therefore, when you perform joint-mobilising exercises, chances are that you are moving the joints that are already flexible, while the stiff areas stay locked in place.

For this reason, people with unstable backs—Types A and B—should avoid doing vigorous spinal-mobilising exercises. They probably won't help. Even if you have a stiff joint, then your body will simply stretch the loosest parts of your spine, possibly making them even more unstable. However, Types C and D, who have a generalised problem with stiffness, will probably benefit from self-mobilisation.

The secret to effective joint mobilisation is to be as specific as possible. A simple guideline is that you should stabilise your spine below the stiff area, then move the parts above it. This strategy should force the target segments to move. While I can't show you how to accurately differentiate one vertebral level from the next, the following exercises will at least guide you toward mobilising the correct region of your spine.

Strengthen your deep stability muscles

The body, with its normal attempt at efficiency, always chooses the easiest way to perform any movement. It's a bit like a lazy factory worker: it doesn't use the best way to perform a task, but the easiest. If the body has two muscles to choose from, it will always use the strongest. As you know, the mobility muscles are frequently stronger than their stabilising counterparts, and so are usually chosen to perform the movement. Because of this tendency, many people find it difficult to *selectively* strengthen their stability muscles. How do we overcome this obstacle?

Luckily, modern biomedical research has again provided us with answers. The key to exercising stability muscles is this: you should try to replicate the role that they normally take in your body, that of a background, low-intensity, almost subconscious use.

If you exercise in this way, then your body will choose the stability muscles, which are best suited for this type of work, rather than choosing a stronger, more active substitute. This replication can be achieved by following four rules.

1. Exercise at very low levels—no more than 30 per cent of your maximum intensity.

Because your body uses the stability muscles for background jobs such as posture maintenance, they are accustomed to being used in a very low-intensity way. If you work too energetically during an exercise, then your body will simply choose a stronger mobility muscle. Therefore, to utilise only the stability muscle, a low-intensity contraction is best. This information should be great news to those readers who are allergic to sweat.

2. Use prolonged holds.
The body will choose the mobilising muscles for quick, sudden tasks, and the stability muscles for slow, prolonged tasks. Therefore, if you wish to facilitate your stability muscles, then you must use very slow, prolonged holds.

Generally, holds of at least five seconds are required before the stability muscles really kick in, so all exercises aimed at increasing joint stability should last at least this long, preferably longer.

3. Don't move.
To selectively emphasise a stability muscle, you should contract the muscle without moving any joints. A simple example is to think of a body builder flexing his or her muscles in a pose—all of their muscles are contracting tightly, but nothing is moving. This type of contraction is called an *isometric* contraction. By using this type of exercise, your body is more likely to use a stability muscle rather than a mobilising muscle.

4. Concentrate.
Your body has undoubtedly developed a strong habit over many years of depending upon the mobility muscles. This habit is so common that it can be considered normal, but nevertheless is undesirable. When performing stability muscle exercises, you must concentrate fiercely to ensure that the nearby mobility muscles are not substituting for a weakened stability muscle. By carefully feeling the target muscle, you can be sure that it is working correctly.

So, to activate and selectively strengthen your stability muscles, you must use very *low-intensity*, *prolonged*, *static holds*, and *concentrate* very closely on the quality of the contraction. Compare this method with mobility muscle strengthening—think of a grunting, groaning, sweating weightlifter—and you'll see the stark difference between the two methods.

In short, if you feel like you are doing almost nothing while you exercise your stability muscles, then you're probably doing it correctly. Conversely, if you find yourself straining, heaving or puffing, then you're definitely trying too hard. Here, you're probably just exercising your mobility muscles, and so you will not gain as much benefit.

Trying too hard is a common problem with these exercises. If you ever find that your progress is slow, the best way to improve is to try less hard! This concept is so foreign to our normal way of thinking, particularly if you are a competitive sportsperson, that you will probably have to regularly remind yourself to take it easy. If necessary, review the above principles, which will help to convince you that gentle contractions are more effective than over-exertion.

To emphasise this point, I usually try not to use the phrase 'strengthening exercises', as it conjures the wrong image. 'Facilitating' or 'awakening' your muscles are terms that more accurately describe the correct process. You are, in essence, trying to *remind your brain that your stability muscles exist*.

Remember, balance—not strength—protects your spine. Please keep all of the information presented above uppermost in your mind as you perform the exercises in the following chapter.

14

Exercises to correct muscle imbalances, joint stiffness and neural tension

Don't just sit there—it's time for work!

Which exercises are best for your spine?

As you know, different spinal injuries require different exercises. I'm sure that you appreciate that the only way that I could assess your particular problem would be to examine you individually. This personalised service would be nice, but its obviously impossible, as at the moment I'm lying on a beach on a deserted Pacific island, sipping a cool beer, spending up big on the $129.23 that I made on the sale of this book.

Luckily, we have a very good substitute to help us decide what type of problem may be causing your spine pain. Your back type—whether it be A, B, C or D—provides us with a serviceable guide in this regard.

In short, types A and B typically have unstable spines that generally lack muscular support. Most of their exercises will therefore concentrate on reactivating their weak stability muscles. Types C and D, on the other hand, are generally very stiff, and so require stretching and mobilising.

By taking note of your neural tension tests, you can also decide whether to include some nerve stretches into your program.

Obviously some overlap will exist, not only between groups but also within the same person's spine. For example, even very stiff spines may still require exercises to strengthen the stability muscles. Think of a stiff knee, which will almost certainly weaken as well, and you'll see why this is so.

Despite any overlap and uncertainty, I'm sure that if you follow the recommended exercises you will be heading in the right direction.

As you will see, the program is variable with regard to not only your back type, but also the amount of time and effort you have to spare, as well as your fitness level.

Each listed exercise will have three levels of ability, through which you can progress as you improve. Don't skip a stage, and definitely don't try to progress too quickly. As mentioned in the last chapter, trying too hard, particularly with the stability exercises, will doom you to failure. Take your time, aim for slow, consistent progress, and you'll do just fine.

As a rule, stay on Level One for at least two weeks. Remain patient, and remember that most of these exercises are *supposed* to feel easy. If, after two weeks, you feel that a particular exercise has become ridiculously simple, then progress to the next stage. Remain on that level of difficulty for at least another two weeks, and then advance to the third and final stage if you are fully confident. By using this conservative method, you will avoid the common pitfall of trying to progress too fast.

Be aware that not all of your exercises will improve at the same rate. For example, you may find that you can advance through your stretching exercises very quickly, while it takes you two months to upgrade your stability exercises. This finding is common, and should not concern you.

Furthermore, I have recommended programs for three different levels of commitment. Those among us who have trouble getting motivated can start with just a couple of the most important exercises, while keener participants can perform a whole routine, leaving no stone unturned.

Again, most people are best served by beginning with a very simple program. In this way, your routine will be easier to complete, and you will develop a regular exercise habit. Sometimes, people who attack their problems with excessive vigour and enthusiasm falter after a couple of weeks. Why not take it easy on yourself for the first few weeks, aim to *never* miss a session, and then build on your commitment once you've established good habits.

While we're talking about commitment, please don't kid yourself that you don't have time for the exercises. I have heard this excuse hundreds of times, and it just doesn't wash. The short programs below take only three minutes to complete. Three short minutes—180 seconds. I'm sure that if you put your mind to it that you could find an extra three minutes in which to relax and do your exercises. If you can't find three spare minutes in the middle of the day, then put your alarm on three minutes earlier, or go to bed three minutes later. Don't blame the kids, or your partner, your boss, or anyone else. In short, if you are struggling to find the time for exercises, then I'd re-examine your motivation and commitment.

Aim to perform at least one set of exercises per day. If you have plenty of time, or if you have chosen a short program, then two sessions per day are better. If you have severe or chronic pain, then three times per day is better still, but any more often than that is, in my opinion, overdoing it, particularly considering the mental 'burn out' factor.

EXERCISES TO CORRECT MUSCLE IMBALANCES

You must *relax* when you do these exercises. You will get nowhere by trying to cram in a quick set of abdominal contractions while eating breakfast and simultaneously dressing for work. Why not spoil yourself— put the time aside, relax, and ease yourself into your routine. Invariably, those who relax while doing their exercises not only gain greater benefit, but also commit to their routine until they are cured.

Importantly, do *not* be tempted to do all of the exercises listed. Remember, what helps one person's back may ruin another's. Please stick to the recommended exercises only.

If you are a borderline category, then you should consult the guidelines below to help you decide which set of exercises to try.

- Borderline AB: The exercises for these two categories are quite similar. In fact, the first two motivation levels are identical. This similarity is because the stability muscles, which are the focus of these two programs, work best in partnership with each other, rather than alone. If you are type AB and wish to do a comprehensive program, then simply omit exercises four and five, which may exacerbate your condition.
- Borderline AC: Try the exercises for type A first. The type A exercises will probably help, but even if they don't provide much benefit, at least they will do no harm. If you have not improved after three to six weeks, then gradually incorporate one exercise from program C each week. Monitor your progress, and discontinue any exercises that increase your pain.
- Borderline BD: Try the exercises for type B first. The type B exercises will probably help, but even if they don't provide any benefit, at least they will do no harm. If you have not improved after three to six weeks, then gradually incorporate one exercise from program D each week. Monitor your progress, and discontinue any exercises that increase your pain.
- Borderline CD: Your spine is stiff everywhere, so you would probably benefit from a generalised stretching program. Simply combine programs C and D together.

Lastly, describing exercises in a book is fraught with difficulties. Many of the exercises are complex to master, and require very subtle techniques. While a barber could theoretically write instructions on how to perform a haircut, in practice it would be very difficult to follow with any great success. I suggest that you seek assistance from a qualified spinal health practitioner if you have difficulty grasping the exercises. OK, I know I'm biased, but in this situation, I reckon that a physiotherapist is best.

Exercises for lumbar flexibility and stability

To design your program using the table below, first decide whether you wish to try the quick, intermediate or comprehensive program. Remember that you can easily increase your commitment level later, when you have established good exercise habits. Then by reading across the top row, identify your back pain type. The numbers in the appropriate box indicate the exercises that form the basis of your program.

For example, suppose you have back type C, and wish to perform an intermediate program. By reading the table, you would perform exercises four, seven, one and two.

Motivation level	Back Type A	Back Type B	Back Type C	Back Type D
Quick Program	Exercises 1 & 2	Exercises 1 & 2	Exercises 4 & 7	Exercises 5 & 6
Intermediate Program	Exercises 1, 2 & 3	Exercises 1, 2 & 3	Exercises 4, 7, 1 & 2	Exercises 5, 6, 1 & 2
Comprehensive Program	Exercises 1, 2, 3, 5, 6, 13	Exercises 1, 2, 3, 4, 7, 14	Exercises 4, 7, 1, 2, 13, 15	Exercises 5, 6, 1, 2, 14, 15

Additional exercises

NEURAL TENSION
Recall the three nerve immobility tests that you completed in Chapter 11. They are listed in the left column in the table on the next page. Then, after reading along the top row to find your test score, add the required exercises to your program.

For example, suppose your score for the Straight Leg Raise test was two, while you scored three points for the Slump test, and your passive knee bend test was clear. You wish to perform the intermediate program. You would add exercise ten, eleven, eight and nine to your list of exercises.

THORACIC SPINE
If you have pain or stiffness in your upper back, then you may find it useful to add exercises eight and nine to your program.

You should now have a list of numbers, which indicate the specific exercises that are most suited to your problem. Don't worry if a few

EXERCISES TO CORRECT MUSCLE IMBALANCES

of them appear more than once; just ignore any repeat references. This list is not necessarily final, as your lifestyle and other factors may indicate some additions or changes. These alterations will become clearer as you continue reading this book.

	1 point	2 points	3 points
Straight Leg Raise	• Add exercise 10 to the comprehensive program	• Add exercise 10 to the intermediate and comprehensive programs • Add exercise 15 to the comprehensive programs	• Add exercise 10 to all programs • Add exercise 15 to the intermediate and comprehensive programs • Add exercises 8 & 9 to the comprehensive program
Slump Test	• Add exercise 11 to the comprehensive program	• Add exercise 11 to the intermediate and comprehensive programs • Add exercises 8 & 9 to the comprehensive program	• Add exercise 11 to all programs • Add exercise 8 & 9 to the comprehensive and intermediate programs • Add exercise 15 to the comprehensive program
Prone Knee Bend	• Add exercise 12 to the comprehensive program	• Add exercise 12 to the intermediate and comprehensive programs	• Add exercise 12 to all programs

Now, by carefully reading the instructions below, you can learn how to perform the exercises that will help you take an enormous leap forward in your mission to permanently rid yourself of back pain.

Exercises to correct spinal muscle imbalances, joint stiffness and neural tension

EXERCISES 1–3: STABILITY EXERCISES
The first two exercises below are to awaken your deep spinal stability muscles. As mentioned in the last chapter, the tone of your deep stability muscles is vital to getting rid of your back pain. Because these two exercises are so important, you must perform them very precisely. To do this, you must rely on your skills of muscle palpation.

What? You don't *have* any muscle palpation skills? Well, I'd better teach you!

Palpation simply means 'using your hands to feel'. When palpating a muscle, you are feeling its tone and hardness to discern whether it is contracting properly. This skill is not easy, and may take a few days to master. Nevertheless, you will be far better able to perform these vital exercises if you are able to use your fingers to differentiate a relaxed muscle from one that is contracting.

A simple place to learn this skill is your biceps muscle in your upper arm. The centre of this muscle is about five centimetres (that's about two inches, for all those readers over the age of thirty-five) above the front of your elbow. The following demonstration assumes that you are sitting in a chair.

First, rest your right wrist in your lap so that your whole right arm is fully relaxed. Really let your whole arm flop. Now use your left hand to feel the tone and hardness of your right biceps muscle. Knead it gently, as though it were a piece of dough, and firmly sink your fingers into the muscle belly. Can you feel how soft and pliable the muscle is?

Now, with your right palm facing up toward the ceiling, lift your hand from your lap. Now, palpate the biceps muscle again. Can you feel the difference? Your biceps muscle is now contracting, and should feel harder, firmer and more toned than before.

Guess what? You've just learned how to palpate for muscle tone. See if you can palpate the different tone in your quadriceps muscle (your front thigh muscle) when your foot is resting on the floor as compared to when you lift it into the air.

When you feel confident that you have mastered the skills of muscle palpation, you should move on to the following exercises.

1. Transverse abdominal muscle contractions
Goal: To awaken and facilitate the deep stability muscles in your lower tummy.

Level One
1. Lie on a firm, flat surface on your back, with your knees bent to a comfortable angle.

EXERCISES TO CORRECT MUSCLE IMBALANCES

2. Relax your tummy muscles, and calm your breathing.
3. Palpate your transverse abdominal muscle. To find it, first locate the bony prominences on each side of the front of your pelvis. Now, slide your fingers about two centimetres (one inch) inwards from the bony points. Sink your fingertips firmly through the top layers of muscle. The deepest muscle, which you can feel with the ends of your fingertips, is the transverse abdominal muscle.
4. Tighten your *pelvic floor* muscles. To do this, pretend that you are urinating, and that you suddenly have to stop. This pelvic floor contraction is important, as these muscles are closely associated with the transverse abdominal muscle. By tightening your pelvic floor, your transverse abdominal muscle will contract automatically. (This effect can be roughly likened to when you bend your little finger—your fourth finger automatically bends as well.)

    You should now verify that your transverse abdominal muscle is contracting by palpating with your fingertips. Do you feel a slight increase in the tension and tone of the transverse abdominal muscle? If so, move on to step five. If not, continue to practice this manoeuvre until you can confidently feel the transverse abdominal muscle tighten.
5. Gently breathe out, then slowly and gently draw your lower tummy inward, without allowing your spine or pelvis to move.

    All of the contraction should occur below your belly button. If your upper abdomen or diaphragm tighten, then you are trying too hard.

    Do not brace your whole tummy, and especially try to avoid the feeling of 'bearing down' as if you were defecating on the toilet. Remember, you are aiming for *a gentle, isolated contraction of just one muscle*.

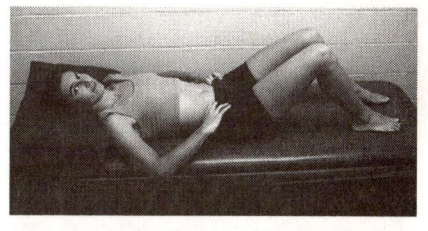

    Here Debbie is hard at work exercising her transverse abdominal muscle. Note the position of her fingers, just inside her front hip bones. She is carefully feeling for the muscle contraction.

6. Allow your breathing to return to normal. Continue to feel for the increased tone in your transverse abdominal muscle for a few seconds. Remember, neither your back nor your upper tummy muscles should move.
7. Relax. Well done, that's one repetition.
8. Repeat ten times.

Level Two

As above, but hold the contraction for five seconds. Note that you should be able to feel the transverse abdominal muscle relax when you let go.

BACK PAIN

Level Three
As above, but hold the contraction for ten seconds.

There are many other advanced exercises for your lower abdominal muscles. But I'm not going to tell them to you. Why? Because if I show them to you, then you'll probably be tempted to try them before your muscles are sufficiently balanced to cope with extra load. Of course, when you feel that you have mastered these exercises, then please see a spinal health practitioner for some further instruction.

2. *Multifidus muscle contractions*
Goal: To awaken the deep stability muscles in your lower back.
Note: Do not be concerned if you cannot perform this exercise at first. As mentioned in the last chapter, experiments have shown that very few people with lower back pain are able to spontaneously contract this muscle. The longer your back has been painful, the more difficult it will be for you to tighten this muscle in isolation. However, your multifidus is so important to your successful rehabilitation that I advise you to persist for at least a month. Seek help if necessary.

Level One
1. Lie on your left side with your knees comfortably bent.
2. Palpate your right multifidus muscle. To find this muscle, use your right thumb to feel for the pointy spinous processes of your lower vertebrae. The multifidus lies directly next to these bumps of bone.

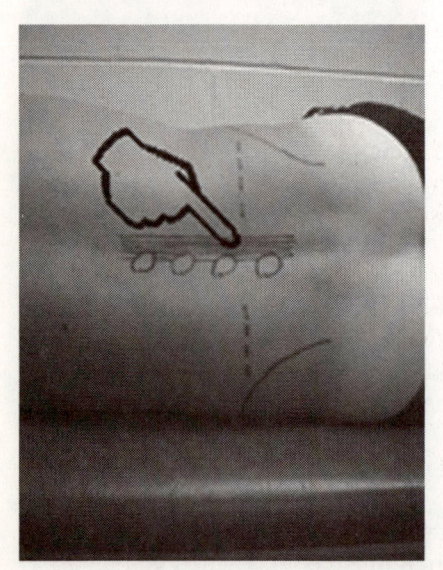

This photograph demonstrates how to find your multifidus muscle. The two curved lines at the sides are the top of Greg's pelvic bones. I hope that you can locate your pelvis bones easily—if not, perhaps you should, ahem, take heed of the advice in Chapter 25 on diet. The round circles in the centre are the spinous processes—those pointy bits that stick out the back of each vertebra. Your multifidus muscle, as indicated by the striped area, lies *directly* next to these pointy bumps.

Your L4–5 area, which is the most frequently weakened area of this muscle, can be found by intersecting an imaginary line (in this case a dotted line) between your hip bones and your spine. The big pretend hand shows the best spot to feel for your multifidus muscle during these exercises.

EXERCISES TO CORRECT MUSCLE IMBALANCES

You should also attempt to locate the most painful, problematic level of your spine. As the L4 and L5 level are by far the most commonly injured, I'll show you how to find these vertebrae. While you are lying on your side, feel for the large pelvic bone that forms your 'hip'. The top of this bone is level with your L4-5 disc, so if you draw an imaginary vertical line from this point, it will intersect your spine at approximately the right area.

3. Keeping your lower back and pelvis *completely* still, simply tighten your multifidus muscle. (It's harder than it sounds.) You should use your thumb to check if the muscle has contracted. If so, it will *slowly* develop a bulge, or feel slightly tighter.

If you can't manage this, then you may find that simultaneously contracting your transverse abdominal and pelvic floor muscles helps the multifidus to contract. Keep trying, but don't overdo it. Remember, your spine must not move at all, not even one nanometre. (OK, I'm exaggerating, but you get the point.)

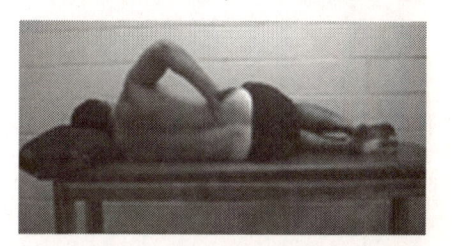

Here Greg is hard at work exercising his multifidus muscle. Note that his thumb is palpating for the increase in muscle tone, which should be very slow and subtle, like a balloon that is slowly filling with air. Nothing else should move if you perform this exercise correctly.

4. Relax. Ten repetitions.
5. Now switch over to your right side and repeat the exercise.

Level Two
Hold the contraction for five seconds.

Level Three
Hold the contraction for ten seconds.

As with the transverse abdominal muscle, there are many advanced exercises for multifidus stability. However, I'm not going to tell you those, either. Sorry about that.

3. *Hip muscle contractions (gluteus medius)*
Goal: To strengthen the muscle that keeps your pelvis level when you are standing, and to generally increase your trunk stability.
Note: To successfully perform the following exercises, your stability muscles (i.e. your transverse abdominal and multifidus muscles) should be in reasonable shape. If you have difficulty maintaining a still, level pelvis while performing the following exercise, then omit it from your program for about three weeks until your stability muscles have regained some tone.

BACK PAIN

Level One
1. Lie on your side, with both knees bent comfortably. Your ankles should be resting on each other, and be roughly in line with your trunk.
2. Tighten your lower abdominal and multifidus muscles as you did in exercises one and two.

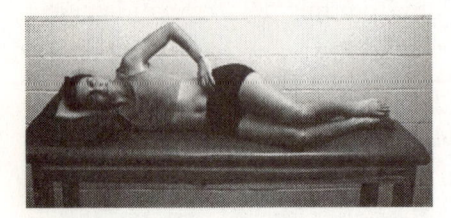

The correct starting position for the hip muscle exercise. Debbie's shoulders, hips, knees and ankles are all level and aligned. Note also that Debbie is palpating her transverse abdominal muscle, just as you did in Exercise 1.

3. Slowly and carefully, lift the top knee about ten centimetres (four inches) into the air, while leaving your ankles resting on each other.

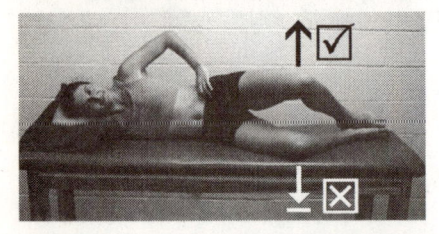

The end of the movement. Note that Debbie's ankles are still in contact with each other, and that her trunk and pelvis have not moved at all.

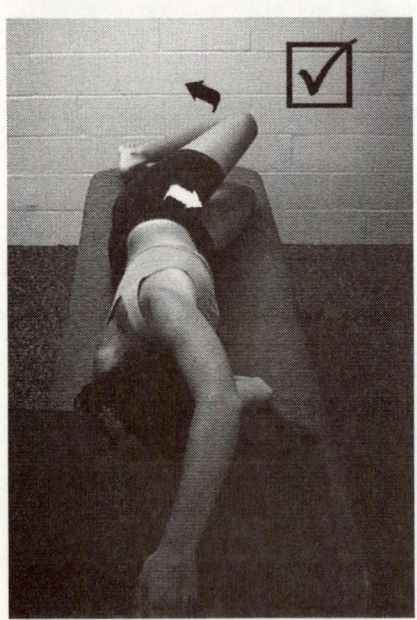

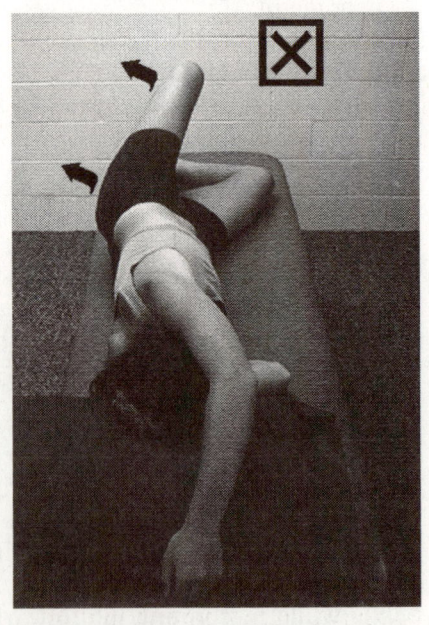

Left: Debbie performing this exercise perfectly. Note that even though her knee has rotated upward, her pelvis has stayed in line with the rest of her body. *Right*: A common but vital error: Debbie's pelvis has rotated backward as she lifts her knee.

EXERCISES TO CORRECT MUSCLE IMBALANCES

Sound easy? Here are the important and difficult parts:

As you lift, you must keep your pelvis and spine *completely still*. In particular, do not allow your pelvis to roll backward.

Keep your bottom leg relaxed. *Do not* push down into the floor with your bottom leg. It's harder than it sounds.

4. Slowly return. Ten repetitions.
5. Repeat on the other side.

Level Two

As for Level One, but lift your top knee as high as you can. Remember, your pelvis is not allowed to move *at all*. Hold for five seconds.

Level Three

As for Level Two, but hold for ten seconds. You can also rotate your pelvis even further forward before you start, which will increase the range of movement of the exercise.

EXERCISES 4–8: JOINT MOBILISATION EXERCISES

4. *Lumbar extension*

Goal: To mobilise your lumbar joints so that they extend backward more freely.

Level One
1. Lie flat on your stomach on a firm surface.
2. Place your hands in a 'push up' position.
3. While keeping your hips on the ground, push up with your arms until you can prop up on your elbows. Keep your back muscles relaxed as you perform this movement. All of the effort should come from your arms.
4. Take a breath in, then further relax your spine as you breathe out. Your lumbar spine should sag toward the floor as you totally relax it.
5. Hold this extended position for five seconds, then slowly return.
6. Ten repetitions.

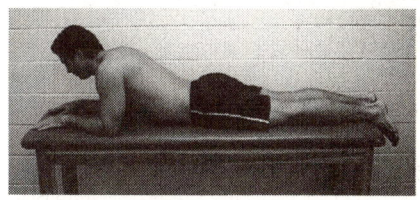

Lumbar extension, Level One

Level Two

As above, except you should extend your arms until your back is fully extended, rather than propping on your elbows. Ensure that your hip bones stay touching the ground.

BACK PAIN

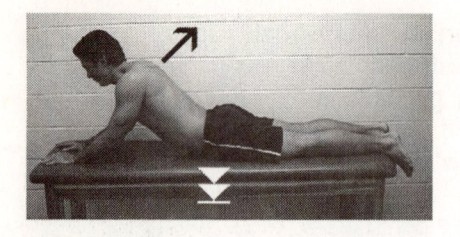

Lumbar extension, Level Two. Note that Greg's hip bones remain on the bench.

Level Three
As for Level Two, but you should fully extend your arms until they are straight. You may allow your hip bones to leave the floor, so that your spine is literally hanging in the air. Remember to completely relax your spine on your outward breath.

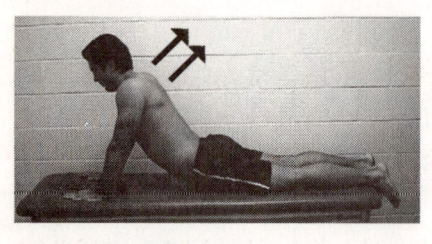

Lumbar extension, Level Three. Greg's arms are now fully extended. His spine is relaxed, and is sagging toward the ground.

5. *Lumbar flexion*
Goal: To mobilise your lumbar joints so that they flex forward more freely.

Level One
1. Lie flat on your back on a firm surface.
2. Pull one knee to your chest, and then bring your other knee up to join it.
3. Breathe slowly out and relax as you hold both knees to your chest for five seconds.
4. Relax and slowly return your legs to the starting position one at a time.
5. Ten repetitions.

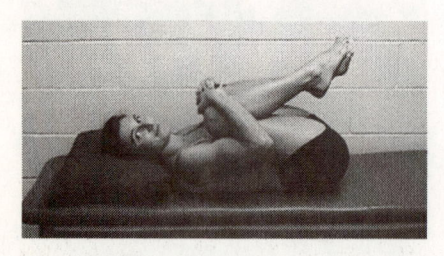

Lumbar flexion, Level One.

Level Two
1. Kneel on all fours on a firm surface.
2. Rock backward so that your buttocks approach your heels.

## EXERCISES TO CORRECT MUSCLE IMBALANCES

3. Relax and hold this position for five seconds.
4. Slowly return to the starting position.
5. Ten repetitions.

Lumbar flexion, Level Two. For Level Three, try to tilt your pelvis, as shown by the arrows. Try to keep your thoracic spine straight when you do this exercise—no easy task, I assure you.

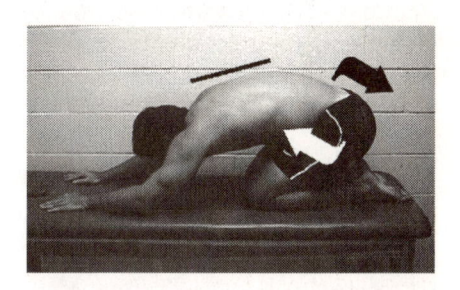

Level Three
As for Level Two, but you should tilt your pelvis backward to increase the stretch on your lumbar spine. You should practice the pelvic tilt manoeuvre in standing before using it in this lumbar spine stretch. To perform a pelvic tilt, tighten your abdominal muscles and squeeze your buttock cheeks together. Tuck your bottom under. The front part of your hips should tilt forward, *à la* Elvis Presley doing a pelvic thrust.

As you perform this pelvic tilt, try to keep your thoracic spine from flexing. Remember, you are aiming to stretch your lumbar area, not your thoracic spine.

6. Lumbar rotation
Goal: To mobilise your lumbar joints so that they rotate more freely.

Level One
1. Lie on your back on a firm surface.
2. Bend both knees up to 90 degrees while keeping your feet on the floor.
3. Breathe out as you gently rotate your knees to one side. Make sure that you keep your knees together at all times.

Lumbar rotation, Level One. Note that both of Greg's shoulder are relaxed, and in contact with the bed.

4. Hold for five seconds, then breathe in as you steadily return your legs to the centre.
5. Perform five rotations to each side.

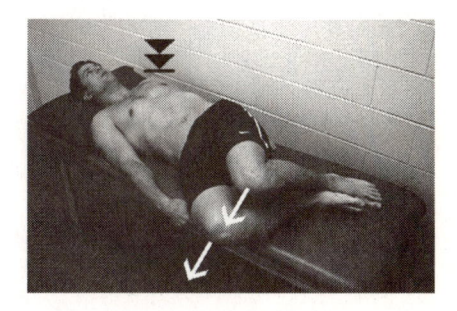

Level Two
As for Level One, but this time straighten your 'bottom' leg. This will allow your top leg to rotate over it. For example, if you are rotating your legs to the left, then your left leg should be straight, and your right knee should twist over your body toward the floor.

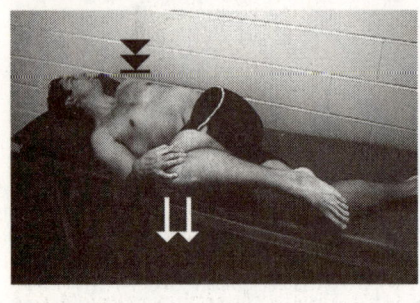

Lumbar rotation, Levels Two and Three.

Level Three
As for Level Two, but use your opposite hand to push your top knee down toward the floor, which will increase the twist in your spine. Rotate your head in the opposite direction to your legs.

7. Lumbar side flexion
Goal: To mobilise your lumbar joints so that they side bend more freely.

Level One
1. Stand with good posture, with your feet comfortably separated.
2. Reach sideways toward the ground with one hand. This should flex your spine sideways.

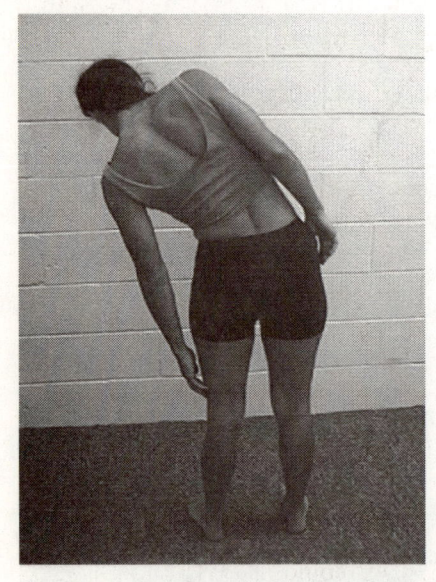

Lumbar side flexion, Level One.

3. Ensure that your movement is a pure sideways bend. Do not allow your spine to bend either forward or backward. Initially, you should use a mirror to check, as spinal movement can be very deceptive.

EXERCISES TO CORRECT MUSCLE IMBALANCES

Make sure that you keep your hips in line with your feet. Don't let your pelvis swing out to the side. Remember, you are trying to keep your pelvis stationary, so that you stretch your spine, not your hips.

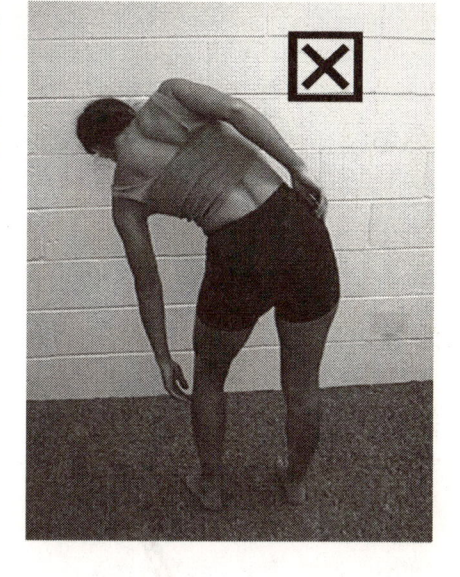

Debbie is making two subtle errors in this photo. Can you spot them? First, she is allowing her left knee to bend. Second, she is bending slightly forward, rather than making a pure sideways movement.

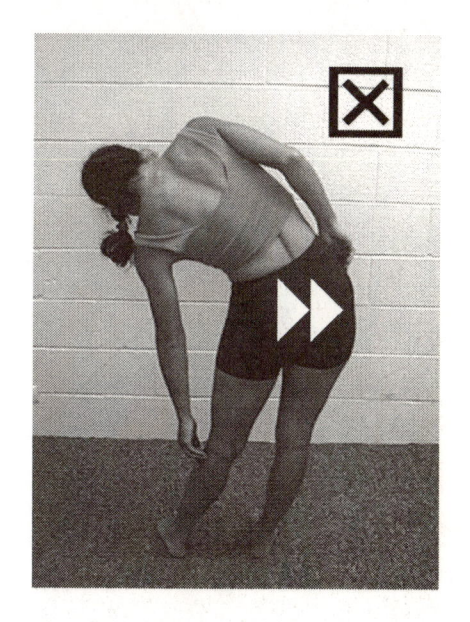

Another error! This time, Debbie is moving her pelvis sideways, rather than keeping it level and in line with the rest of her trunk. As a result, her hips are doing most of the stretching, rather than her lower back. Compare the tilt of Debbie's pelvis to the correct photograph opposite on the previous page, and you will see a subtle difference.

4. Relax and allow gravity to stretch your spine.
5. Hold five seconds, then slowly return to the starting position.
6. Repeat five times each side.

BACK PAIN

Level Two
As above. You can reach over with your top arm to increase the intensity of the stretch.

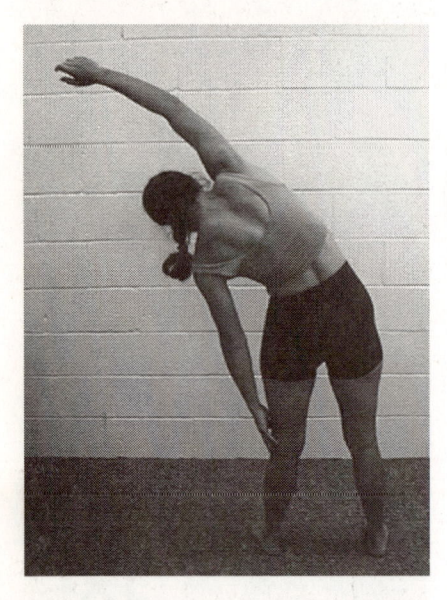

A beautifully executed lumbar side bend, Level Two.

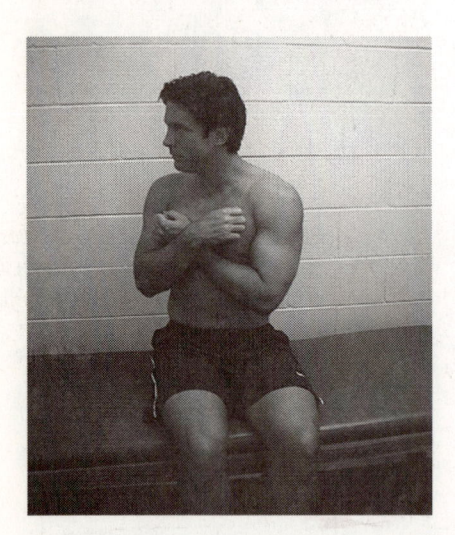

Thoracic rotation, Level One.

Level Three
As for Level Two.

8. Thoracic rotation
Goal: To mobilise your thoracic joints so that they rotate more easily.

Level One
1. Sit with a good posture on a solid bench or table.
2. Cross your arms loosely across your chest, then rotate your body to one side until you feel pain or stiffness.
3. Relax in this position for five seconds, then steadily return to the starting position.
4. Five repetitions in each direction.

Level Two
This exercise is similar to Level One, but requires extra concentration. You are going to attempt to rotate each part of your spine separately, using your hand position as a guide.

1. Sit with a good posture on a solid table or bench.
2. Place your hands on your hips, just below your ribs. Rotate your trunk to the side, but allow spinal movement only in the section below your hands.

EXERCISES TO CORRECT MUSCLE IMBALANCES

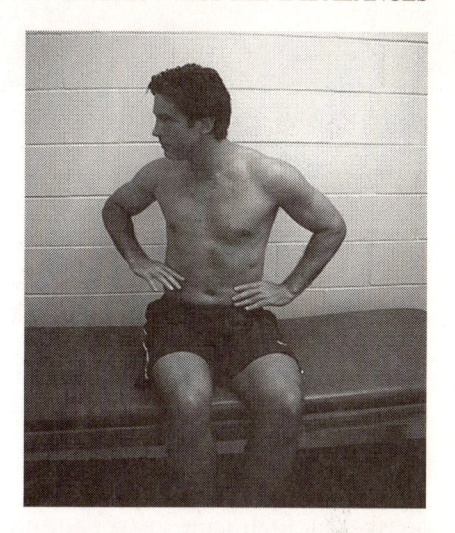

Thoracic rotation, Level Two. Greg is using his hands to guide his movement. In this picture, his hands are level with the bottom of his rib cage, and he is rotating only that part of his spine below this point.

3. Keep the lower part of your spine rotated, and move your hands up to the middle of your ribs. Now further rotate this part of your spine.

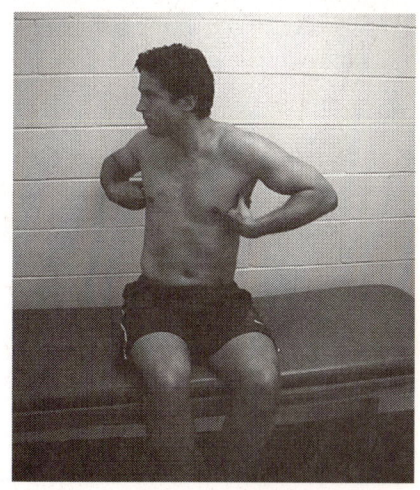

Now Greg has moved his hands up higher, and is rotating the next part of his thoracic spine. In this way, he can ensure that each area of his thoracic spine is sequentially moved, rather than just the joints that felt like moving.

4. Hold this degree of rotation, and move your hands up to your armpits. Then rotate this section of your spine.
5. Finally, fully twist your shoulders and neck. Your whole thoracic spine should now be fully coiled. Slowly return to the starting position.
6. Repeat five times in each direction.

This exercise may seem difficult at first. With practice it will become smoother, and will eventually be as seamless and natural as Level One.

Level Three
As for Level Two, but you should pull yourself around using your arms at the end of the movement.

9. Thoracic extension
Goal: To mobilise your thoracic joints so that they extend more easily.

For each of these exercises you will require a firm, padded roll. To make one, take an average-sized bath towel, fold it in half lengthwise, then roll it tightly to form a firm cylinder. Secure it with tape or rubber bands.

When you have practiced these exercises for a few months, you may wish to progress to a firmer roll: a hand towel wrapped around a rolling pin, for example.

Level One
1. Sit in a high back chair with the roll positioned horizontally behind the lower part of your thoracic spine (i.e. level with the bottom of your ribcage).
2. Place your hands behind your head.
3. Relax and breathe out as you lean backward. Push your chest outward, and feel the pressure of the roll on your spine as you extend back over it.
4. Hold for five seconds, then relax.
5. Move the roll a few centimetres higher, then repeat. Continue this process ten times, by which time the roll will be near the top of your thoracic spine (i.e. almost at your neck).

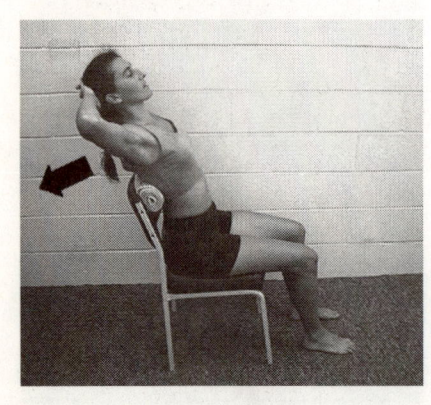

Thoracic extension, Level One.

Level Two
1. Lie on your back on a firm surface. Bend your knees to 90 degrees.
2. Place the roll under the lower part of your thoracic spine (i.e. level with the bottom of your ribcage). Allow your arms, head and buttocks to rest on the floor.
3. Relax and breathe out, and allow your spine to extend over the roll.
4. Hold five seconds, and then relax.
5. Move the roll a few centimetres higher, then repeat. Continue this process ten times, by which time the roll will be near the top of your thoracic spine (i.e. almost at your neck).

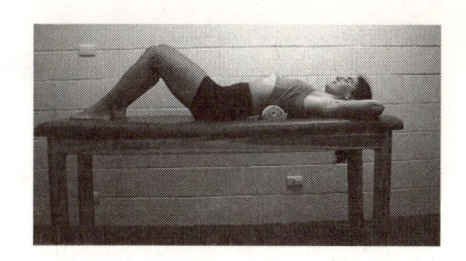

EXERCISES TO CORRECT MUSCLE IMBALANCES

Thoracic extension, Level Two.

Level Three
1. Lie on your back on a firm surface. Bend your knees to 90 degrees.
2. Place the roll under the lower part of your thoracic spine (i.e. level with the bottom of your ribcage).
3. Using your hands behind your neck, gently lift your head a tiny distance off the floor. Simultaneously lift your buttocks a tiny distance off the floor. All of your upper body weight should now be resting through the rolled towel under your spine.
4. Relax and breathe out, and allow your spine to extend over the roll.
5. Hold five seconds, and then relax.
6. Move the roll a few centimetres higher, then repeat. Continue this process ten times, by which time the roll will be near the top of your thoracic spine (i.e. almost at your neck).

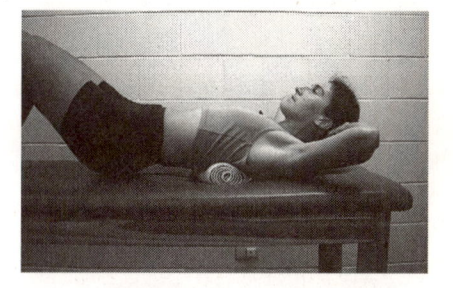

Thoracic extension, Level Three. Note that Debbie's head and bottom are slightly raised from the table. This movement can be difficult to master, as you must simultaneously relax your spinal muscles.

EXERCISES 10–12: NERVE-LOOSENING EXERCISES

Note: Nerve stretches are a vital exercise for many sufferers of back pain. However, nerves sometimes have an adverse reaction to stretching, occasionally becoming very sore, tender and inflamed. Therefore, I suggest that you perform these exercises *very gently* for the first three sessions, and note any disagreeable reactions. If stretching the nerve seems to make your problem worse, then discontinue them for three weeks, then try again.

You can try these techniques without any holding time, relying on movement alone to increase the nerve's mobility. This is the nerve 'flossing' technique to which we referred earlier.

BACK PAIN

10. Sciatic nerve stretch
Goal: To loosen the sciatic nerve that runs down the back of your thigh.

Level One
1. Lie on your back on a firm surface, with both legs flat.
2. Using a towel around your right foot, lift your right leg into the air until you feel a gentle stretch. Ensure that you keep your right knee perfectly straight, and that your left leg stays flat on the floor. Keep your right leg in the midline, or even slightly across your body. In other words, do not let your leg rotate or move outwards.

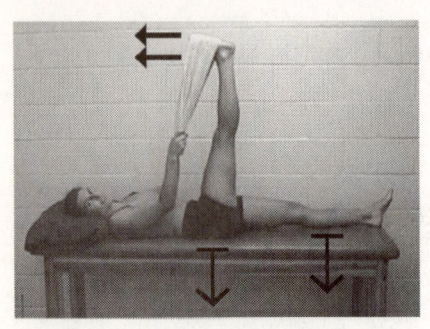

The straight leg raise stretch. I'm sure that you are just as flexible as Debbie, right? Right?

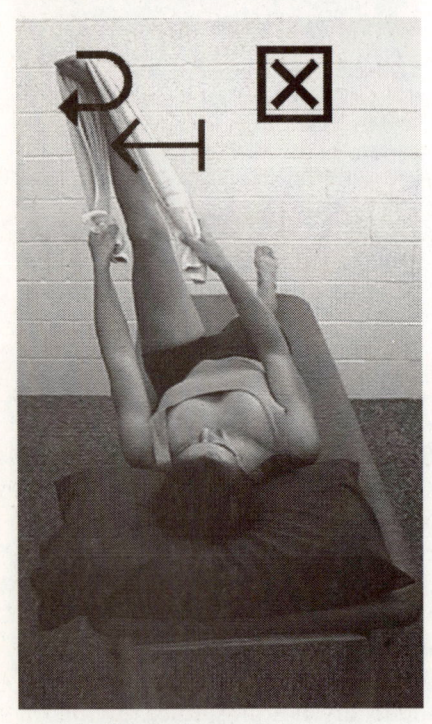

Here Debbie is making two common mistakes, as indicated by the arrows. First, she is twisting her leg outward. Second, she has allowed her leg to drift away from the midline. To prevent these errors creeping into your technique, you must ensure that you keep your foot straight, and your leg in line with the rest of your body.

3. Relax and hold five seconds, then slowly return to the starting position.
4. Repeat five times, then repeat a further five times on your left leg.

Level Two
As for Level One, but pull firmly rather than gently. Hold for ten seconds.

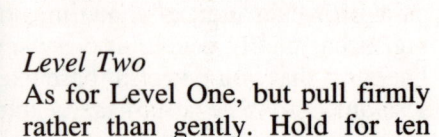

Level Three
As for Level One, but pull very firmly. Hold for fifteen seconds.

EXERCISES TO CORRECT MUSCLE IMBALANCES

11. Slump stretch
Goal: To stretch the dura and other nerve connective tissue.

Level One
1. Sit on a firm surface, such as a table. Preferably, the surface should be high enough so that your feet are clear of the floor.
2. Allow your back to fully slump into a 'C' shape.
3. Let your neck bend forward so that your chin is on your chest.
4. Relax and hold there for five seconds.
5. Five repetitions.

Level Two
1. Sit on a firm surface, such as a table. Preferably, the surface should be high enough so that your feet are clear of the floor.
2. Allow your back to fully slump into a 'C' shape.
3. Bend your neck forward so that your chin is on your chest.
4. Straighten your right knee, so that your right leg becomes horizontal, or straighten just as far as you can.
5. Hold for five seconds, then relax.
6. Five repetitions, then a further five repetitions on your left leg.

Level Three
1. Sit on a firm surface, such as a table. Preferably, the surface should be high enough so that your feet are clear of the floor.
2. Allow your back to fully slump into a 'C' shape.
3. Bend your neck forward so that your chin is on your chest.
4. Straighten your right knee, so that your right leg becomes horizontal, or straighten just as far as you can.

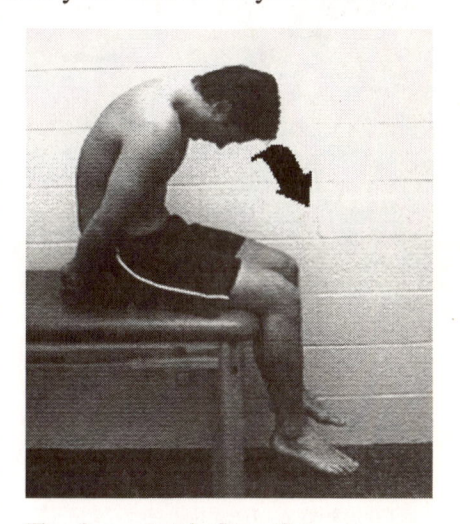

The slump stretch, Stage One.

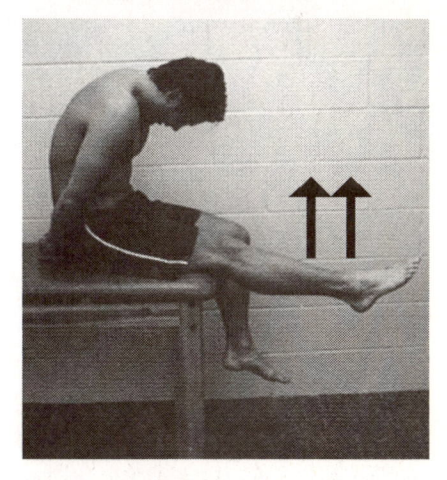

The slump stretch, Stage Two. Yes, I know it pulls behind your knee, but do it anyway.

133

BACK PAIN

5. With your right leg extended, pull your right foot and toes back toward you as far as possible.

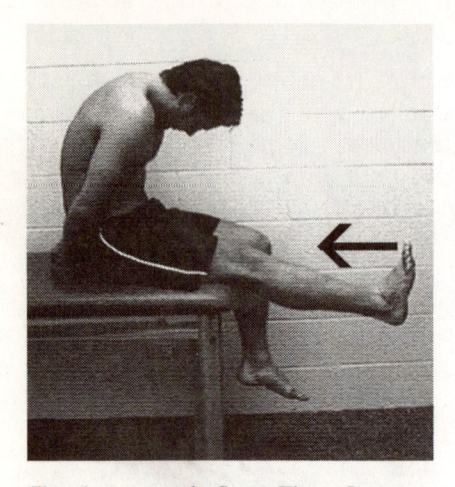

6. Hold for ten seconds, then relax.
7. Five repetitions, then a further five repetitions on the left side.

The slump stretch, Stage Three. Ignore that pulling feeling in your calf muscle, if you can.

12. Femoral nerve stretch
Goal: To stretch the femoral nerve that runs down the front of your thigh.

Note: This exercise requires flexible knees. If your knees are stiff or injured, then this exercise will probably not be effective. Of course, it may help your knees, but that's another story.

Level One
1. Lie on your tummy on a firm surface.
2. Bend your right knee up until you feel a gentle pull at the front of your thigh. Use a tie or belt around your ankle to facilitate this, if necessary.
3. Keep your back flat and relaxed on the floor. Do not allow it to arch. Also, ensure that the front of your right hip joint remains in constant contact with the floor.

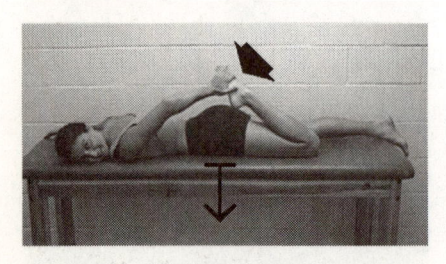

4. Relax and hold for five seconds, then slowly return.
5. Repeat five times on each leg.

If you felt a cramp in the back of your right thigh when performing this exercise, then you probably used your hamstring muscles to bend your knee. To avoid this cramping feeling, use your hands to produce the stretch, and relax your leg muscles. Use a tie or belt around your ankle, if necessary.

The prone knee bend stretch. Note how Debbie's hips remain in contact with the bed, and that her spine is not overly arched.

Level Two
As for Level One, but pull firmly rather than gently. Hold for ten seconds.

EXERCISES TO CORRECT MUSCLE IMBALANCES

Level Three
As for Level One, but pull very firmly. Hold for fifteen seconds.

EXERCISES 13–15: MUSCLE STRETCHES

13. Front thigh stretch
Goal: To stretch the iliopsoas muscle that runs between your spine and the front of your hip joint.

Level One
1. Lie on your back on a firm surface, such as a table. Your pelvis should be aligned with the edge of the table, with both legs over the edge.
2. Pull your left leg up to your chest, and hold it there with your arms.

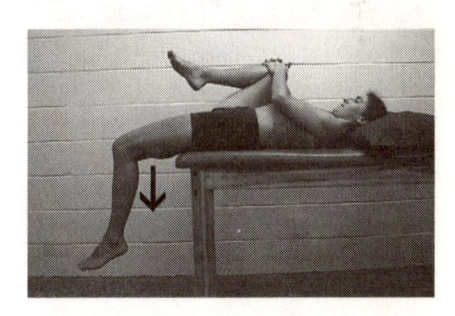

The front thigh stretch for the iliopsoas muscle.

3. Allow your right leg to hang freely. When you fully relax, gravity will pull your leg downward, producing a mild stretch at the front of the thigh.

    Do not allow your lower back to arch off the bed. You may worsen your condition if you do.

This is an example of what *not* to do. In this photo, Debbie's spine has lifted off the bed. This error will completely ruin the effectiveness of the stretch, so be very diligent in avoiding it. You can maintain a correct position by pulling your upper leg firmly into your chest.

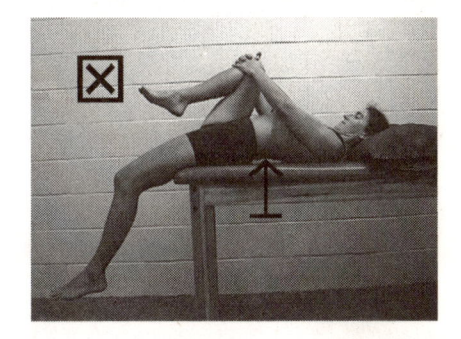

Also, make sure that your thigh stays in line with the rest of your body. Don't allow it to rotate, or move sideways.

135

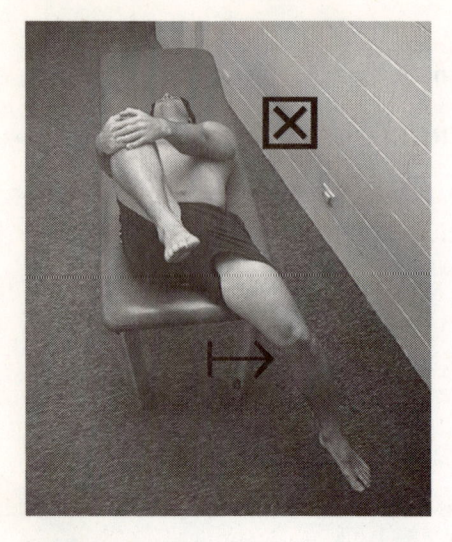

Here's another way to hash up this stretch. Greg has let his leg drift sideways, away from the midline. Please ensure that you keep your leg in line with your body when you perform this stretch.

4. Five repetitions on each side, holding for ten seconds.

Level Two
As above, except use a two kilogram (about five pound) weight on your right knee or ankle to increase the intensity of the stretch.

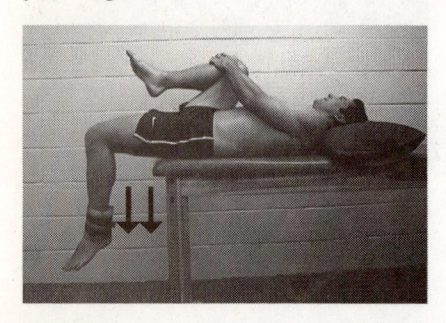

The front thigh stretch, using a small weight (say, two to five kilograms) around your ankle to increase the intensity of the exercise. Don't forget to relaaaaax.

Level Three
As above, but use a five kilogram (ten to fifteen pound) weight around your knee or ankle.

14. Back thigh stretch
Goal: To stretch your hamstring muscle, which will allow your hips to bend further.

Level One
1. Lie on your back, with your left leg flat and your right knee bent.
2. Place both hands behind your right knee. Use your hands to stabilise

your thigh as you straighten your right knee as far as you can. Your leg should be close to vertical.

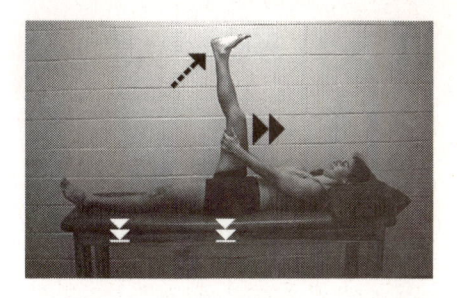

A back thigh stretch for the hamstring muscle—Levels One and Two.

3. Five repetitions on each side, holding for ten seconds.

Level Two
As above. You can increase the intensity of the stretch by stabilising your left leg. Either have someone else hold your thigh, or somehow wedge it under a couch.

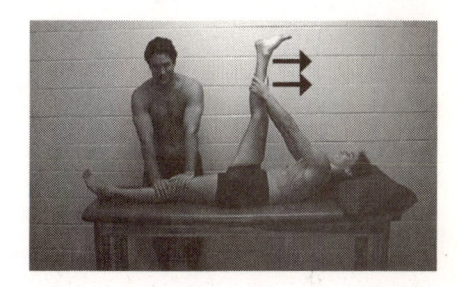

A back thigh stretch, Level Three, with a partner. Aren't they having fun!

Level Three
As above. You can further strengthen the stretch by using your hands to pull your right thigh further backward.

15. Bottom muscle stretch (piriformis)
Goal: To stretch the deep hip muscles in your bottom. This exercise sometimes helps to relieve buttock pain, and sometimes helps to release tension from the sciatic nerve.

Level One
1. Lie on your back with your legs flat.
2. Pull your right knee up to your chest, while keeping your left leg on the ground.
3. Bend your right knee to 90 degrees.
4. Grasp your right ankle with your left hand, and your right knee with your right hand.
5. Simultaneously pull your right knee toward your left shoulder, and

BACK PAIN

pull your ankle around toward your left ear. (Not *in* it, just toward it!) You should feel a stretch in your buttock area.

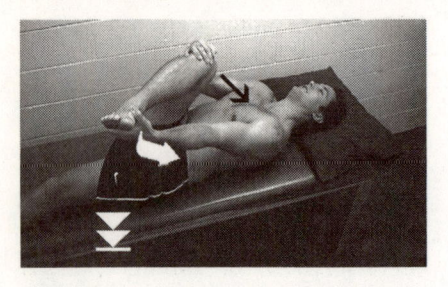

A piriformis stretch. Note how Greg is not only pulling his right knee toward his left shoulder (the black arrow), but is also pulling his ankle around toward his left ear (the white arrow). His left thigh remains flat on the bed. If you get confused, just try to twist yourself into a pretzel and you won't be too far wrong.

6. Five repetitions on each side, holding for ten seconds.

Levels Two and Three
As above. Make sure that you hold your knee firmly toward your chest as you twist your leg. Do not allow it to move away.

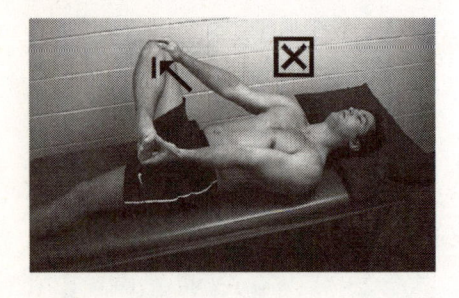

In this photograph, Greg has not pulled his right knee far enough toward his left shoulder. This error results in an ineffective stretch.

Well, what are you waiting for?

15
Safer sitting
Sit up straight? What rubbish!

'Sit up straight.'

You've probably been told to 'sit up straight' dozens of times in your life. From parents to teachers to well-meaning grandparents, you've no doubt received this advice on many occasions. Sit vertically, use a hard straight chair, concentrate on your posture, and you'll look after your back, right?

Wrong.

Correct sitting posture has nothing to do with 'sitting up straight'. What is more, a stiff, hard, squared-off chair is not much good for your back, and trying to continually think about your posture while concentrating on other tasks is a waste of time. Where does all this bad advice come from?

In this chapter, we are going to debunk these outdated myths. Furthermore, we will explore ways for you to sit more efficiently, and so take an enormous amount of strain off your lower back.

Poor sitting posture is one of the greatest single causes of back pain. Many people, particularly those with sedentary jobs and lifestyles, are sitting almost every waking moment. Many people sit at work for eight or nine hours, then sit for another hour or so in the car. They also sit during meals, and then finish their spine-destroying day by sitting in front of the television or computer for another few hours. This twelve hours or so of sitting is repeated every day, typically with a very poor posture in an unsupportive chair. No wonder their spines degenerate.

To illustrate how damaging prolonged sitting can be for your back, try this simple experiment. Grab your left index finger with your right hand, and pull it backwards. Keep pulling until you feel a slight stretch at the front of the finger joint. Don't extend it so hard that it hurts; just use enough pressure so that your finger is stretching. Now hold it there. Keep holding . . . keep pulling . . .

. . . for the rest of the day.

Then, when you awaken tomorrow morning, I want you to start pulling your finger backwards again. Hold onto it for all of tomorrow as well, and then repeat the experiment every day for the rest of the week. No, do it for the rest of the year.

If you actually managed to perform this absurd experiment, I am sure that you would not be surprised if your finger became very sore. You would expect that the ligaments would not only become overstretched, but that they would also develop scar tissue, and become inflamed and raw. In short, your finger joint would accumulate a lot of microtrauma. This outcome is so readily imaginable that nobody would dream of doing something as stupid as stretching their finger for a whole day, much less an entire year.

Yet that is exactly what you are doing to your lower back when you sit with a poor posture!

When you sit slumped in a chair, with your lower back unsupported, your discs and ligaments are stretched to their limit. Combine this poor positioning with the compressive force of your body weight, and the high intradiscal pressures associated with sitting, and you can begin to imagine the huge strain that sitting places on your lower back. When you continue this force for many hours per day, for weeks, months or decades on end, you have a sure-fire technique to ruin your spine.

Mother Nature did not design our lower backs with prolonged sitting in mind. I doubt that prehistoric humans spent much time sitting about on rocks, nattering about the latest cave painting exhibition, when the bisons were due, or what a shame it was that they didn't have tails. No, for most of our evolution, our ancestors were too busy chasing after food to have time for idle sitting.

Let's now look at techniques to avoid the build up of microtrauma that destroys so many people's lower backs.

The first set of advice will be for all back types: A, B, C and D. After that, we'll look at some further advice for types B and D (backs that hurt in flexion situations). If you are not sure, or if you are borderline (type AB, or CD for example) then you should also read and follow the advice for types B and D.

Advice on sitting for all back pain types: A, B, C and D

If your job or lifestyle demands prolonged sitting, then a good chair is essential. Sure, a decent seat can cost a lot of money. But so does a week off work, lying in bed with a ruptured disc.

What's more, a good chair will last a lifetime. If you have another 30 years of life remaining, then you probably have about another 100,000 hours of sitting left. Even if you buy a ridiculously expensive, ergonomically designed, fully adjustable, top-of-the-range chair, it's very little, spread over several decades, especially if it saves years of pain, stiffness and frustration.

Trying to self-correct by thinking about your sitting posture is next-to-useless. Having to continually think about your posture while concentrating on other tasks—be it working, eating, or watching even the most banal television soap opera—is doomed to failure. Even if you were able to concentrate on your posture ten times per day for a minute at a time—no easy task, believe me—then you would still only be in a correct position for a paltry two per cent of the time. The other ninety-eight per cent of your sitting hours would be spent straining your ligaments and ruining your discs.

Can you see that *thinking* about your posture is essentially useless? Sure, you will probably have to break a few bad habits. But please understand that by using a good chair in the correct manner, it will *automatically* hold your spine in a reasonable position. In short, don't even bother trying to continually think about your posture. It won't work. Just make sure you have a good chair, break a few bad habits, then sit back, relax, and let the chair do all of the work for you.

So during the following discussion on efficient sitting, I have assumed that you have a good, supportive chair. If not, then you'll have to use your accrued knowledge to evaluate your current crop of chairs, or those in the furniture shop display floor, to see if any of them are suitable for the very important job of protecting your spine.

Two simple rules for more efficient sitting

Over the years, I've heard dozens of theories about how to sit correctly. Most of them range from the useless to the unattainably complicated. However, I believe that you will easily attain a more efficient sitting posture if you follow two simple rules.

1. Lean into your back rest, and
2. keep your bottom at the back of the seat.

So let's now look at these two simple rules to discover why they are so important, and see how easy they are to achieve.

(1) Lean back into the backrest
If a competition was run to see who could make the worst, most unsupportive chair, the winning design would probably look something like a stool. The most obvious design fault for a stool is that it has no backrest.

Yet perversely, even when our chairs do have a backrest, many people 'forget' to use it. They sit or slump forward on the chair, usually totally disregarding the under-used backrest. If you sit without using the backrest then you might as well be sitting on a milk crate.

BACK PAIN

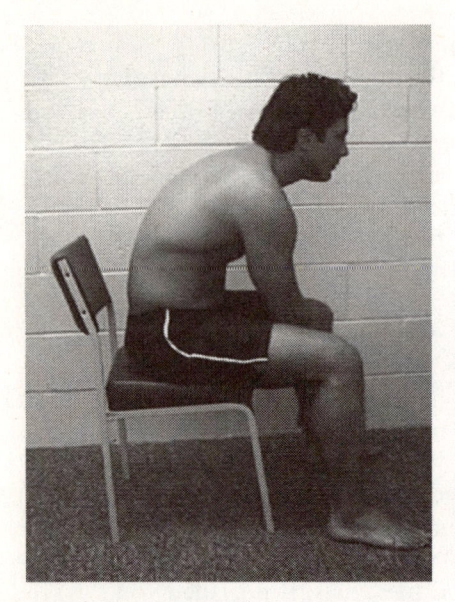

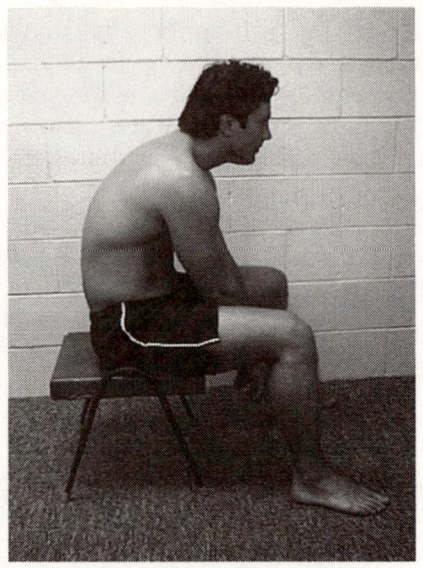

How to ruin your spine in one quick lesson: Sit like this. Note that although the chair in the left photo has a back rest, Greg is not leaning against it. He may as well sit on an old stool, as in the right photo, for his posture is identical. The moral of the story: even a very good chair is useless, if you don't use it properly.

So, to repeat what should already be obvious: you must always lean into your backrest when sitting.

In fact, you should take this one step further, and lie against the backrest. When I say 'lie', I am not implying that you should be recumbent, staring at the ceiling instead of the computer screen, or into the eyes of your no doubt very attractive dinner partner. I am simply suggesting that your shoulders and upper spine should be leaning on the backrest, as well as your lower spine.

A relaxed, 'lying' sitting posture is more easily achieved if the backrest is tilted at an accommodating angle. I suggest that a backward slant of 20 degrees is a good starting point, which you can adjust to suit yourself.

Note that this angle of tilt is greater than is typical; most standard chairs have five to ten degrees of backward tilt, while many have no tilt at all. I cannot think of a good reason why this is so, as a bigger backward tilt is not only better for your back, but more comfortable as well.

Some health practitioners promote the idea that an upright, 90 degree posture is the only way to sit correctly. I cannot see any good anatomical reason for this advice. Ninety degrees only gets a mention because it is a squared-off right angle. Unfortunately, the human body is not designed with such neat coincidences in mind.

How does this slightly altered posture help your back? First, lying against the backrest is a simple, effective way to reduce the pressure inside your lower back discs. Recall from Chapter 4 that disc pressure is only 25 mmHg when lying, but as high as 70 mmHg when sitting. So by making your sitting posture a little bit more like lying, you lower the intradiscal pressure. Research supports this theory: one study found that when the top part of the seat was tilted back by 20 degrees, the disc pressure reduced by 20 to 30 per cent.

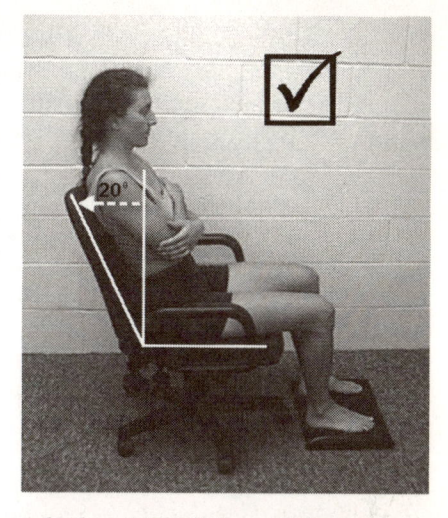

A back rest tilt of about 20 degrees is optimal for efficient sitting. Forget the old rule of 'sit up straight'. With a 20-degree backward tilt you can 'lie' against the backrest, and let it do all of the work for you.

Second, this habit helps to keep your joints in a more neutral position. Slumping or bending forward in your seat forces your back into a greater degree of flexion, meaning that your spine loses its lordosis—its natural inward curve. This position stretches and strains the joints, which can be very damaging when maintained for long periods. Think of the finger-pulling experiment, and you will see why keeping your joints in a neutral position is so important.

Third, lying against a tilted backrest decreases the leverage effect of your upper body weight, meaning that the chair does the supporting work, rather than your joints and muscles. One research project found that when the top part of the seat was tilted back by 20 degrees, the required muscle activity was reduced by 30 to 40 per cent.

Many people claim that they cannot adopt this laid back posture because they have to work over a desk. It is impossible, they claim, to work effectively while sitting back against your chair. To these cynics, I have one thing to say: rubbish!

All that is required is a little reorganisation of your desktop and you'll manage easily. Slumping forward over a table or desk is simply a bad habit that you have developed over many years. Like all bad habits, it can be difficult to correct. However, with persistence you will find that you can work just as effectively, probably even more so, when you lie back, rather than slump forward, on your chair.

If you must sit forward for short periods, fine. Changing your posture for a few minutes will probably do you good anyway. However, for most tasks, including reading, keyboard work, television watching and talking, a laid-back sitting posture is easily achieved. You can find further information on work stations and ergonomics in Chapter 19.

Obviously, you cannot effectively 'lie' against your chair if it has only the usual half-height backrest. Back pain sufferers from around the world should unite, and lynch, pillage and plunder those manufacturers who produce chairs with half-sized backrests. (Only kidding). For although most chairs these days have low back rests, a full-length support is far preferable for avoiding back strain. So please, try to buy, beg or borrow a chair that has a full-length backrest.

Furthermore, a full height backrest protects and supports your thoracic spine. Although this book is primarily about low back pain, the effects of sitting on the thoracic spine should not be underestimated. A slumped-forward sitting posture places so much stress on this area that almost every sedentary worker has some degree of thoracic disc degeneration.

As we discussed in Chapter 9, the thoracic spine can directly cause pain and stiffness in the lumbar area. Furthermore, stiffness and degeneration in the thoracic spine places more strain on your lumbar area, with the likelihood of an increased rate of degeneration. A full-length backrest will look after this other vital area of your spine.

In short, forget everything that you've heard about 'sitting up straight'. (Ring your primary school teacher and tell her she was wrong, if it makes you feel any better.) Avoid straight, hard chairs with a vertical backrest. Instead, tilt the backrest at an angle of about 20 degrees, then lie into your chair and let it do all of the hard work. Try to use a full-length backrest, rather than the more normal half-height rest. Avoid stools more fiercely than you avoid 'friends' who sell Amway.

(2) Keep your bottom at the back of the seat
If failing to lean on the backrest is the cardinal sin of sitting, then letting your bottom slide forward is a close second. This rule is particularly important for your lumbar spine, as it is left unsupported in mid-air when your bottom slides away from the backrest.

The best way to automatically keep your bottom in place is to make sure that the seat width, from front to back, is correct. Particularly, the seat base must not be too wide. Most ordinary office and table chairs are fine in this regard. Conversely, most lounge chairs, easy chairs and sofas fail dismally.

If your seat base is even slightly too wide, then the front edge of the seat will push into the back of your knees. When this happens, your natural, subconscious response is to slide your bottom forward.

Unfortunately, this movement draws the lower back away from the protective sanctity of the backrest, leaving your spine bowing in mid air.

In this situation, many people find they are more comfortable using a footstool, or a 'pouffe', as they were called in the good old days. Some back injuries, particularly type B and D spines, do not respond favourably to the use of footstools. Even more at risk are people with tight nerves. Can you recall the Straight Leg Raise test and the Slump test that you performed during Chapter 11? If you scored any points during these tests, then you probably have tight nerves, meaning that a footstool is likely to exacerbate your pain. Therefore, if you have tight nerves, or have back type B or D, don't use a footstool, OK?

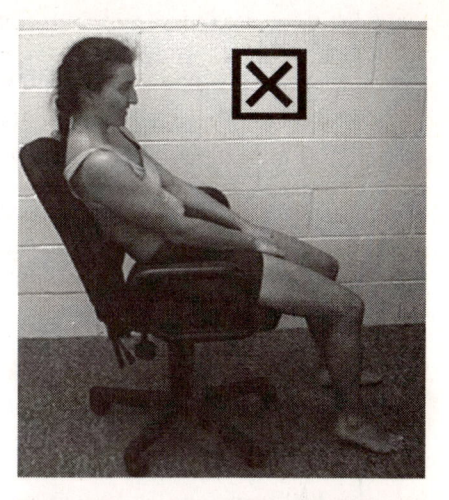

If you allow your bottom to slide forward on the seat, then your lower back will leave the back rest. This unsupported posture is bad news, as it will result in accumulated microtrauma and eventual injury.

On the other hand, if you have back type A or C and you do not have tight nerves, then you should have no problems using a footstool. It might even help.

OK, enough talk of pouffes, let's get back to chairs. I suggest that you perform this simple test on any chair on which you intend to bestow the privilege of supporting your spine. Sit down, and push your bottom back into the seat as far as it will go. Really push it back hard. Now check to see how much space is between the back of your knees and the front edge of the seat.

A gap of about two to four centimetres (one to two inches) is perfect. If the gap is less than this, or if your legs are touching the chair, then the seat base is too wide. My guess is that within about half an hour your bottom will start sliding forward, and your lumbar spine will lose the support of the backrest.

The other most important feature of the chair is its height from the floor. Although a five-year-old child might look cute sitting on a big person's chair with their legs merrily dangling in the air, most pragmatic adults don't go for this look. We like our feet on the floor—which, I suppose is a fair and reasonable thing.

If your chair is too high, you will have a natural inclination to

BACK PAIN

slide forward so that your feet can touch the floor. In this situation, your lower back is again left to fend for itself, unsupported, and pressured down upon by about 1/20 of a tonne of human flesh. To avoid this, simply make sure that your seat is of a height such that your feet can comfortably touch the floor when your bottom is snugly back in the seat.

However, another word of warning to those of you who are type B or D: Don't try to put the seat too low. This has the effect of decreasing the angle between your hips and back, and so pulling your back into a more flexed position. As you know, type B and D spines do not like to be held flexed for too long. So types B and D have a delicate balancing act with their seat height; not so high that your feet can't touch the floor, but not so low that it forces your knees any higher.

Conversely, types A and C will probably be more comfortable with a lower hip-back angle. If you are type A or C, then you may wish to set your seat height lower than is customary. Failing this, a footrest such as a telephone book will lift your legs slightly higher, which will also afford your back a more comfortable posture.

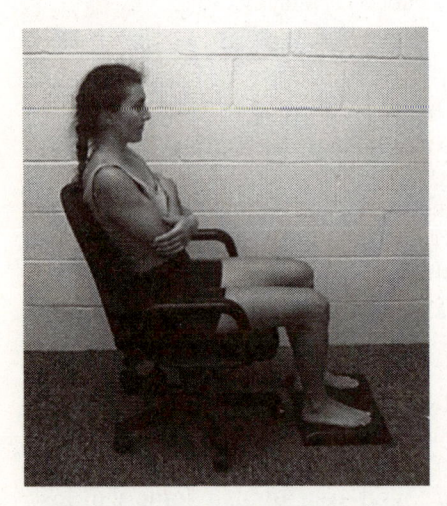

This is the perfect sitting posture if you have a type A or type C spine. (Types B and D, hold on, your picture is coming soon.) Note that Debbie's feet are flat on the floor, with her knees slightly higher than her hips. She is using a low foot rest to facilitate this position. Her bottom is at the back of the chair, and she is leaning her whole spine against the back rest, which is tilted at about 20 degrees.

To summarise, you must keep your bottom at the back of the seat. You will find this far easier if the seat base is narrow enough to accommodate your legs. Correct height is also necessary, particularly for types B and D. Types A and C can set their seat heights slightly lower, and may use a footrest if they wish.

Starting now, get into a lifelong habit of supporting your spine when you sit.

A few other points about sitting posture

BREAK THOSE BAD HABITS
As you can deduce, I believe that a good, correctly adjusted chair is the secret to an efficient sitting posture. However, you may have developed some bad habits from years of poorly adapted seats. As with most habits, you will probably find that breaking them is frustratingly difficult. For example, when you are lounging on a heavily padded sofa, halfway through not only the late movie but also a bottle of wine, your bottom will almost inevitably slide forward. Or when you have been studying hard at the computer (i.e. playing computer games) for hours on end, and you've completely forgotten that your backrest even exists.

A few simple techniques may help you break these habits. First, use a cue, such as a commercial break, to readjust your position in the chair. In the car, a red light can serve the same purpose. Many people do this subconsciously anyway. With practise and persistence for a few weeks, the new habit becomes ingrained, and you will automatically check your posture each time something breaks your thought pattern. Some clever people I know have organised their computer to give them a reminder every thirty minutes or so.

To help break a strongly ingrained bad sitting posture, you might want to wrap an old scarf, tie, or whatever, around the back of the chair, and then loosely knot it in front of your hips. (I sometimes use a football club scarf that my wife bought me after we won the 1987 premiership.) Essentially, you are creating a seat belt to restrain your bottom from sliding forward. This method is not as drastic or as difficult as you might imagine. The knot or belt buckle can be undone in an instant, and nobody will even notice it. After a week or two of restrained sitting, discontinue using the seat belt, by which time you should find it easier to break your old habits.

Note that these techniques subtly differ from continually thinking about your sitting posture, which, as you have already seen, is so difficult as to be useless. You are simply trying to get rid of an old habit by occasional repositioning. The difference is that in this case, the chair is providing the correct posture, not your muscles and joints.

DON'T STAY SEATED FOR TOO LONG
This tip is just commonsense. Holding any posture for too long is bound to be harmful. Use little cues (a commercial break, for example) to move around, stand up, take a short walk, or even perform a few back exercises.

GETTING IN AND OUT OF THE CHAIR
Some people find that rising from a chair is more painful than is sitting. Much of this discomfort is no doubt due to the couple of hours or so

BACK PAIN

of microtrauma that has just accumulated in their spine. By sitting with a supported posture, you will probably find that this transitional pain diminishes.

However, some people, particularly those with type B spines, may still experience problems with these types of transitional movements. If so, you may wish to try this simple technique. When you wish to stand up, wriggle your bottom forward to the edge of the seat. Then turn to one side, and pull your feet beneath you. Using the arm rests and your leg muscles, push yourself into a standing position.

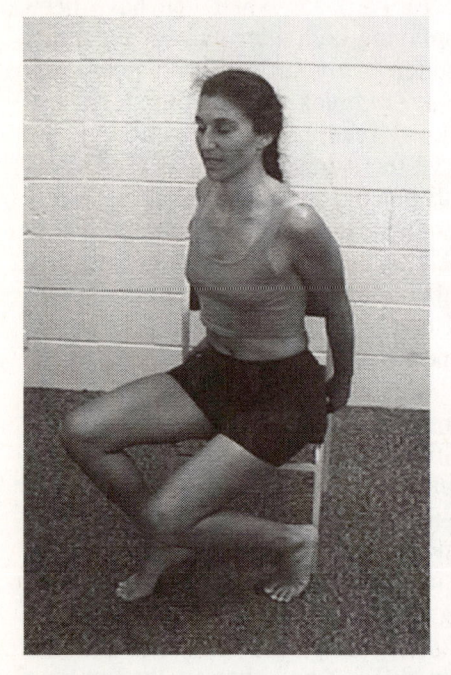

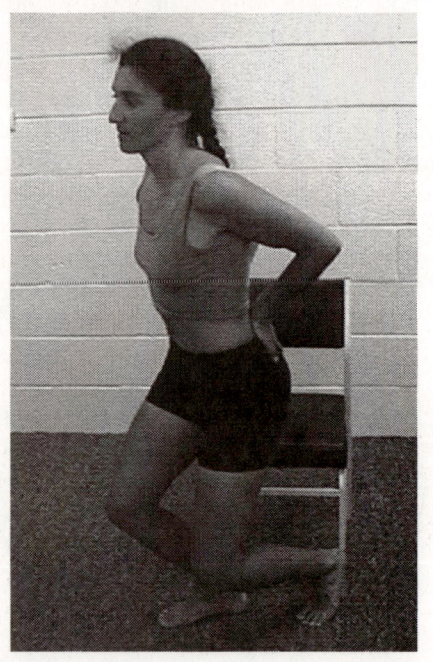

The two photographs above show a safe method for arising from a chair. In the photo on the left, Debbie has moved forward to the edge of the chair, and has turned sideways so that her left leg is almost underneath her. Then, as shown in the right photo, she uses her strong leg muscles to push into standing, supporting her spine as she does. By using this method, Debbie is able to maintain the inward curve in her lumbar spine at all times.

By using this technique, you will keep your back in a neutral position, rather than the overflexed movement normally associated with rising from sitting. Similarly, some find that sitting down into a chair is painful. If so, use this sideways entry technique in reverse.

A FEW MORE WORDS ABOUT CHAIRS

You no doubt already realise the most important features of a good chair: a full-length backrest, tilted backward at about 20 degrees, and suitable seat base width and height. Below are a few more pointers to consider.

- The chair should have armrests.

  Studies have shown that sitting is more efficient when the chair has armrests. They also make it easier to stand up and sit down.

- The chair should be suitably covered.

  The seat base should be comfortably padded, as the bits of bone in your bottom that bear your weight are, for some reason, rather pointy. A silly design feature, if you ask me. If the seat is too hard, then you will tend to slide your hips forward to relieve the pressure on the pointy bits, which will overflex your spine.

  If you have a thin, bony physique, then you should use heavier, softer padding. Those of you who are—how do I say this politely?—well-rounded in this area need use only thinner padding, as you already have your own.

  In all cases, the seat surface should not be slippery. High friction will help to keep your bottom where you left it: hopefully in the correct position at the back of the seat base. Some ergonomic chairs have dual density foam inside the seat base: soft at the back, and firm at the front. This excellent idea helps to keep your bottom at the rear of the seat . . . where it belongs.

  On the backrest, types B and D should use firm or minimal padding. However, types A and C can get away with softer or thicker covering.

- The angle of tilt of the seat base.

  Some ergonomic chairs have an adjustable tilt on the seat base. Should you tilt the seat base forward or backward? Some researchers have suggested that a forward tilt of five to ten degrees is beneficial to help to open the hip angle, and so allow the lumbar spine to assume a more neutral position. However, the forward tilt encourages your bottom to slide forward, which in my opinion negates any other benefits.

  Other authors advocate a slight reverse tilt, on the basis that it encourages your bottom to remain at the back of the seat. This advantage may be useful for types A and C, and complements a lower seat height. However, as a backward-tilting seat base would push the lumbar spine into too much flexion for types B and D, those types would be better served by keeping the seat base flat.

- Ensure that your chair is suitable to your environment.

  For example, consider the manoeuvrability of your chair. The world's best, most perfectly adjusted chair is worthless if you cannot reach frequently used desk drawers. Also, wheels or castors are sometimes useful, such as in an office, while at other times they can be a nuisance. So ensure that you consider the layout of your home or office before making any new purchase.

- Are 'kneel chairs' any good?

My answer to this question comes in two parts, with the first part being a resounding 'yes' and the second part being an unequivocal 'no'. Kneel chairs are fine in theory, as they help to align your spine in a more neutral position, and also eliminate worries about seat width and height. However, many of these chairs do not have a back rest, and so allocate much of the stress and strain to your back muscles and joints. They are often impractical, and are difficult for people who sit and stand frequently. In addition, you have to have strong, healthy knees to use one for a long period.

Therefore, when all things are considered, you're probably going to be more suited by a normal, high back-rested ergonomic chair. However, if you meet all of these criteria:
- your knees are healthy
- you don't have to get in and out of the chair too often
- this type of chair suits your work area, and
- the kneel chair has a full length back rest, preferably one that tilts backward

then a kneel chair may do you good.

IN THE CAR

Cars have the nasty habit of shaking, vibrating and transmitting a whole range of other forces to the body. Therefore, it is even more important that you maintain good sitting posture in the car.

Luckily, most car seats these days are adjustable, so a correct seating alignment is readily achievable. Just follow the rules outlined above, and I'm sure that you'll manage just fine. Specifically, you should observe the following familiar guidelines:

- Tilt the seat backward by about 20 degrees.
- To reach the steering wheel from your new lying-back position, you may have to slide the whole seat forward.
- The seatbelt is a wonderful device for habit breaking. A firmly tightened lap belt will stop your bottom sliding forward, while the shoulder strap will encourage your upper torso to lean against the backrest.

Then, with the car seat looking after your back, you can turn up the stereo (not *too* loud), switch on the cruise control, and travel in comfort.

Further sitting advice for back types B and D *only*

As a type B or D spine, you probably already realise that sitting is a high-risk activity for your spine. All of the above advice is vital to help decrease the pressure on your back. However, you probably require extra help to prevent your sitting posture from worsening your back pain.

Recall from our earlier discussions that the lumbar spine—the lower back—has an inward curve called a lordosis. In this natural concave position, the joints and discs are in a protected state. As a type B or type D back, your spine is vulnerable if you lose this lordosis.

So when sitting, particularly for long periods, it is vital that you maintain this lordosis. How do you do this effectively? The secret is to ensure that something is supporting the lordotic curve in your lower back. We're going to refer to such things as a *lumbar support device*.

I was going to hereafter refer to a lumbar support device as an LSD, but as these initials are already taken not only by a popular 1960s hallucinogenic drug but also a trendy mechanical gizmo thing on a car, I'll just stick with the full name.

A lumbar support device is not a complicated structure. Many commercial examples are available, ranging from simple foam cylinders to woven frames. The underlying principle is that when you insert one behind your lower back, it maintains your lordosis while you sit.

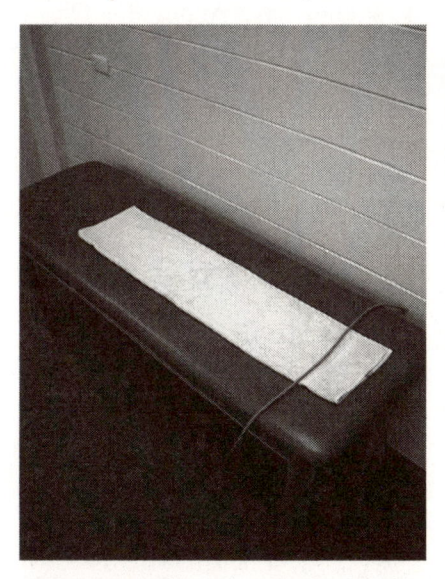

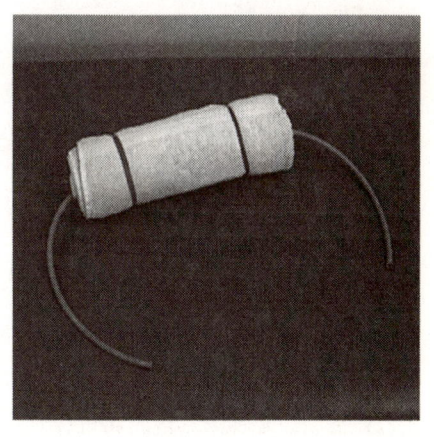

How to make a lumbar support device in two easy steps. First, fold a towel in half lengthwise, and lay a length of rope across one end. Then tightly roll the towel, and secure it with rubber bands. Woo hoo—your own lumbar support device!

Probably the easiest way to obtain a lumbar support device is to make one from an old towel. Simply fold a towel in half lengthwise, then tightly roll it to form a cylinder. Tape the roll firmly, or secure it with a few rubber bands. Hey presto! Your own lumbar support device.

If you are making a roll from a towel, then a length of rope or an old stocking laid across the towel before you start to roll will prove useful. This will enable you to tie your lumbar roll onto your chair so that it automatically supports your back when you sit. This might be a good job for that fluorescent lime green necktie that your Aunty Ethel gave you for Christmas five years ago.

To use simply insert the lumbar support device behind your lower back. Then relax. Don't try to arch your back over the roll. Just sit naturally, and it will automatically hold your lumbar curve in a more correct position.

I suggest that you buy or make a few lumbar support devices, and leave them on the chairs in which you normally sit. Have one in your office chair, one in front of the television, and another in the study. Don't forget the car.

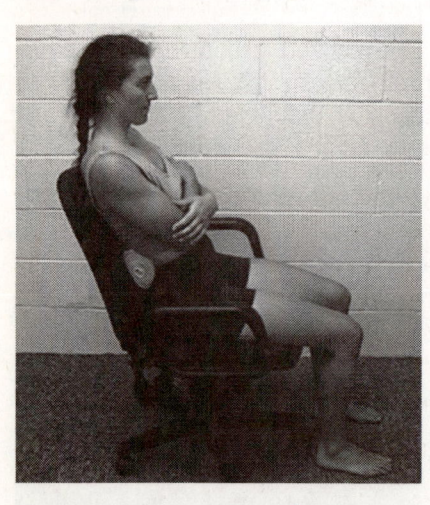

The perfect sitting posture if you have a type B or type D spine. Note that Debbie's feet are flat on the floor, with her knees slightly lower than, or level with, her hips. Her bottom is at the back of the chair, and her lower spine has extra support from a lumbar support device. Debbie is leaning her whole spine into the back rest, which is tilted back at about 20 degrees.

The size and firmness of the lumbar support device will depend upon a few factors. First, your size. A petite little old lady will not require a lumbar roll as large as would, say, Andre the Giant, my favourite 1970s wrestling champion.

Second, people with high F-E scores, whose spines really detest being held in flexion, should generally have firmer or larger lumbar support devices. The larger and firmer the roll, the less flexion it will permit. If you have a low or borderline F-E score, then a smaller or less firm lumbar roll will suffice.

Third, the nature of the chair has an important influence on your choice of lumbar support. A soft, heavily padded lounge chair needs a large, firm device. However, you would probably find the same roll extremely uncomfortable were you to use it on a hard-backed wooden chair.

As a general guideline, a simple lumbar roll should be about ten centimetres (four inches) in diameter, and about thirty centimetres (twelve inches) long. These measurements can be adjusted according to the guidelines above.

Periodically, gimmicky-looking lumbar support devices appear on the market. These gizmos have strange shapes and sizes, with some virtually requiring an instruction book in order to use them. One example is a padded belt-like structure, which you loop around your knees and lower back, using the weight and pressure from your legs to hold your lordosis in place. Another example is a cuff that you wrap around your back, and inflate until you have the correct level of support.

Nothing is intrinsically wrong with any of these devices. As long as they consistently help you to maintain the curve in your lower back, then they are fine. However, consider a few points before spending your hard-earned dollars on a commercial product. First, is it simple to use? Any device that requires more than one second to apply will quickly irritate you, particularly if you sit and stand frequently. Second, can the device be readily used in different situations, including the car? Third, could you do the same job with a simpler, cheaper device?

If you ask yourself these questions, you'll probably conclude that a simple foam roll, or an old, rolled-up towel does the job as well as anything. These are cheap, simple and effective. Why spend money on a whiz-bang gizmo that's probably going to end up gathering dust in the cupboard under the sink, next to the waffle-maker and those empty coffee jars that you thought you'd use some day?

Simple lumbar rolls are readily available. Most spinal health practitioners and chemists stock them, or can order one for you. As mentioned earlier, if possible you should buy a few, in different sizes, and leave them in your usual sitting places. Do it today.

One common item that doubles effectively as a lumbar support device is a good old hot water bottle. A firmly filled hot water bottle is about the right size, and has the added advantage of providing warmth, which is a particularly good for type D backs.

What doesn't make a good lumbar support device? Pillows. A pillow is far too vague, broad and soft to effectively support your lordosis. Sure, it's more comfortable, but it won't help your back. Please don't kid yourself that shoving a pillow on the couch, and occasionally scrunching it behind your back, is supporting your spine. It's not.

You may find that you feel slightly uncomfortable for the first few days of using a lumbar support device. This feeling is normal and expected. In fact, if you *don't* feel slightly uncomfortable, then you're probably doing something wrong. However, do not worry, as the minor

BACK PAIN

discomfort will quickly pass. The lumbar support device should flatten slightly, conforming to your spine, and your back will soon become used to being held firmly in position.

Within two or three weeks, you will probably start to feel uncomfortable and hideously unsupported if you are *not* using a lumbar support device. When you automatically think this way, you will know that you have progressed a long way toward pain-free living. Give yourself a gold star.

16

How to lift and bend more efficiently

What else can you do while you're down there?

They say that you know you are getting old when you bend down to tie up your shoelace and think 'what else can I do while I'm down here?'

Many people who present to their spinal health practitioner for treatment of lower back pain can recall first hurting their back while lifting. Lifting is often, to use a bad analogy, the straw that breaks the camel's back. Just one isolated bad lift can tear a previously weakened joint, leading to days, weeks, even years of pain and frustration.

Furthermore, repetitive incorrect bending or lifting can cause a critical accumulation of microtrauma. Although any *particular* bend or lift does not do much damage, the cumulative effects of many lifts can destroy your spine. A little experiment will help you to further clarify this concept.

Grab a coat hanger, and cut off a short length of wire. We're going to pretend that this wire is a little person, albeit an extremely skinny one. Now bend the wire in the middle, as if our little skinny person is bending at the lower back, and then straighten it again. Inspect the wire. Does it still look normal, healthy and strong? Probably, yes. One lift did not *appear* to hurt our friend.

Now bend and straighten the wire again. Is the wire still OK? Unless you're the type of person with fingers so strong that people hate shaking your hand, then the wire still probably looks fine. Our friend's back still *looks* uninjured. However, if you were to examine the wire with a powerful microscope, you would see that you had already inflicted some tiny, infinitesimal injuries on the wire. Microtrauma!

If you don't believe me, then keep bending the wire. Bend and straighten, bend and straighten, bend and straighten. If you have the patience to repeat this inane activity for, say, an entire television commercial break (i.e. about twenty minutes), then you will see what happens. The microtrauma will accumulate until the wire weakens to breaking point. Eventually, the wire will snap.

Although you did not inflict any traumatic or violent acts on the wire, it is now clearly injured. If this piece of wire had feelings and emotions, then this one would be experiencing a lot of pain. Your lower back is the same. Repetitive lifting and bending inflict microscopic injuries on your spine, which accumulate if your body does not have a chance to heal them completely. Then one day, after the most seemingly trivial incident, it snaps.

The enormous stress that causes the microtrauma is revealed by disc-pressure measurements. Probes inserted into the discs of living subjects reveal that the pressure inside a disc rises by 85% following a simple forward bend. Adding a 20-kilogram weight, even when it was lifted with a good technique, shot the pressure up by about 300%. Worst of all was a poorly executed lift, during which the pressure inside the disc escalated by a whopping 500%!

Obviously, you have little margin for error when dealing with such high pressure. A slightly faulty technique or pre-existing degeneration may be all that is required to injure your back.

Following is some advice on how to avoid these pitfalls. However, *do not interpret this advice as meaning that you should never forward flex your spine*. Please don't become paranoid about bending your back. Backs are made to bend. In fact, they depend on regular movement to stay healthy.

Occasionally I examine patients who were told decades ago by their doctor 'don't bend your spine or you'll do a disc'; advice that they faithfully followed ever since. These people's spines are usually so stiff that their F-E and S-U scores are off the scale, and they have a lot of trouble regaining normal flexibility.

This advice is not intended to make you move rigidly or stiffly. Leave that to those tower guards in London who stand perfectly still all day, not moving a millimetre, not even if you pull a silly face right in front of their eyes. In short, do not be afraid to perform so-called spine-destroying actions such as bending forward from the waist and touching your toes. One or two toe touches will do you no harm whatsoever.

So how do we avoid injuring our lower backs in high-risk bending and lifting situations? Three techniques will help you to lift more efficiently.

1. Stabilise your spine.
2. Use a correct lifting technique.
3. Avoid lifting where possible.

Let's now examine these three areas in detail.

(1) Stabilise your spine

Any extra support that you can provide your lumbar spine when you are lifting is a huge advantage. There are two ways to do this.

First, you can wear an external brace, weight belt or corset. However, reliance on external support has many disadvantages, not the least being that you may not have it handy when required.

Furthermore, and this is my main objection, wearing a brace does not fix your problem. It's cheating. Although this shortcut may sometimes be the best and easiest way to help some people, for most of the population, which probably includes you, there is a far better way. So for now we'll forget about external supports—don't worry, we'll come back to them in Chapter 29—and instead concentrate our energy on a preferable method of stabilising your spine: from within.

By using your abdominal and back muscles in the correct way, you can provide natural support for your lumbar spine. Disc-pressure studies have shown that a good tummy muscle contraction lowers the intra-discal pressure by up to half. Not only that, you can't leave your tummy and back muscles in the front seat of the car when you go to pick up your shopping, as can happen with a brace.

Therefore, rule number one, for all spine types, is this: *contract your transverse abdominal and multifidus muscles when you lift.*

Sound difficult? You're right, it is a bit tricky. Hopefully, you've already taught yourself how to perform these muscle contractions. If not, I suggest that you return to Chapter 14, and thoroughly learn exercises 1 and 2. The detailed instructions will give you a better idea of where the muscles are situated, and how to best contract them. This knowledge will come in very handy, not only when you lift, but also in many other aspects of controlling your back pain.

By contracting these two muscles when you lift, you will provide direct muscular support for your lumbar joints and discs. I suggest that for the next three months, while your muscles are regaining their tone and balance, that you do this consciously. In other words, you should make the effort to self-brace your back by contracting your transverse abdominal and multifidus muscles every time you lift.

Why only three months? Once you awaken and strengthen your transverse abdominal and multifidus muscles, they will start to contract *automatically* during stress situations. You won't even have to think about tightening your muscles, as this will happen naturally. This automation is not a fallacy, nor is it a pipe dream of spinal health practitioners. Research has shown that this effect exists.

Recall the study in Chapter 12, in which subjects were asked to repeatedly raise and lower their arms while the researchers monitored their stability muscles. This study showed that the muscles of back pain sufferers did not *automatically* stabilise their spines. However, after training their stability muscles for a few months, the same subjects were

BACK PAIN

retested. Lo and behold, the stabilising muscles subconsciously contracted during arm movements.

It is as though your brain simply needs to be reminded, through regular exercise and correct use, that the stability muscles exist. Once this has occurred, your mind subconsciously recruits these muscles, which not only protects your back, but also maintains their tone, meaning that they become even better able to support your back next time they are called upon. This 'vicious cycle' is actually beneficial!

So please ensure that you contract your stability muscles every time you lift. Try to use an isolated contraction of just those two muscles, if possible (as described in the exercises), rather than simply tensing your whole stomach and back. If you frequently lift, then I would advise you to add transverse abdominal and multifidus muscle exercises to your program if they are not already included.

(2) Use a correct lifting technique

Unless you live in an isolated cave on top of the Himalayan mountains, I'm sure that you've already been indoctrinated in the rules of correct lifting: bend your knees, don't twist, keep your back straight, blah, blah, blah.

These old chestnuts are fairly accurate. Nevertheless, I would like you to read along while we delve deeper into these rules of safe lifting. Not only will you discover why they are important, but also we will refine some of the advice so that it is more applicable to your back type.

BEND YOUR KNEES
In other words, get your bum low, keep your head up.

There are two absolutely spectacular reasons why you should bend your knees when you lift. The first reason uses anatomy, while the second uses physics. Don't let either of these big-sounding topics scare you.

The anatomical reason has to do with the shape of the lumbar spine during bending. When you lift by flexing your spine forward rather than bending your knees, your lumbar spine loses its natural inward curve, its lordosis.

When you lose your lordosis, the jelly-like centres of your lumbar discs are forced backwards. When this motion is combined with the high intradiscal pressures associated with lifting, it is easy to imagine how the nucleus could either bulge backwards, or prolapse its way through the annulus altogether. Of course, you not only hurt the discs when you lift in this way, but you also strain the facet joints, ligaments, muscles and the sacro-iliac joints.

HOW TO LIFT AND BEND MORE EFFICIENTLY

Another vulnerable structure during a poorly executed lift is the sciatic nerve. If you bend forward with straight knees, you not only increase the pressure in your spine, but you simultaneously stretch your sciatic nerve. If you're trying to give yourself an old-fashioned dose of sciatica, then a straight-legged lift is a great way to go about it.

The second spectacular reason that you should bend your knees when you lift concerns the physical effects of leverage. The effects of leverage can be easily envisaged by considering a seesaw. When two children play on a seesaw, a heavy child can counterbalance a lighter child if he or she sits closer to the fulcrum, or middle point, of the plank. This balancing occurs because the lighter child, by virtue of a greater distance from the balancing point, has greater leverage.

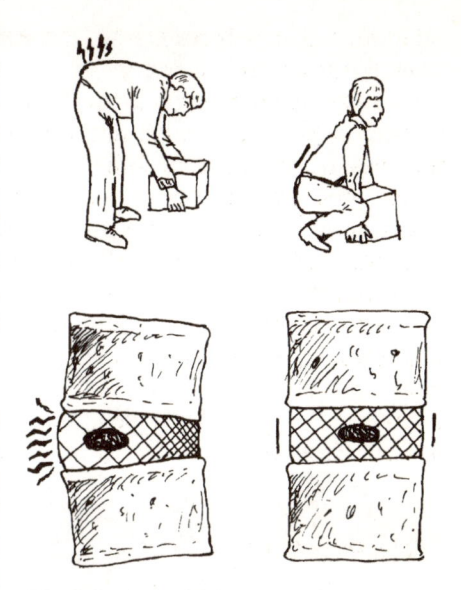

The left picture shows the effects on your discs of a poorly executed lift. Can you see that a poor lifting technique not only tightens and strains the back fibres of the disc, but also forces the nucleus backward, heightening the probability of a bulge or herniation? The picture on the right shows the more favorable outcome of a correct lifting technique.

So when lifting, the closer you hold an object to your spine, the less leverage it has against your back. Consequently, objects that you hold close are far easier to lift, and exert less pressure through your spine, than objects that you hold at arm's length. This leads us to another rule of lifting, which is so important that I'll type it in italics: *always hold objects that you carry as close to your body as possible.*

One other tip also becomes important when we consider the effects of leverage. *Keep your back as vertical as possible.* If you maintain a vertical spine, then the torsional effects of your upper body weight are greatly reduced. However if you allow your spine to become horizontal when you bend, then your spine must not only support the weight of the object, but also the combined mass of your trunk, arms and head.

Let's now look at an example that illustrates these points, with apologies in advance to any biomechanists out there who are horrified at my overly simplistic explanation of the following situation.

Suppose we have two people about to lift a 50-kilo weight. We'll call them Dumb Derek and Smart Simon. (At this point, I should

BACK PAIN

apologise to my mate Derek. I don't think you're dumb at all, it's just that your name sounded good next to the word 'dumb'. To my other mate Simon, I offer the same message, but in reverse.)

Anyway, Dumb Derek decides to lift the weight without bending his knees, meaning that the object is, say, about one metre from his lower back. Not only that, but Dumb Derek's spine also has to contend with the weight of his upper body, which we'll say is also 50 kilograms.

In contrast, Smart Simon bends his knees, and holds the weight close to his body as he stands, meaning that the weight is only 20 centimetres away from his spine. To show this situation diagrammatically, we'll do what real physicists do, and draw stick figures.

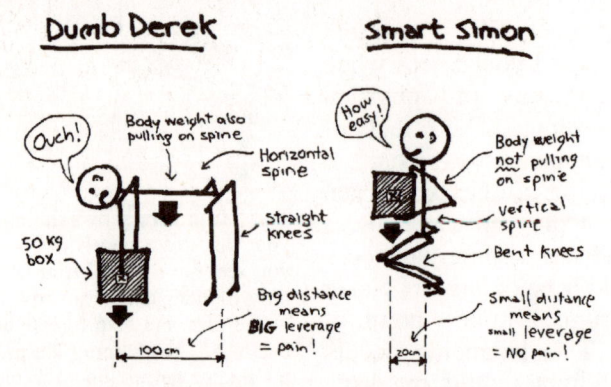

A physicist's drawing of lifting biomechanics.

We can roughly calculate the force that is working through each person's spine by simply multiplying the mass of the object by the distance from each person's lower back. Smart Simon has only 10 units of force pulling his spine into flexion. However, Dumb Derek's has a whopping 75 units of force trying to pull his back down. That's 750% more strain. Ouch!

So you can see that not only is poor Dumb Derek likely to injure his spine, but is also going to work more inefficiently, tire more quickly, and have a lower maximum lift.

Are you starting to see why lifting with bent knees is so important? Moreover, can you see why keeping your back vertical, and holding any objects close to your spine, is smarter? Not only do these techniques stop your spine from being overstretched, but also they make a lot more sense mechanically.

DON'T TWIST

Can you remember our short lesson on disc anatomy in Chapter 2? Recall that the outer fibres of disc, the annulus, have a criss-crossed orientation. This crossover pattern ensures that the fibres always pull

HOW TO LIFT AND BEND MORE EFFICIENTLY

tightly around the jelly-like nucleus, regardless of which way you rotate. As one set of fibres loosens, the other fibres automatically tighten. In a well-used spine, this arrangement works wonderfully.

However, if you bend and then twist your spine, things start to go wrong. You've already learned that flexing your lumbar spine will force the nucleus backward, and simultaneously stretch the back fibres of the disc. If you add a twist while you are bending, then you doubly tighten half of the fibres. Not only that, but as the other fibres are now loose, the tight fibres must contain all of the disc pressure by themselves.

Think about it. Not only are the annulus fibres being stretched and pressured, but half of them are doing all of the work. Of course, the same theory applies to the joints and muscles when you twist while lifting. Only half of them will be fully participating. If you add some weight and repeat a few dozen times, then you are at short odds to be lying in bed with an aching back by tomorrow.

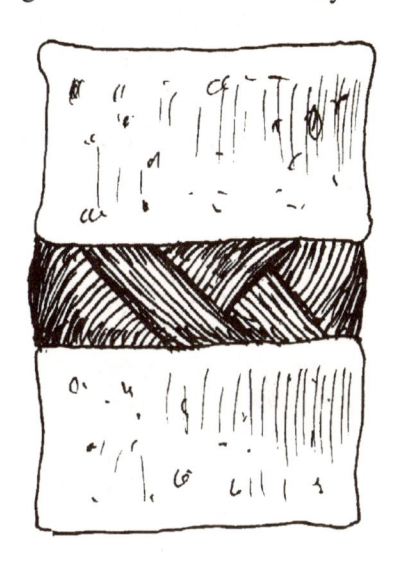

The criss-crossed orientation of the fibres of the annulus, which holds the nucleus in place.

A far better way is to avoid twisting when you lift. Instead, pivot on your feet to change direction.

By swivelling on your feet, you can keep your spine in a neutral position, ensuring that your entire back supports the weight. I'm sure that you can master this technique with just a little practice and concentration.

Here's another tip from the same stable. *When picking up an object from the ground, make sure that your body is already pointing in the direction that you intend to travel.* In this way, you won't have to twist, nor will you have to turn around while carrying an awkward or heavy load.

So in general, try not to twist when lifting. It is a known 'danger activity' for all spinal types. Studies have shown that of all the advice that applies to lifting, this tip is perhaps the most important.

KEEP YOUR BACK STRAIGHT

While the above two 'old wives' rules' are correct, this third rule could use a bit of a spit and polish. 'Keep you back straight' provides only a very loose understanding of what you should really be doing. Let's change this vague statement into a more precise hint: *when lifting, you must position your spinal curves in their most protected state.*

The most protected state of your spinal curves depends upon your back pain type. If you are in doubt, or if you are borderline, then follow the instructions for types B and D, which are more likely to help.

Paradoxically, both sets of hints draw from the experience of Olympic weightlifters, who, not surprisingly, know a thing or two about lifting. Besides, who am I to argue with a bunch of big, beefy blokes, each of whom can lift half a tonne above his head?

LUMBAR SPINE POSITIONING DURING LIFTING FOR TYPES B AND D ONLY

As a type B or D spine, your lumbar spine prefers to be held in its natural lordotic curve. As lifting is such a high-pressure activity, you must ensure that you maintain this inward curve of your lower back at all times.

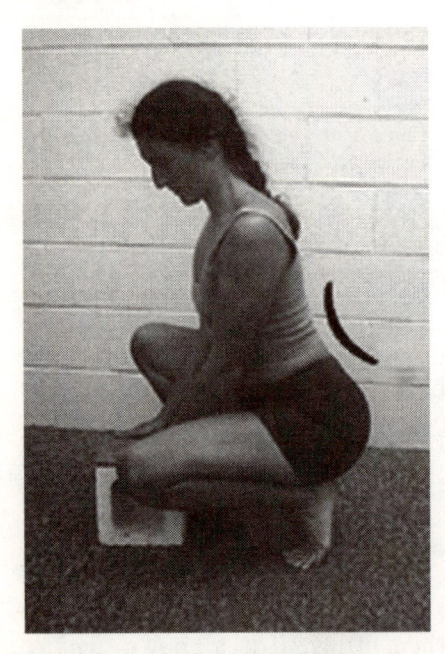

The correct lifting technique for a type B or type D spine. Note the inward curve in Debbie's lower back—the lumbar lordosis.

The easiest way to maintain this position is to 'lock' your back when lifting. By a locked back, I mean that your lordosis is held in a tight curve, which does not allow your back to flex forward at all.

Picture an Olympic weightlifter. Many of these athletes find that by locking their spines into a fixed, extended position, they can safely lift massive weights, time after time. Obviously, some weightlifters do suffer from back pain. However, this probably occurs because they do not have a type B or D spine.

When you hold your back in this fully lordotic position, an *isolated* contraction of your transverse abdominal and multifidus muscles is an important skill to have perfected. This isolation is so important because the other stomach muscles tend to tilt your pelvis, meaning that they pull your back into a rounded, less safe position. However, your transverse

HOW TO LIFT AND BEND MORE EFFICIENTLY

abdominal and multifidus muscles will simply stabilise your spine, without any undesirable tilting or repositioning.

If you're a type B or D, then you need not read the next section. However, our discussion on safe lifting continues after that.

LUMBAR SPINE POSITIONING DURING LIFTING FOR TYPES A AND C ONLY

As a type A or C spine, your lumbar spine does not like to be held in a position of extension. However, as you now realise, lifting is a very dangerous activity when performed with too much flexion. So back types A and C have a delicate balancing act when positioning their spines for a lift: not too much flexion, but without an excess of extension.

Weightlifters are often taught to lift with their spine in an arched, fully lordotic position. However, about one quarter of all serious weightlifters develop stress fractures in their lower vertebrae—a classic type A or C injury. This percentage is much higher than the rate of this injury in the general population. My guess is that this problem arises so frequently because the injured lifters probably had type A or C backs.

A better way for these weightlifters—and for you—to lift is to use a neutral lumbar curve. You must not allow your back to flex forward, but should not let it lock into a fully lordotic curve either.

For this balancing act, you will require well-developed transverse abdominal and multifidus muscles, working in tandem with each other. By co-contracting these muscles, which are on either side of your spine, you will prevent your spine from moving. Mastering this technique will require some persistence, and perhaps even some practise in front of a mirror. I'm sure that with a little bit of dedication you'll manage this just fine.

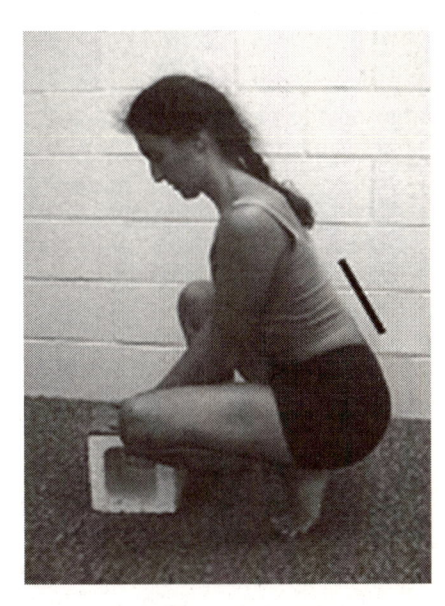

The correct lifting technique for a type A or type C spine. Note that Debbie's lower back is flat, rather than locked into an inward curve.

(3) Avoid lifting where possible

This hint is an extension of commonsense. In general, you should plan a different way of transporting an object rather than lifting or carrying it by yourself. For example, you could:

- push it along the ground
- use a trolley
- ask someone else to give you a hand
- slide it up a ramp
- pay someone else to lift it
- leave it where it is (my personal favourite).

Why chance injuring your lower back, when a few seconds of imaginative planning may allow you to avoid the lift all together? I'll give some more specific hints in this regard in Chapter 19 when we discuss how to ease the burden of work and household chores.

Summary of safe lifting

After reading this chapter, you should have a solid foundation of knowledge on the principles of safe, effective lifting. Let's summarise them here for clarity. To lift safely, you should:

1. Contract your transverse abdominal and multifidus muscles.
2. Use a correct lifting technique:
   - Bend your knees (bum down, head up).
   - Carry all objects as close to your body as possible.
   - Keep your back vertical.
   - Don't twist when lifting; pivot on your feet instead.
   - When picking up an object, stand with your body pointing in the direction of travel.
   - Position your spinal curves in their most protected state:
     –Type B and D use a locked back method.
     –Type A and C use a neutral spine method.
3. Avoid lifting if possible.

Next, we'll look at another potentially stressful group of activities for some lower backs, standing and walking.

17

Ways to walk and stand without straining your spine

How to remain on just two legs without causing spinal pain

The advice in this chapter is primarily directed at those people with type A and C backs. You should also take note if you are in a borderline category such as AB or CD. Although most people who are type B or D rarely experience pain while walking or standing, the principles of spinal stability outlined below will not do you any harm, and are worth your consideration.

Two postures frequently lead to pain during walking and standing. Let's look at these two postures individually to discover why they cause back pain, and how to avoid them.

Bad posture number one—sway back

As you know, the natural position of the lumbar spine is in an inward-curving lordosis. However, problems can arise during standing or walking if this curve is exaggerated. This exaggerated curve is technically known as a *hyperlordosis*, but is more commonly referred to as *swayback*.

Physical problems, such as a stress fracture or disc weakness can also cause problems during upright stance. In these cases, the stability muscles are not supporting the joints firmly in place, and so rendering them vulnerable to the effects of posture and gravity.

So how do we hold the lumbar spine in a more correct position, and so avoid worsening any instability or hyperlordosis? The answer lies deep within your belly ... yes, that's right, your transverse abdominal muscle. Of course, your multifidus muscle in your spine lends a helping hand as well.

If you have been ignoring everything that I've said so far, then you may not yet have tried the first two exercises in Chapter 14. If so, I suggest you try them now. You require well-toned transverse abdominal and multifidus muscles if you are going to rid yourself of pain during standing and walking. If this sounds like you, then I suggest you add these exercises to your program if they are not already included.

BACK PAIN

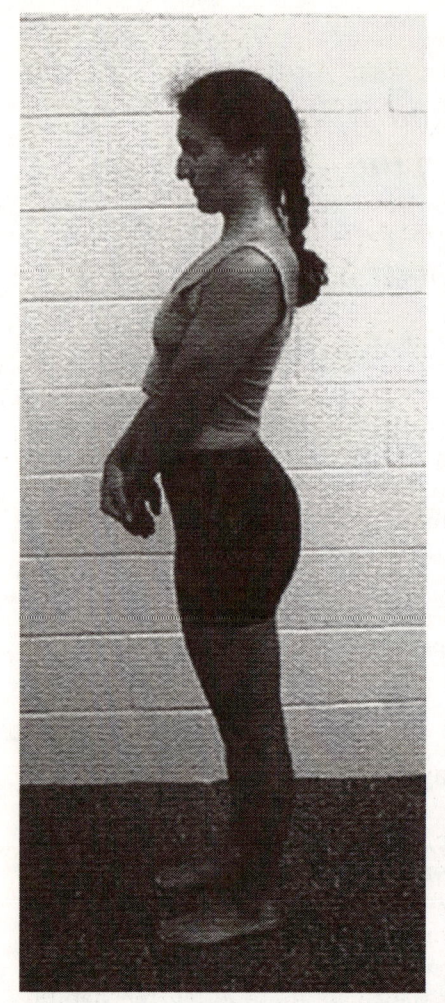

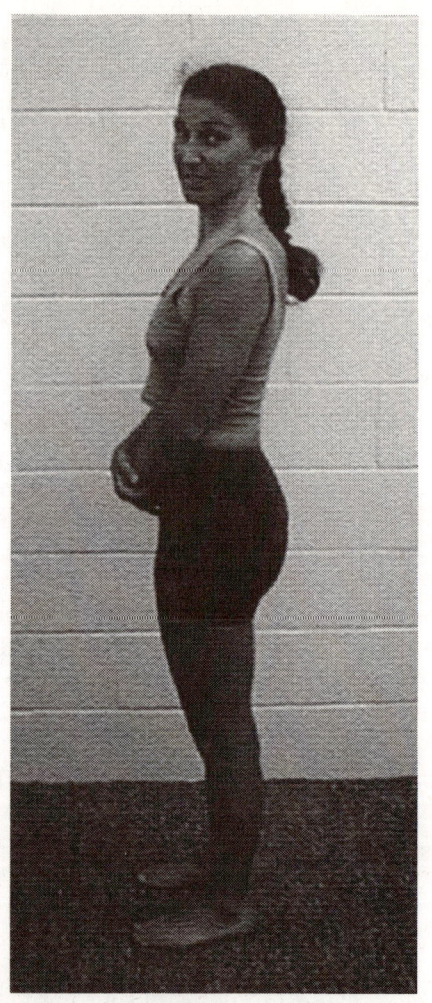

The photograph on the left depicts an exaggerated lumbar lordosis—commonly referred to as a 'swayback'. This poor standing posture will quickly lead to aches and pains if maintained for too long, especially for back types A and C. The photograph on the right shows a flatter, more normal curve, which can be achieved by strengthening your tummy muscles, and stretching your front hip muscles.

Once you have control over these muscles, you have mastered a large component of the problem. Simply by using a gentle, background contraction of your stabilising muscles when standing or walking, you will not only support your spine internally, but will help to prevent gravity from pulling your lumbar spine into an exaggerated curve.

As with lifting, I suggest that you perform this low-level contraction consciously for the first three months. Start by practising the contractions when standing still. Use set times each day to remind yourself, such as cleaning your teeth, showering, or preparing each meal. Standing in a bank queue is an excellent time to practice, as you'll probably have about half an hour of idle time to fill. Feelings of back pain also serve as a more-than-useful reminder to try some gentle muscle contraction.

After a month, you should start on the more difficult task of stabilising your spine while walking. Begin by using a cue to intermittently activate your stabilising muscles. For example, telephone poles can serve as a cue to alternately tighten then relax your stabilising muscles as you pass them.

Of course, you won't have to think about this muscle contraction forever. As mentioned previously, the muscles will soon realise that they are supposed to be contracting, and will function automatically. At this point, your lower back pain during standing will rapidly diminish.

One other muscle that deserves attention if you suffer from pain during standing and walking is the front hip muscle, the iliopsoas. If this muscle is tight, then it pulls your spine into an exaggerated, swaybacked curve. If you suffer with this pain during prolonged standing, then I suggest that you add exercise thirteen to your program if it is not already included.

Bad posture number two—dropped hip

Some people, particularly, those with type A backs, develop a very unstable standing posture that relies on taking the body weight through one leg, while dropping the pelvis on the other side. This dropped-hip posture is the way your body avoids using weak or tired postural muscles.

A dropped-hip standing posture twists the spine into an unnatural sideways curve. As you know, constantly stretching ligaments and discs soon leads to accumulated microtrauma, and eventual injury.

A similar process occurs during the walking cycle. Those people with weak postural muscles subconsciously 'drop' their hip when walking, or during other similar activities such as climbing stairs. Runners with this problem look uncoordinated and, well, floppy. This effect may be so subtle that it can only be detected through careful video analysis, or may be so obvious that the entire gait looks like an unstable waddle.

If your pelvis continually drops, even by just a few centimetres, it stretches and strains your spine. When repeated day after day, step after step, then damage gradually accumulates to breaking point.

BACK PAIN

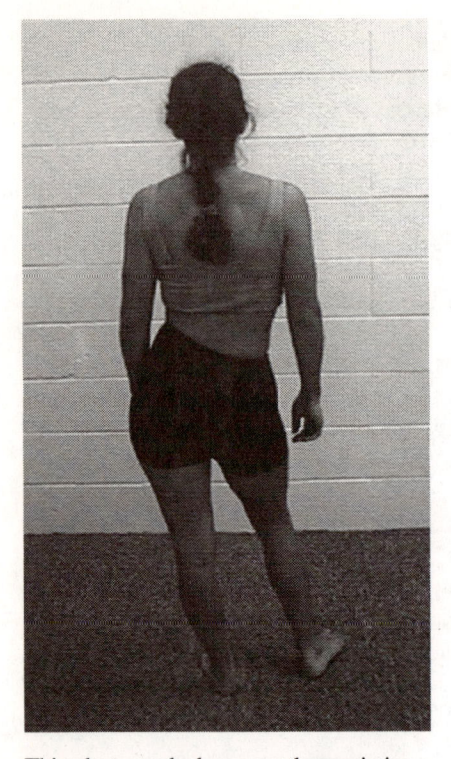

This photograph shows another variation of poor standing, in which Debbie has 'dropped' her right hip. This type of posture is common among people with weakened hip stability muscles, and frequently causes pain during prolonged standing.

Obviously, you should avoid this unstable pattern of standing and walking. The best way to achieve this improvement is, of course, to strengthen your postural muscles. As you know, the transverse abdominal and multifidus muscles stabilise your lumbar spine. In the case of this hip-dropped pattern, another muscle assumes great importance. Sitting deep inside your hips, under your buttocks, this vital postural muscle is called the *gluteus medius*.

The gluteus medius connects your pelvis to the top of your thigh bone. Its usual function is to hold your pelvis level when you stand on one leg, and to hold your body upright during the 'stance phase' of walking or running. A weakness of this muscle manifests as a dropping pelvis during any of these activities.

Exercise 3 in Chapter 14 explains how to reactivate and strengthen your gluteus medius muscle. Like all postural exercises, it is initially difficult to master, and requires lots of concentration. However, I am sure that once you have mastered this exercise that your standing posture will improve ... and, of course, your pain will disappear.

If you experience pain while walking or standing, and you are not already performing exercise three, then I suggest that you add it to your program. This exercise is a 'must' if you find yourself regularly standing with a dropped-hip posture.

A few more notes on standing posture

When using the above postural techniques, don't expect the improvement to arrive after the first twenty minutes. Have some patience! You have probably been inadvertently misusing your lumbar spine and its stability muscles for your entire life. Obviously, a lifetime of postural bad habits takes a long time to correct, so you'll need persistence.

Luckily, after a while, the stability muscles will learn to contract by themselves. If you work calmly and regularly on your stability muscle exercises, and frequently correct your poor standing and walking habits, then this automation should be starting to work within three months. At this point, your back will have a solid base of muscular support, and your pain will start to disappear. Not only that, but as you've fixed the cause of your problem, it will probably stay away ... forever.

Footwear

Some spinal health practitioners make a lot of fuss about footwear. 'High heels,' they exclaim, 'will ruin your spine!' While I can see some minor advantages to having flat, supportive shoes, I can't really see why occasional use of high heels leads to doom and gloom for your spinal pain.

Medical folklore says that high heels change your centre of gravity, forcing your spine into a mechanically undesirable position. I must admit that I haven't tried walking in high heels (not on a regular basis, at least) but I fail to see how they would dramatically alter your centre of gravity, apart from lifting it an inch or two higher.

If you feel that your footwear may be causing or exacerbating your back pain, then you should test yourself with a little experiment. Simply wear your high shoes as often as possible for one week, and observe the results. Then, the following week, restrict yourself to flatter shoes and compare. You can then make an informed decision for yourself.

Concerning sports shoes, the market is changing too constantly to provide you with any specific advice as to which brands to choose or avoid. Here, you should be guided by the advice of a competent podiatrist, or, as a last resort, a trained sports shoe salesperson.

However, I have one word of warning: do not buy shoes that feel excessively soft underfoot. Shoes with large, soft, heavily padded heels often cause more damage to your back than do harder-soled shoes. This paradox has been demonstrated experimentally, and occurs because soft shoes alter the normal stress-absorbing mechanisms of your body. Allow me to explain.

When running, your body uses many subtle movements to dissipate the enormous stress of footfall. For example, your knee buckles slightly, your spring-like foot arches stretch, and your hips joints rotate ever so slightly. These automatic reactions combine to create a natural shock absorption system for your lower back.

However, overly soft, padded shoes trick your legs into thinking that all is well. The tiny shock-absorbing movements disappear. In this case, all of the force is transmitted up your rigid leg, straight into your lower

BACK PAIN

back, making you vulnerable to injuries such as stress fractures, facet joint degeneration and sacro-iliac joint sprains.

Other ways to rest your back when standing

If you must do a lot of standing and walking, then you may find that certain positions help temporarily ease your pain. Some of them are very unobtrusive; no one need even know that you are in pain. All of these positions have one thing in common: they reduce the hyperlordosis in your lumbar spine. Here are some positions to try.

- Use a footrest.
  Using a footrest is a simple way to help avoid the build-up of postural strain on your lumbar spine. In particular, those people with back type C will find it useful, as a foot rest will draw the lumbar spine out of its exaggerated lordosis, relieving pressure on the overworked joints.

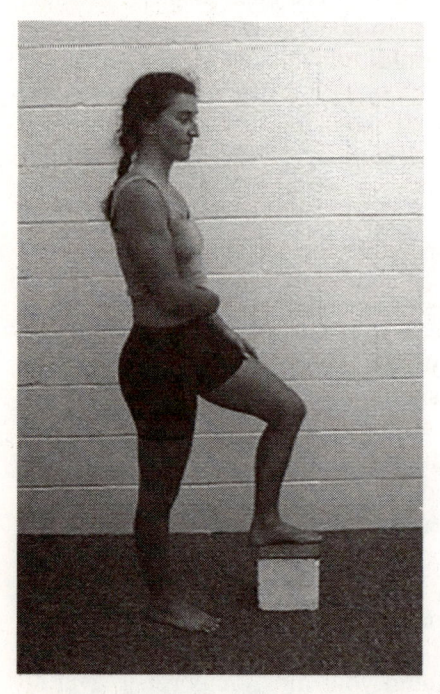

Standing with a footrest will lessen the curve of your lumbar spine, temporarily relieving the pain of swayback.

Almost anything can serve as a footrest. Anything solid, non-slip and about ten centimetres (four inches) high will do. A thick telephone directory will suffice in a pinch. If you are standing near a bench, then opening a cupboard door will allow you to rest one foot upon the lowest shelf.

A footrest may also relieve some pain from those people with type

A spines. However, while the footrest may help reduce the hyperlordosis, it also encourages an awful hip-dropped posture. In this case, the footrest will probably do more harm than good. If you have a type A spine, then I suggest that you avoid using a footrest until your muscles are stronger, and your pelvis has the strength and stability to remain level.

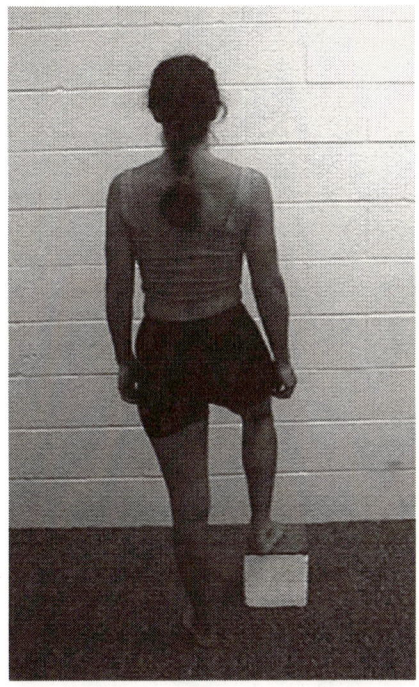

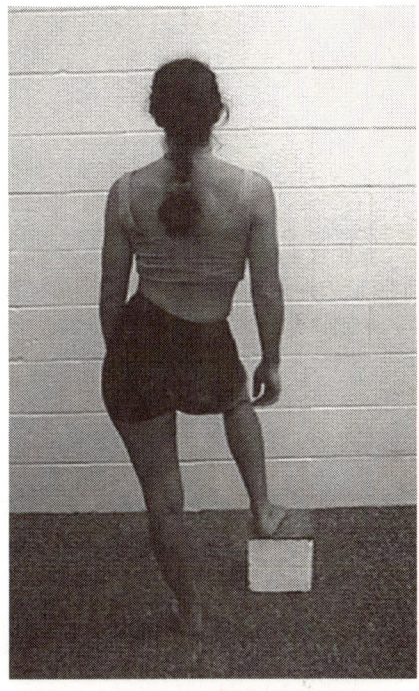

The right and wrong way to use a foot rest. In the left photo, Debbie's hips and pelvis are level, meaning that her spine is held in a neutral, protected position. However, in the right photo, her hip has dropped, dragging her pelvis and spine out of alignment. As you can see, using a foot rest does not automatically ensure that your spine is protected.

- Lean your lower back against a wall.
  Stand with your feet comfortably apart, with your heels about thirty centimetres (one foot) from the wall. Lean back against the wall, then slightly bend your knees. This movement should flatten your lumbar spine against the wall, providing it with support and stability. This is an excellent posture in which to practise contracting your transverse abdominal and multifidus muscles.

- Stand with one hip flexed.
  Stand with your back to a wall. Then simply bend one knee to about 90 degrees, and rest the sole of your foot against the wall. This posture is a way of providing yourself with an imaginary footrest.

BACK PAIN

As such, it is vital that you maintain a level pelvis when in this position, which you can achieve by contracting the gluteus medius muscle on your weight-bearing leg.

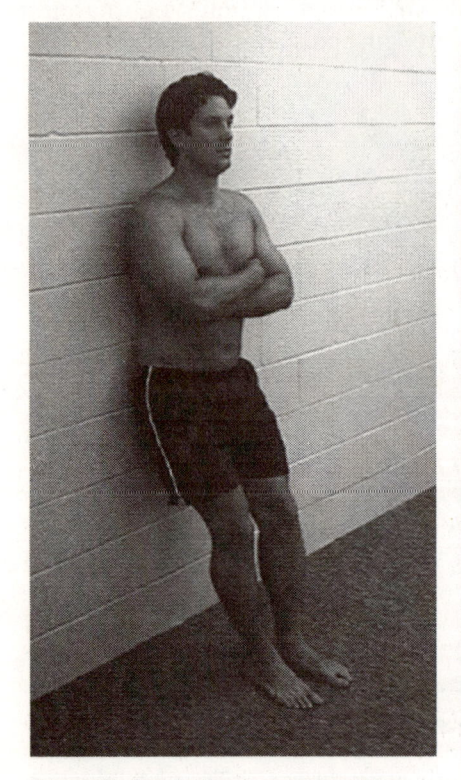

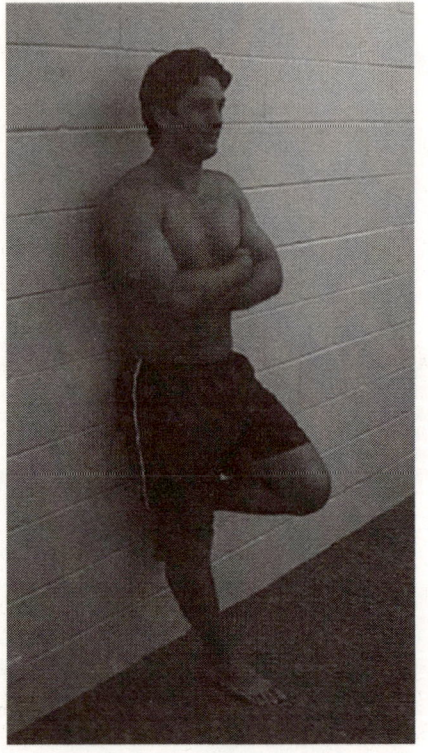

The wall sit, which may temporarily relieve standing-related low back pain.

A one-legged wall stand, which combines a wall sit with a foot rest.

- Lean forward onto a bench or shopping trolley.
  By leaning forward onto a bench or shopping trolley, you pull your lower back into slight flexion. This posture is useful to ward off the stress from hyperlordosis.

- If all else fails—have a seat!

Summary of standing and walking posture control

- Use your transverse abdominal and multifidus muscles to prevent hyperlordosis.
- Strengthen your gluteus medius muscle to avoid hip-drop posture.
- Remain patient, practise hard, and do your stability exercises.
- Use simple rest postures to temporarily relieve pain if necessary.

18

Simple tips for lying and sleeping

There's a bit about sex in here too

Many people with back problems find that their pain and stiffness is at its worst first thing in the morning. Is this morning pain due to a bad mattress, or poor lying posture? Well, to be honest, not necessarily.

Injuries to other parts of the body—a sprained ankle, for example—are also frequently stiff and sore upon rising in the morning. Obviously, a sprained ankle has nothing to do with your mattress, nor would it be adversely affected by your sleeping posture.

Furthermore, most back structures are relaxed when you are lying. Disc-pressure measurements show that intradiscal pressure is lowest when you are recumbent.

Nevertheless, your sleeping posture and your mattress do have a role to play in the management of your lower back pain. There are two good reasons why you should scrutinise your sleeping arrangements. First, sleeping is a very prolonged activity. Most people average about eight hours of sleep per night—2,920 hours per year—so even a minor imbalance or imperfection can magnify into a noticeable problem. The second reason that sleeping is an important consideration for your spine is very simple: we all have to do it.

So let's look at various elements of sleeping and lying, and discover how our backs are likely to respond. By the way, there's a bit about sex in this chapter too. (That should keep you reading.)

Sleeping positions

Some sleeping positions suit some spinal types, while hurting others. How do you know which is best for you? Below are eight common positions for sleeping and resting, each of which is accompanied by recommendations for each spinal type. Most of the information should be self-evident.

1. Flat on your side
Position: Lying on your side, with your knees comfortably bent, and level with each other. Most people find it more comfortable if they use

a pillow between their knees. Note that the hips are slightly flexed, and that the shoulders and pelvis are aligned.

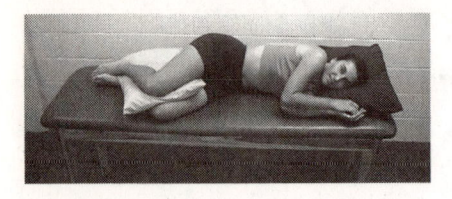

Recommended for: All back types.

Comments: This position, which holds the spine in a neutral, supported alignment, is ideal for all back pain types, either for sleeping or for short rests. If you have back pain, then this is an ideal position to adopt while lying.

Flat on your side.

2. *Twisted on your side*
Position: Lying on your side, with your uppermost knee lying across your lower leg so that it rests on the mattress. Note that the shoulders and pelvis are not aligned.

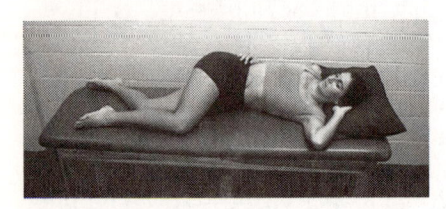

Recommended for: No-one.

Comments: While this sleeping position is very common, it is not necessarily the safest. The extra spinal twist causes a prolonged stretch to your joints and discs. In particular, types A and B should avoid this position. Posture number one, flat on your side, is very similar, and is a preferred alternative for all.

Twisted on your side.

3. *Foetal*
Position: Lying on your side with both knees pulled close to your chest.

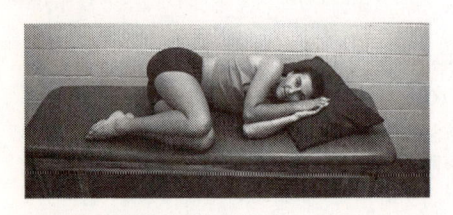

Recommended for: Types A and C.

Comments: The high degree of lumbar flexion may help ease the pain of those with back types A or C.

Those with type B pain will probably find that this position makes their pain worse.

The foetal position.

Type D people may find it useful to help stretch their back, and may use it for short rests of up to five minutes' duration.

4. Prone

Position: Lying flat on your tummy.

Recommended for: Types B and D for short periods only.

Comments: The high degree of lumbar extension may help ease the pain of those with back types B or D.

People with type A pain will find that this position makes their pain worse, and should avoid using it completely.

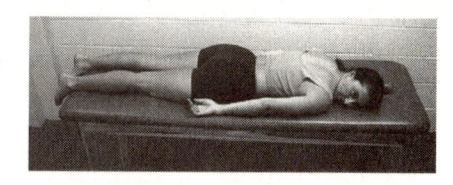

Prone lying (lying on your tummy).

Type C sufferers should also avoid it for long periods, but may find that up to five minutes in this position helps to stretch and loosen their spine.

This position should be avoided by anyone using a very soft mattress, as the degree of extension may be too extreme.

In general, anyone wishing to rest in this position should consider using position five as an alternative.

Note that lying prone places enormous strain on neck joints, and for this reason you should avoid using it for long periods such as overnight. Prone lying should also be avoided by anyone with a history of neck pain or stiffness, headaches or dizziness.

5. Prone with pillow

Position: Lying on tummy, but with a pillow under the hips.

Recommended for: Types B and D, or as an alternative to position four for types A and C.

Comments: The pillow has the effect of reducing the amount of extension in your lumbar spine as compared to position four. Types B and D should find this position comfortable.

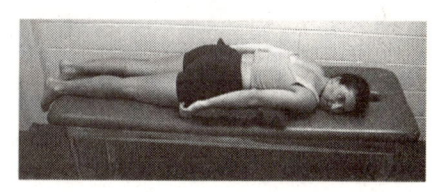

Prone lying with a pillow under your tummy.

This position is also useful as an alternative for types A and C when prone lying is necessary, such as when receiving a massage.

Lying prone with a hip pillow is also an acceptable substitute for position four for types B and D if their mattress is very soft.

As with normal prone lying, this position should be avoided by anyone with neck problems.

6. Supine

Position: Lying flat on your back.

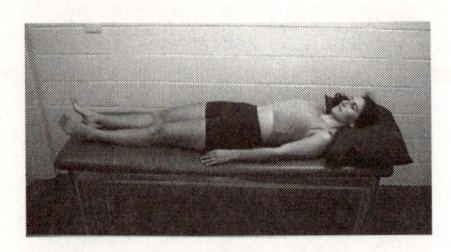

BACK PAIN

Recommended for: Types B and D.

Comments: Lying supine on your back encourages your spine into extension. Therefore, types B and D may find it restful.

Types A and C should avoid it, particularly if they also have stiff front hip muscles. A better alternative is position (7), below.

Supine lying (on your back).

7. Supine with knee pillows

Position: Lying flat on your back, with a couple of pillows under your knees.

Recommended for: All back types.

Comments: This position holds the spine in a neutral position. As such, it is an ideal position for all back pain types, particularly when combined with a firm sleeping surface.

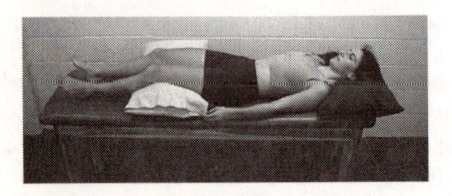

Supine lying with pillows under your knees.

8. The 90-90 position

Position: Lying on your back, with your lower legs resting on a chair or padded box. Your hips and knees should both be flexed to 90 degrees, with the back of your knees holding a tiny bit of your bodyweight. This should slightly elevate the lower part of your bottom from the bed.

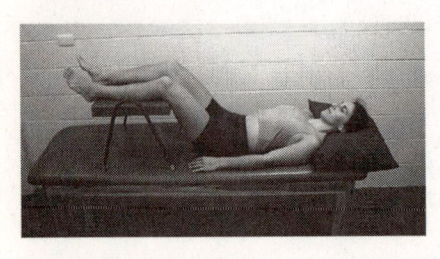

Recommended for: Types A and C, and anyone suffering from recent-onset back pain of any type.

Comments: Some sufferers of acute, severe lower back pain, as well as types A and C, find that the gentle traction effect of this technique helps to relieve their pain.

The 90–90 position.

While not useful for sleeping, this position is handy for other tasks such as reading or relaxing.

Mattresses and sleeping surfaces

Mattresses are made to feel good, not necessarily for support. Manufacturers realise that you may only spend a few minutes testing each bed in the furniture showroom before deciding upon a purchase. They have to make each mattress comfortable, instantly comfortable. This comfort usually often comes, unfortunately, at the expense of long-term support.

When choosing a mattress, you should generally aim for one that feels slightly too firm. You will quickly adapt to the extra hardness, and your back will thank you for it.

However, different back types respond to different firmnesses. If, like most people, you sleep on your side or on your back, then a softer mattress will tend to allow more lumbar flexion. Using this assumption, we can make some recommendations for each back type. If you are a borderline case, then err on the side of firmness.

- Type B spines require lots of support, and therefore a very hard mattress; for example, a futon, or fifteen-centimetre (six-inch) dense foam mattress.
- Type D backs also require firm support. A dense foam mattress, or firm commercial product will do the job nicely.
- Type A backs can tolerate a slightly softer surface, such as a firm or ordinary commercial product.
- Type C spines can luxuriate in a more giving, softer, surface, such as a standard commercial mattress. Just don't go overboard on the softness!

Of course, even the best, firmest mattress in the world is useless if it sits atop an old, wilting base. If you suspect that your base may be inadequate, then try laying your mattress directly on the floor for a few nights. If you find that this extra firmness helps lessen your pain and stiffness, then you can be confident that a harder base will improve your spine in the long term. At this stage you could try the old 'plywood under the mattress' trick. Or maybe even buy a new bed!

By the way, don't forget to rotate and/or flip your mattress every six months or so. Commonsense will tell you that this will not only help it to support your spine more evenly, but will also prolong its useful life.

Waterbeds are a tricky proposition with respect to lower back pain. If you wish to use a waterbed, then ensure that it is firmly filled. Use the guidelines above to further adjust for your back type.

Occasionally, beanbags, hammocks or couches are used for sleeping or resting. These 'beds' allow and encourage a very high degree of lumbar flexion, and so are not suitable for many people's spine. If a spinal health practitioner had been shipwrecked on Gilligan's Island, they would have made a fortune. I'd like to bet that the whole crew had terrible lower back problems after years of sleeping on old, sagging hammocks.

Specifically, type B spines should avoid hammocks and beanbags, while type D backs should chose firmer surfaces where possible. However, type C backs will find them fine for short periods, as will type A spines. I must admit, however, that I often break my own rules in this regard, particularly on lazy Sunday afternoons during cricket season.

Sex and back pain

I must admit that I never dreamt that I'd be giving advice on sex. All this advice I am about to dispense on sex positions obviously makes me a sex expert, of which I am rather proud. I might even advertise it on my business cards.

On the other hand ... hmmm. I'd better get on with the advice.

Put simply, if you're an A or a B then you should stay on the bottom, with your unstable back supported firmly on the bed (or floor, carpet, kitchen table, beach or whatever surface you may be using).

However, if you're a C or a D then you need all the stretching and movement you can get, so you'd probably be better on top. What a fun way to exercise!

I tried to talk the models into a few demonstration photographs. Debbie thought that it was a great idea, but Greg was a bit nervous about the whole nude thing. Sorry about that, readers.

How to overcome early morning backache and stiffness

Many people, especially types C and D, find that their back is at its absolute worst when they first arise in the morning. This stiffness may or may not be due to an unsupportive mattress. Either way, below are a few tips to make those first few minutes a bit easier.

Exercise before you arise
In Chapter 14, we outlined exercises to increase the flexibility of your spine. In particular, exercises four to twelve, which stretch your joints, muscles and nerves, may be useful. Early morning, before you even get out of bed, is an excellent time to do these exercises, for a few reasons.

Simple tips for lying and sleeping

First, your pain and stiffness will abate far more quickly if you perform some slow, gentle stretching techniques. Second, you are less likely to injure your spine in the early part of the day if you have already stretched. Third, the early morning is an excellent time for habit forming. Not only are you less likely to be disturbed during this time, but waking up is something that you do at least once per day. Use that alarm clock as a reminder to do your exercises, and you'll never forget.

Use heat
One effective way to reduce morning backache and stiffness is to use a heat source such as an electric blanket. Small, back-sized electric heating pads are also commercially available, which make an ideal companion for your spine on a cold winter's morning.

However, an electric blanket is not the most desirable bed partner on a breezeless, 25°C summer night, with the humidity hovering around a cosy 90 per cent. In this case, the following trick will help. By connecting the heat blanket to an electric-timer switch, you can program it to activate an hour or two before you awaken. In this way the blanket generates heat only in the cooler hours of the morning, and will have nicely warmed your spine by the time you arise.

Arising from your bed
If your back is acutely painful, or if you have severe instability as indicated by a very low S-U score, then you may find that the process of getting out of bed is very difficult. Under these extreme circumstances, you may wish to try the following technique.

- If you are lying on your back, shuffle yourself across to about 30 centimetres (one foot) from the edge of the bed. Bend your knees to about 90 degrees.

- Now, tighten your lower tummy and multifidus muscles, and 'block roll' onto your side. When performing a block roll, your back should stay stiff, like a log; your neck and upper back should twist at the same rate as your lower back.

- Your kneecaps should now be just over the edge of the mattress. When you are ready to sit, slowly straighten your knees until your ankles are on the edge of the mattress, and tighten your tummy muscles again.

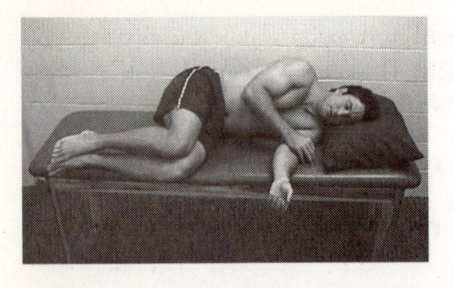

On your marks... Greg has positioned himself ready to stand. He now tightens his stability muscles before proceeding.

- Then, drop your ankles over the edge. Your lower legs will now serve as a counterweight as you push yourself into sitting. That's the hardest part over.

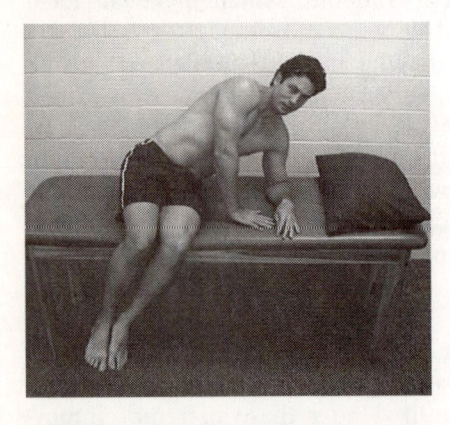

Get set... With his legs acting as a counterweight, Greg pushes himself into a sitting position. He uses his tummy and spinal muscles to stabilise his spine as he does.

- Next, wriggle your bottom forward to the edge of the mattress, and pivot around on your bottom so that your feet are underneath you. From this position, you should be able to keep your spine vertical as you push yourself into a standing position.

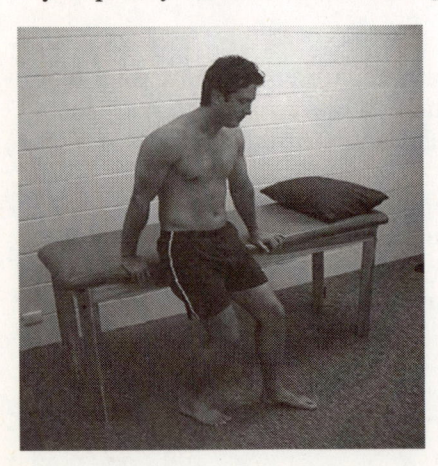

Go! Greg has moved his bottom forward to the edge of the bed, and has pulled his feet back underneath him. He can now keep his spine in a neutral position as he uses his leg muscles to stand.

Trust me, it's not as difficult as it sounds, although you may require one or two practice runs to get it right. If you have trouble getting *into* bed, then you can use the same procedure in reverse.

Summary

You have seen how certain sleeping positions will suit different types of back problems. Mattresses, too, can be tailored to suit your individual spine. Finally, some gentle exercises and heat can make those first twenty minutes far more comfortable.

More advice on sex? Don't ask me, I'm just a physiotherapist.

19
Easing activities of daily living
Principles + commonsense + imagination

During the proceeding four chapters, we have dealt with four of the main stress situations for your spine, namely:

- sitting
- lifting and bending
- standing and walking
- lying and sleeping.

After reading and digesting these sections, you should now have a grasp of the fundamentals of back care.

However, your daily life is undoubtedly composed with far more complexity than just these basic activities. Sometimes, applying your knowledge to everyday tasks can be difficult, as the demands and pace of normal life interfere with your concentration. To help you succeed in this process, this chapter will give examples on how to apply the principles of back care to activities of daily living. The big word for this process is *ergonomics*, the study of work.

In short, we're simply going to combine the basic principles of back care with some good old commonsense, and add a dash of imagination. Hopefully, these good habits will soon become second nature, not consciously planned movements.

However, please don't interpret the following advice as inferring that you should never flex or extend your spine, and that to do so would invite lifelong pain. Your spine *needs* movement to stay healthy. Flexibility is one of the essential principles of spinal rehabilitation.

However, you should use your spine cautiously in a few situations, as described in the following list.

1. Caution is required with any activity that is **highly repetitive**.
Think of the wire-bending experiment in Chapter 16. The outcome of this little investigation, in which you can easily break a length of wire using gentle but constant bends, illustrates the potential danger of repetitive tasks.

Some examples of highly repetitive tasks include stacking shelves at

EASING ACTIVITIES OF DAILY LIVING

a supermarket, shovelling cement on a building site, or bowling a cricket ball for hours on end.

*2. Caution is required with any activity that is **prolonged**.*
Remember that silly finger pulling experiment in Chapter 15? That demonstration showed how a gentle force can become very destructive if you maintain it for long enough.

Examples of activities that use prolonged postures include television watching, desk work, lecturing, leaning over a bench, crouching in a confined space such as under a low house, or painting a ceiling.

*3. Caution is required with any activity that is **heavy**.*
This rule is self-evident. You *cannot* carry a piano down the stairs by yourself. Cumbersome lifting also falls into this category.

*4. Caution is required when you perform an activity that is known to be **dangerous**.*
The previous chapters outlined several positions that are hazardous for almost everyone with a painful spine. Lifting with a twisted, bent spine is one example. Prolonged sitting on an unsupportive chair is another. You should use extra caution if your circumstances force you into a risky situation.

*5. Caution is required when you are performing any activity that is **unsuitable** for your back type.*
As you know, each back type will respond differently to a given situation. I'm sure that you have started to develop an appreciation of the activities that are most damaging to your back type.

For example, type A and C backs will become painful if you lie on your tummy, as they don't like being held in extension. Conversely, type B or D spines won't last long if you sit without a lumbar support, as they hate being held in flexion.

Using your newfound knowledge, you should start to develop an awareness of what constitutes an unsuitable activity for *your* back. Then, when confronted by such a situation, you will realise *in advance* that extra caution is required.

The rest of this chapter will provide numerous examples to help reinforce the principles of efficient spine use, as well as providing some hints and tricks on how to avoid unsuitable postures or positions.

In between these high-risk situations, bend however you like. You're not a robot.

BACK PAIN

Hints on how to perform daily activities without hurting your spine

MANAGING YOUR JOBS
Break all tasks up into manageable portions. Don't try to weed the whole garden, or spring-clean the entire house, in one backbreaking session per year.

Furthermore, try to alternate jobs that require extension, such as cleaning high windows, painting a ceiling or trimming high hedges, with jobs of a flexed nature, like planting at ground level, bath cleaning or swabbing the deck. (What is 'swabbing' anyway? Is there anything else that you 'swab' besides a deck?)

USING TOOLS OR APPLIANCES
When doing jobs such as raking or vacuuming, Types B and D should use long-handled tools or appliances so that they can remain as upright as possible.

Conversely, types A and C may find that regular-length tools and appliances allow them to 'lean' into their work, and subsequently give them less pain.

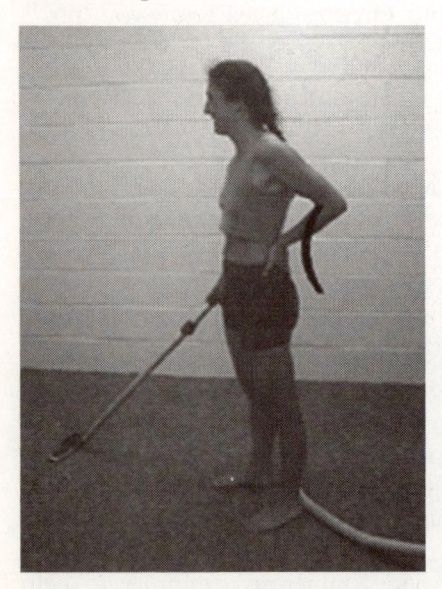

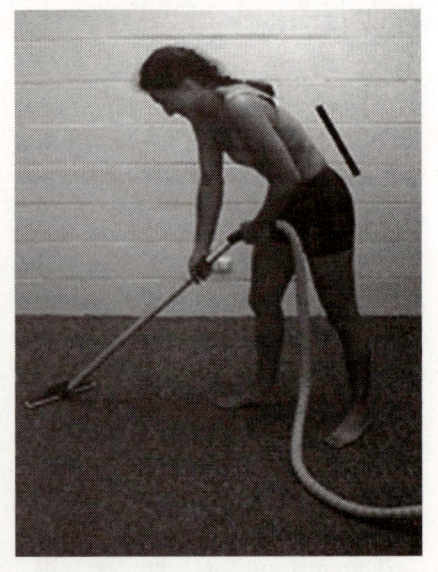

The left photograph shows the ideal working posture for spinal types B and D: upright, with the inward curve maintained in your lumbar spine. You can see why long-handled tools are important in this situation. By contrast, back types A and C may be more comfortable with the posture shown in the right photograph, which uses a slight forward bend of the lumbar spine.

All back types should swap the tools from one hand to another occasionally, which will ensure that you are not repetitively stressing one side of your back. Try to become ambidextrous with appliances.

Push-style brooms and straight-topped rakes might be better than the fan-shaped whisk types. The straight shape is better because the required action does not depend on repetitive twisting.

PUSHING TASKS

When pushing objects such as a mower or pram, types B and D should stand as close to the object as is comfortably possible. This position allows a more upright posture, and so helps avoid prolonged forward leaning.

On the other hand, types A and C may find that they feel more comfortable with the hand piece set lower, which will encourage a slight forward lean.

All types of spines will probably find it easier to move across a hill, such as when mowing a lawn, rather than up and down.

BENCH WORK

Types B and D should keep their workbenches as high as possible to prevent prolonged bending or hunching over work. If the bench is low, then you should bend your knees, or stand with feet astride, so that you are closer to your work. This posture is easy to maintain, and is an excellent habit to prevent prolonged spinal bending.

As a last resort, types B and D may find it useful to support their spine by taking some of their weight through one arm, particularly when doing one-handed tasks such as painting or dusting.

Types A and C may find it useful to place a brick or telephone directory under the work space to use as a footrest. Remember to keep your pelvis level, as discussed in Chapter 17. Alternatively, you can open a cupboard door, and use the bottom shelf as a handy footrest.

Types A and C should also consider sitting as an alternative to standing at a bench. Many tasks—ironing, for example—can be performed just as easily in a sitting position. A swivel chair is usually more practical in this setting than is a fixed-base chair.

STORAGE

All back types should try to store heavy or frequently used items at waist height. In particular, types B and D should avoid storing heavy items down low. Types A and C should avoid storing heavy items in high places.

BACK PAIN

CARRYING
If carrying dirty, sharp or prickly objects, ensure that you are wearing protective clothing. As you know, carrying the load close to your body will decrease the stress on your spine. Protective clothing will allow this to be done without inviting trouble from your washer-person.

Alternatively, you should try to arrange your tasks so that carrying is not necessary. For example, use a clothes trolley, rather than lugging about a heavy laundry bag. Use a wheelbarrow to transport unwieldy garden tools.

HEAVY YARD WORK
When performing heavy work, such as shovelling, all back types should ensure that their knees are bent, and that their stability muscles are working. Treat each action like a separate lift.

Specifically, try to stand with your body pointing to the destination of your shovel-load, so that you can avoid rotating. If twisting is essential, then keep your back firm and pivot on your feet instead. Take a few small steps around with your feet, if necessary.

If you are using a wheelbarrow, then place it in the direction of travel before you fill it. Start to fill it over the front wheel, so that the heaviest part of the load is well forward.

JOBS AT GROUND LEVEL
To prevent repetitive bending, Types B and D should kneel on all-fours to perform jobs at ground level, such as weeding or stacking low shelves. In this hands-and-knees posture, gravity tends to pull your spine into extension, not flexion, which should be more comfortable for your spine.

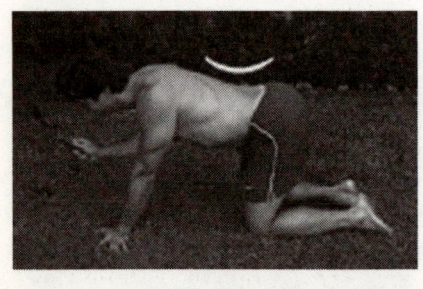

This hands-and-knees posture is ideal for back types B and D when performing ground-level tasks. Note that gravity naturally pulls Greg's spine into slight extension, affording it some degree of protection.

Types A and C will probably find that half kneeling (one foot and one knee on the ground) is the most comfortable position in which to perform low-down tasks. By leaning forward and taking some of the weight through one arm, the spine can be maintained in a position of supported flexion.

EASING ACTIVITIES OF DAILY LIVING

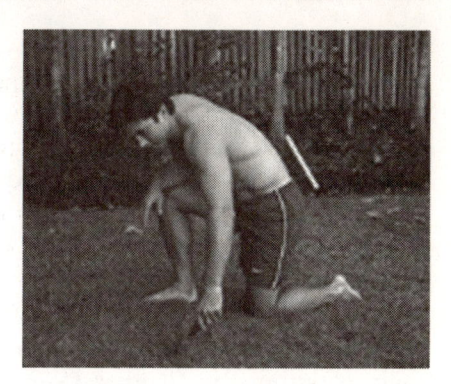

This half-kneeling posture is ideal for back types A and C when performing ground-level tasks. Note that Greg's spine is straight, rather than locked in an inward curve, which should be more comfortable for type A and C spines.

An even simpler solution for all back types is to organise the task at waist height. For example, a bench or table is a far more sensible place to sort laundry than is the floor.

HIGH TASKS
When performing high jobs, such as cleaning windows or trimming trees, types A and C should use a stepladder or a sturdy box, rather than arching their back to reach high. Alternatively, the high object, such as a clothesline, can be lowered so that high reaching is unnecessary.

WORKING ON THE CAR
When working on the car engine, all back types, particularly B and D, should lean against the front of the car. A short plank of wood, padded on both sides by an old towel, provides a useful leaning platform. Alternatively, a knee resting on the bumper can provide some additional support.

When changing a car tyre, push down on the wheel brace rather than trying to pull up on it. During all such jobs, make use of leverage, such as an old pipe over the end of the brace, to lessen your own exertion.

COOKING
If you are cooking a large meal in a heavy pot, then place it on the stove before adding the ingredients. A few small trips are easier than is one precarious, heavy lift.

Use your biggest, heaviest pots on the front burners of the stove. That way, if any awkward leaning lifts are necessary, at least they can be done on smaller, lighter pots.

WASHING
Types B and D may find that a top-loading washing machine requires less bending than does a front-loading model.

A high wall-mounted drier is excellent for types B and D, while types A and C would be more comfortable with a waist-high setting.

When pegging clothes onto the line, all back types should ensure that the clothesbasket is in front of them, not to the side. This positioning will help negate any unnecessary repetitive twisting. As mentioned earlier, types A and C should keep the line height low to avoid repetitive high reaching.

WORK STATIONS—SITTING AT A DESK
First, and most importantly, ensure that you have a good, supportive chair as outlined in Chapter 15.

A document holder is a useful addition to any desktop. By holding your documents or books vertically, you will find it far easier to maintain a laid-back sitting posture. Buy one today. At a pinch, you can even nail a large bulldog clip or two to your desk, or into an adjacent wall. Use the clips to support your reading material.

Your computer screen should be set high enough so that you do not have to tilt your head down to look at it, as a flexed neck posture encourages a rounded, slumped back. Touch-typing is a valuable skill. Touch typists can look forward, rather than down at the keyboard, which facilitates a correct sitting posture.

To find the correct height and position for your keyboard, begin by sitting in your chair with an efficient, relaxed posture. Allow your shoulders to relax, and hang your arms loosely by your sides. Now bend your elbows to 90 degrees. Your keyboard should sit directly below your fingers.

Most computer work stations today have adjustable shelving, and a slide-out section for the keyboard. By altering these components, most people can arrange their work station to a comfortable position.

If you have an old-fashioned flat top desk and/or a strained budget, then a few telephone books and a thin sheet of timber can be fashioned into a serviceable ergonomic work station. These designs will sit fashionably beside your bulldog-clip document holder, and will nicely complement your rolled-towel lumbar support device!

Employment

Many people find that their job is their major source of lower back irritation. A simple test is to ask yourself this question: is my back any better when I am on holidays? If so, then your job may be the wrong type of activity for your spine. If this is the case, then you have, broadly speaking, four ways of alleviating your situation.

Easing activities of daily living

1. Change your work duties.
Many workplaces now have multi-tasking, or offer a variety of duties to its employees. Already you should have a solid idea of which types of movements and postures are best for your spinal problem. For example, if you have a type B or D spine, then standing tasks will probably suit your spine better than will sitting jobs.

By reviewing the principles outlined in the last five chapters, you will hopefully identify at least one task in your workplace that is suitable for your spine. Then, it's just a *simple, straightforward matter* of asking the boss if you can change.

Beg, plead, bargain, train, upgrade, whatever you have to do. Remember, you're spine is at work probably about forty hours per week—far longer than any other activity—so it will greatly benefit if your daily routine is agreeable.

Remind your boss of the benefits of suitable duties, such as less sick pay, increased productivity, and reduced chance of a compensation claim. Any wise employer will listen to sensible, calm, well-argued reasoning. You may even be able to baffle your boss with some oblique references to your L4-5 spondylolisthesis, the subsequent nerve root compression, and to the unsuitability of the ergonomic arrangement for such an unstable injury. Or whatever . . .

If these techniques do not work, then buy him or her a copy of this book for their next birthday, subtly bookmarked to this page. If even this effort fails, you will have to resort to strategies two, three or four.

2. Rearrange your work tasks so that they are more suited to your spine.
If circumstances force you to remain on the same pain-producing task, investigate if you can alter the job set-up so that it better suits your spine. For example, if you have a type A spine, and your job normally involves a standing position, you may be able to sit on a tall chair instead.

Perhaps other devices—longer-handled tools, a document holder, or a better chair, for example—would make your job easier on your spine, and increase your productivity as a bonus. Your boss might even pitch in for some of the cost. You'll have to use the principles that you have learned in this book, along with some imagination and lateral thinking, to create a more suitable work environment for your spine.

3. Change your spine so that it can handle the task.
This book is dedicated to this topic. By using exercises, posture control, elimination of bad habits, and dozens of other techniques that you will later learn, you may be able to change the condition of your spine so that it can handle the task without discomfort.

As a last resort, you could use techniques such as taping or bracing to temporarily support your spine.

4. Get a new job.
If all else fails, and you have chronic, constant pain, then you may choose to look for employment that is more suitable. Please take into account your back pain type. Remember, not all physically demanding jobs are bad, and sedentary jobs are not necessarily better for your spine.

I hope that you can now see the myriad ways that you can alter your activities of daily living to better protect your spine. I suggest that you now take a few minutes to list any tasks of yours that are repetitive, prolonged, heavy, dangerous or unsuitable for your spine.

Then, using the principles that you have learned, suggest a solution. Try a few of them out over the next few days, and see how you go.

Keep this list handy, and build on it as you read the rest of this book. The ideas will prove useful when, in the final chapter, you design your own rehabilitation strategy to banish your back pain forever.

20

The effects of stress on your spine

How dinosaurs and the tribe next door cause your low back pain

If the symptoms of stress were all the same, we would realise that we were dealing with a disease far worse than the bubonic plague, AIDS, and the common hangover all rolled into one.

While doctors and other experts cannot precisely determine a figure, many feel that about half of all the pains and illnesses in today's society are due to stress. Others argue that this percentage is too low. Why do we tolerate such a devastating plague with such seemingly little response from health authorities and practitioners?

One reason that stress-related problems receive such scant attention is that they do not present themselves as straightforward diagnoses. Stress appears in many different forms, and underlies a multitude of seemingly unrelated conditions. For example, if an elderly widow goes to the doctor with an upset stomach, she may be diagnosed with an ulcer, not with 'stress'. When a fifty-year-old executive presents with chest pain, he is diagnosed as suffering from angina, not from 'repressed anger'. And a housewife may be told she has dermatitis when she develops itchy skin, not 'anxiety'. Yet these cases, and thousands of others just like them, were probably caused or exacerbated by stress.

Similarly, when you see a spinal health practitioner about your sore back, they will usually examine your spine, not your head. Fair enough, too. Yet while a joint, disc or nerve may be causing your current pain, it is possible that your high stress level over prior years caused your spine to degenerate in the first place.

Another reason that stress is so often ignored by health practitioners is that it is such a complex area. When we talk about the causes of stress in the next chapter, you'll see that they are almost impossible to define as simple, identifiable situations. Because the reasons are hard to pinpoint, they are difficult to treat objectively.

Because of these complications, the training and research into stress management is largely ignored by medical and other mainstream health training facilities. Consequently, stress-related illnesses are usually handled poorly by all but a few dedicated practitioners. Often, the time is spent—for better or for worse—on more immediate problems and solutions. Stress is usually put into the too-hard file, which may help to explain why anxiety, tension and their related symptoms are epidemic.

In the next few chapters, we'll be looking at many aspects of stress, including how it causes pain, why it affects us, and how to decrease it. Then we'll also discuss some more abstract qualities of stress, such as how the power of the mind can help your total wellbeing. I make no apologies for the in-depth nature of the following discussion, as the extra emphasis on relaxation will help to balance the lack of attention it usually receives from spinal health practitioners.

Of course, I'll be concentrating on the aspects of stress that relate directly to back pain. If, after having read the next few sections, you feel that stress is contributing to your problem, then I urge you to do further research on the subject.

Are you stressed?

I wonder if at this point you are thinking 'I'm not stressed... none of this really applies to me'. Before you decide to skim over the next four chapters, you should be aware that most people who are stressed don't even realise it. This unintentional ignorance occurs because stress builds so gradually and insidiously that you are usually unaware that it is happening.

Furthermore, the demands and pace of modern life mean that *most* people are stressed, and so we come to accept a high level of stress as normal. After all, if our parents and siblings are stressed, our work colleagues are stressed and our friends are stressed, then we don't even realise that we are uptight. Yet then we are surprised or annoyed when we fall ill, or our backs start to ache again.

Another reason that you may not realise how much tension you are carrying is that stress does not always show itself in an obvious way. If you don't eat, you become hungry. If you don't drink, you feel thirsty, and tiredness will soon let you know if you've been missing sleep. However, our bodies are not so good at telling us that we should be relaxing. The signs can be subtle, varied, and sometimes nonexistent until it's too late. For all of the above reasons, many people are simply unaware that stress is contributing to their problem.

Stress can cause not only spinal pain, but can alter moods and attitudes, and even create real, measurable physical changes in the body. Read through the following list, and see how many of these signs and symptoms are familiar to you.

COMMON EFFECTS OF STRESS ON THE MIND	COMMON EFFECTS OF STRESS ON THE BODY
• alcoholism	• angina or other heart pain
• apprehension	• arthritis

- cigarette smoking
- depression
- drug dependence
- fatigue
- feelings of anxiety
- headaches
- insomnia
- irrational fears/phobias
- irritability, impatience
- lack of motivation or energy
- lack of concentration
- a short temper
- obsessional behaviour
- panic attacks
- asthma
- cold sores, mouth ulcers
- constipation or diarrhoea
- fibrositis, aching joints
- frequent bouts of the 'flu
- increased or irregular heart rate
- migraines
- nausea or other tummy upsets
- sexual problems
- shakiness
- shortness of breath
- skin problems of all types
- stomach dyspepsia, reflux or ulcers
- stuttering

Anything sound familiar? If so, then my bet is that at least some of your back pain is stress-related. So let's now look at stress in more detail, and discover how it affects our minds and bodies. You can then apply this knowledge to help reduce or obliterate your back pain.

The fight-or-flight response

You may be wondering exactly how stress causes back pain, as the relationship at first seems tenuous. Many people rightfully ask questions such as 'How does the tension/anger/anxiety that I feel toward my boss/partner/situation translate to back pain arising from my discs/joints/muscles? The two problems seem so removed from each other.'

The question of how our mind affects our body is difficult to answer precisely. Science has come a long way in the past few millennia, especially the last one hundred years. However, our understanding of life, the universe and everything still has a couple of big holes in it, one of which is the workings of our own brain, whose mechanisms remain largely mysterious. As such, any questions regarding how the mind influences the body are most accurately answered with a simple statement: I dunno.

Of course, empirical evidence—studies that examine the relationship between one thing and the other, without really suggesting a mechanism—shows a clear link between stress and back pain. Many people need no convincing of this link at all, as the only time that they feel back pain is when they are anxious.

Nevertheless, we can postulate a couple of ideas as to how anxiety and emotional tension affect the body. To appreciate both theories, and to comprehend the stress process altogether, you must understand a reaction called the *fight-or-flight* response.

The fight-or-flight response is a prehistoric reaction of the body to prepare it for battle (a fight) or to run away from danger (the flight). (Some authors have suggested that another 'F' word be added to denote preparation for sexual activity, but as this is a family book, I'll leave that one out.)

When our prehistoric ancestors were faced with danger, their brains reacted by activating a special part of their nervous system, and by instantly releasing hormones. These two responses stimulated the release of adrenalin and other chemicals, which then altered the function of many bodily structures to prepare for battle, or to run away. These same responses persist to this day.

For example, the fight-or-flight response causes your body to minimise the activity of your digestive processes, instead channelling blood flow to your muscles. It causes your heart rate to accelerate and your respiration to deepen, preparing your cardiovascular system for sudden action. Your pupils dilate to let in extra light, and sometimes your hairs even stand on end in an outdated attempt to make you appear bigger and more fearsome. All of these responses are rapid, reproducible, and are automatically stimulated by the perception of danger.

During prehistoric times, these responses were appropriate. The fight-or-flight response played a vital role in preparing the body to avert danger. Without these reactions, our ancestors would probably have perished in the dangerous, hostile place that was prehistoric Earth.

However, the threat of physical danger is very rare in modern society. Sure, most of us are concerned for our physical wellbeing a few times during our life. However, most of us generally meander through life without the threat of being eaten by a dinosaur, or being scalped alive by a warrior from the tribe next door. But in today's society, these physical dangers have been replaced by another source of stress.

Computers.

Computers that break down. Computers with incompatible software. Computers whose hard drives crash on a regular basis, taking with them at least five chapters of this book that I have forgotten to back up. Did I mention computer keyboards that lose the 'E' key? (Ar you sur that I didn't mntion that bfor?) Oh, and while I'm talking about stress situations, could I add 'when patients turn up late for appointments', plunging my carefully planned afternoon into disarray? Humid weather—I hate that, too. Worst of all is when the city council phone machine puts you on hold for twenty minutes, and then tells you to call back later. And paperwork. And meaningless registration fees. And ...

Sorry about that rant, I got carried away. Can you see that, although we no longer have many physical threats in our lives, these dangers have been replaced by hundreds of new stress agents?

However, our body still uses the same old way of coping with stress:

THE EFFECTS OF STRESS ON YOUR SPINE

the fight-or-flight response. So guess what happens when (pick one that applies to you):

(a) Your parents come home from their holiday a day early. Unfortunately, you had a few (hundred) friends around last night, and now have thirteen seconds to complete about nine hours of cleaning.
(b) You discover that your wife has thrown out your favourite 'Adam and the Ants' T-shirt that you've kept since high school.
(c) Your overweight, leering boss, who has been looking you up and down since you started work in the typing pool, asks you to stay after work to help him with some 'urgent business'.
(d) Your baby daughter, who is now fifteen, is going out on her first date. Her partner, a scrawny, pimply seventeen-year-old with a bad moustache, picks her up in a van.
(e) You're late for an important meeting, and find yourself stuck on a single-lane road behind a little old lady in a Volvo.

Guess what happens in these, or any one of a million other, stressful situations. That's right, your body initiates a fight-or-flight response. Adrenalin and other stress hormones flow through your arteries, your muscles tense, your heart and breathing rates increase, and your pupils dilate. In short, your body undergoes responses that would have been appropriate 40,000 years ago, but are utterly useless when dealing with today's aggravations.

Furthermore, stress today is probably more constant than it once was. In our prehistoric days, the threat of physical danger would usually pass quickly, so our systems could return to normal. However, in today's fast-paced, everchanging, sue-or-be-sued society, stress situations attack us virtually every waking moment. Our bodies live with a constant, low-grade fight-or-flight response, which gradually degrades our mental and physical wellbeing.

The fight-or-flight response is, in short, the *physical manifestation* of mental stress. Let's now look at how it can cause lower back pain.

Muscular tension as a cause of back pain

The first theory relates to muscle tension. Recall our discussion on muscle imbalances in Chapter 12, when we referred to two groups of muscles: the mobilising muscles and the stabilising muscles.

If you were about to be speared through the buttocks by the horn of a raging *triceratops* dinosaur, which group of muscles would you rather have ready to fire? Would you rather that your body used:

(a) the stabilising muscles, which securely hold the joints in a correct position, and maintain a good posture, or
(b) the mobilising muscles, which will help you to run away?

If you said 'a' then you would have made a very nice entree for the triceratops. However, if you thought that the mobilising muscles would be more useful in this situation, then I congratulate you for a correct response.

Can you guess what happens to your mobilising muscles if you are constantly tense and anxious? That's right, your body holds them on full alert, ready to produce fight-or-flight at a moment's notice.

Many people carry stress in their mobilising muscles. Hunching, tight neck and shoulder muscles are a common example. Another frequently observed example are the jaw muscles, which, as any dentist can tell you, often become tight, causing nocturnal teeth-grinding. (Providing yet another holiday in the Whitsunday Islands for the dentist.) And, of course, many people develop tightness in their lower back mobilising muscles.

If the mobilising muscles are frequently or constantly held in this highly reactive state, they gradually develop extra tone and strength. Meanwhile, the stabilising muscles lie relatively quietly. After some time, the two muscle groups develop an imbalance. You know what happens next: the muscle imbalance causes degeneration in nearby joints, eventually leading to pain and injury. *Voilà*, your stress has given you back pain!

The 'gate theory' of pain

The second theory of how stress affects back problems concerns your perception of pain. You may have noticed that when you are anxious, you experience pain more vividly than when you are relaxed. For example, consider a low-grade headache, which seems to throb with extra intensity when you are upset.

This difference in perceived pain occurs even though the physical pain signals arising from your body are identical. In other words, the same amount of pain hurts more when you are stressed than when you are relaxed.

This effect works in reverse as well. A calm, peaceful mind perceives less pain than does an active mind. Some people—Himalayan yogis, for example—can meditate and relax so deeply that they feel no pain at all. As one Yogi said with complete seriousness: 'I feel pain ... but it does not hurt.' Wouldn't that be nice! Deep hypnotherapy can produce the same results, and can be so effective that deeply relaxed, hypnotised people have undergone surgery without anaesthetic.

Obviously, our state of mind can alter our pain perception. To understand how this effect occurs, you must appreciate a simple mechanism known as the *gate theory* of pain.

Recall from Chapter 9 that pain messages from an injured structure travel up a nerve, and then join the spinal cord, through which they travel up to the brain. When the message enters the spinal cord, it must cross over a small joint, known as a *synapse*. To get a rough picture, think of a synapse as being like an electrical switch that joins two wires together.

The relationship between the spinal cord nerves and the peripheral nerves is not necessarily one-to-one. The synapse area in the spinal cord has the ability to allow many, just a few, or almost none of these incoming messages up the spinal cord. Of course, if the signals cannot pass up the spinal cord, then they do not register in the brain as pain.

The spinal cord acts like a gate—hence the name 'gate theory'—in allowing only a varied number of signals up at a time. In effect, the spinal cord has the capability to control how many pain sensations you are experiencing, which, of course, dictates your level of discomfort.

How does the gate theory relate tension to back pain? It is possible that mental stress opens more gates in your spinal cord. In prehistoric days this response would have been useful, priming the spinal cord to receive signals from the limbs. In this way, the caveperson's reactions would have been very responsive and sensitive—useful qualities in a dangerous situation.

You have probably noticed that your nerves become 'edgy' when you are tense, and that you become overly responsive to stimulation that would not normally affect you. For example, if you are stressed and someone claps his or her hands, you startle. However, if this same noise occurred when you were relaxed, you would barely notice it. This hypersensitivity is a simple example of how the fight-or-flight response primes your nerves to receive even the smallest signals.

If you are stressed, the fight-or-flight response opens many spinal cord gates, meaning that more of the pain messages ascend to your brain. In this way, stress can cause minor back pain to feel awful, and an otherwise bearable injury can become intolerable.

Sometimes a vicious cycle can develop, in which your back pain causes you to feel stressed, which increases your perception of the pain. Naturally, the extra discomfort makes you even more anxious, which further heightens your pain, and so on.

In summary, the fight-or-flight response, although inappropriate to many modern stress situations, has a powerful effect on your daily life. It impairs your physical wellbeing because the tension in your mobilising muscles ultimately creates muscle imbalances, leading to joint wear and tear. Furthermore, you will experience pain with more intensity when you are tense than when you are mentally relaxed.

Let's now look at another important area: your *physical tolerance to stress*. The next chapter will show you in simple terms how your stress level and your physical tolerance to stress affect your health.

21

Your physical tolerance to stress

Why some people are always well, while others are continually crook

Ill health and wellbeing seem to affect people in a vastly disproportionate manner. For example, you probably know a few 'hypochondriacs' who are frequently sore or sick. They're always suffering from a cough or a cold, their back is constantly sore, and they visit a health practitioner virtually every week. Even worse, they regularly provide you with an avalanche of unrequested details about their numerous maladies.

Equally, I'm sure you've also met people who rarely have any aches or pains, and never catch any bugs that are going around. Are these people just lucky? Between these two extremes are a vast majority of people, who have occasional problems, and intermittent aches and pains. Ask yourself now to which group do *you* belong?

Why does health vary so much from one person to the next, even though we are all subject to similar everyday hazards? The answer may well lie in how we physically tolerate stress.

Consider the first graph on the next page. Suppose that the dotted line represents your *stress level*. As you'd expect, it goes up and down in response to life's challenges. Sometimes things are going well, and stress is minimal. Other times, life doesn't seem as easy, and our anxiety increases. As you'd expect, the dotted line on the following graphs goes naturally up and down, just as does the stress of life.

The solid line represents your *physical tolerance to stress*. This line represents your body's constitution. It is influenced by factors such as diet, exercise, disease, genetics and sleep.

The height of this line represents the amount of stress that your body can physically handle before it breaks down. When you are sleeping soundly, eating sensibly and exercising regularly, your physical tolerance to stress rises. If you skip meals, work too hard or drink too little, er, sorry, I meant drink too much, your physical tolerance may fall. As you'd expect, this line also creeps slowly up and down.

When the dotted stress level is above the solid line of your physical stress tolerance, injury, pain or illness are imminent. At times such as this, your mind and body simply cannot cope with the degree of stress to which you are subjecting them. Something *must* give.

YOUR PHYSICAL TOLERANCE TO STRESS

As shown in the last chapter, our bodies have a variety of ways of pointing this out to us, including headaches, skin problems, depressive disorders, and, of course, back pain. Let's look at some fictitious cases—we'll use three of the Seven Dwarfs—and see in general terms how our bodies react to excessive stress, and to the general way that we are treating them.

First, consider the case of Happy, who we'll represent in Graph One. Happy has a very high stress tolerance, and a very low stress level. Even during periods of high anxiety, his body and mind remain within their capacity to cope. Consequently, Happy is almost never sick, has no chronic pain, and comfortably copes with his lot in life.

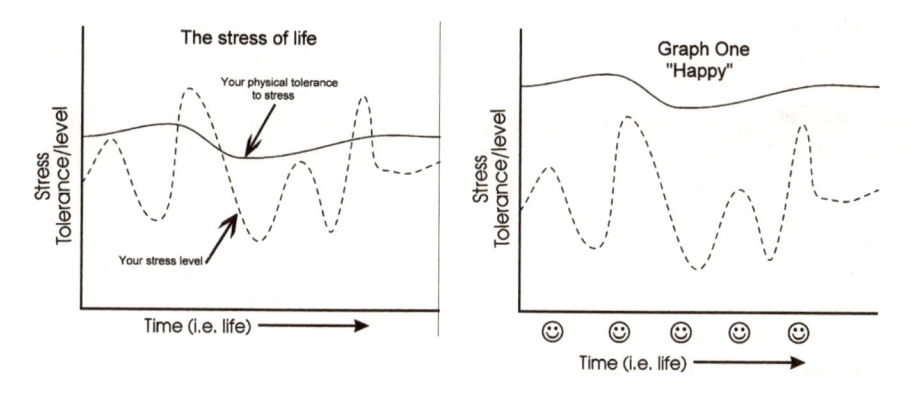

Graph Two represents another person/dwarf, Grumpy. Grumpy's stress level is typically very high, while his stress tolerance is unfortunately very low. As a result, Grumpy's body and mind are in a constant state of disrepair. He drinks alcohol excessively, is often sick, suffers frequent bouts of depression, and has very low self-esteem. Grumpy has also suffered from a chronic, generalised backache for ten years, which he blames on his job.

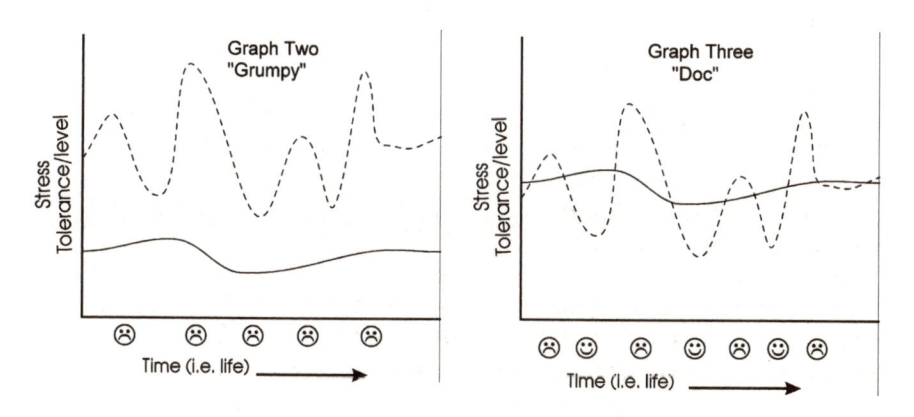

BACK PAIN

Obviously, both Happy and Grumpy are extreme examples, although Grumpy's case may be more common than you think. Other people are more closely represented by Graph Three, which we'll call Doc. Doc's stress tolerance is fairly steady, but, like most of us, his stress level fluctuates from week to week. During the periods in which Doc's stress level rises above the capacity of his body to cope, something collapses.

Therefore, Doc feels unwell occasionally, and his lower back plays up from time to time. Rarely does he associate any of his symptoms directly with stress. Instead he blames other more tangible factors for his problems, such as the weather, food poisoning, the wicked witch, or any one of a thousand other causes of minor maladies.

Now, let's look at how these situations can change. Let's suppose that, as shown in Graph Four, Doc increases his stress tolerance. Now, even during stressful times, his body is able to cope without breaking down.

The same effect occurs if Doc lowers his stress level, as shown in Graph Five. Again, his body rarely reaches the point of breakdown, and as such he is happier and healthier. Funnily, his back seems remarkably well during these times, which he attributes to a magic potion that his fairy godmother brewed last summer.

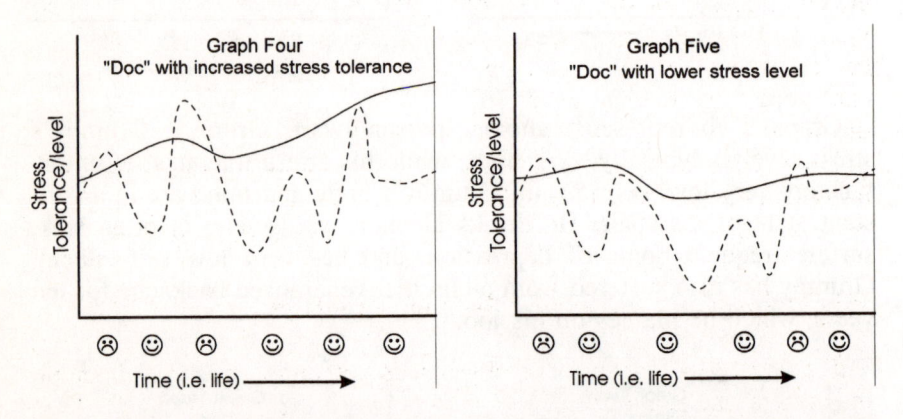

Naturally, these affects also occur in reverse. For example, consider Happy again, and suppose that his physical stress tolerance decreases, as in Graph Six, or his stress level increases, as in Graph Seven. In either of these situations, Happy will feel the physical and mental detriments of stress. He will become sick, or depressed, or maybe develop aches and pains in his back.

200

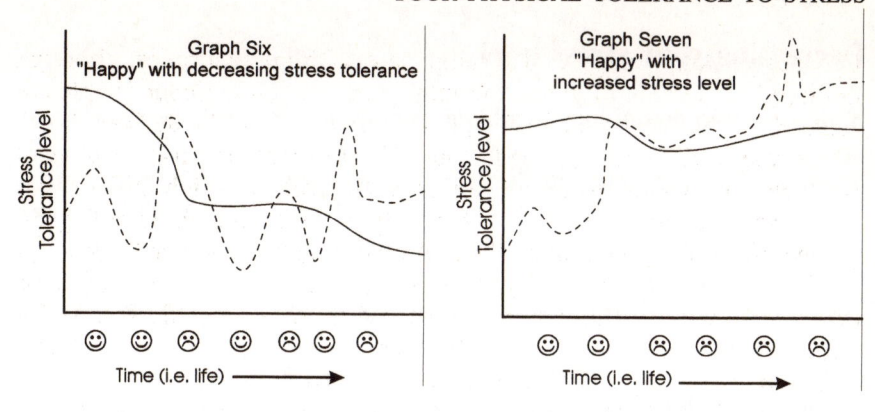

Graph Six — "Happy" with decreasing stress tolerance

Graph Seven — "Happy" with increased stress level

Finally, back to poor old Grumpy. Grumpy's best hope is to decrease his stress level *and* increase his stress tolerance, as shown in Graph Eight. Not an impossible task, but he's going to require a lot of dedication and persistence to work his way out of his present situation.

Can you see that although life still has its difficulties, stress doesn't have to effect us? By learning to either decrease our stress level, or increase our tolerance to stress, we can create a situation in which we can cope, no matter what life throws at us.

How do we take these two important steps? Let's find out.

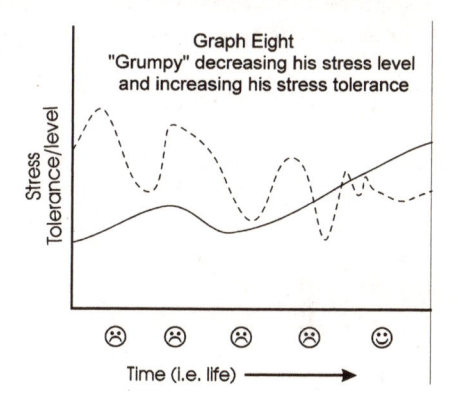

Graph Eight — "Grumpy" decreasing his stress level and increasing his stress tolerance

Increasing your physical tolerance to stress

The secret to increasing your physical tolerance to stress can be summarised in one sentence.

Listen to your mother.

That's right, just do all those things that your mother always told you to do: eat properly, get plenty of sleep, exercise regularly, blah blah blah. Of course, if your mother regularly advised you to take up heroin, then you can ignore that last piece of advice.

In later chapters, we'll be looking at how you can balance your overall health more effectively. You will learn not only how to use agents such as diet and exercise to increase your physical stress tolerance, but to directly improve your back pain as well. A double benefit!

Decreasing your stress level

You have two techniques available to help you to decrease your stress level.

First, you could change the things that stress you. The other technique is to change yourself, so that external situations and happenings do not make you as stressed. Here, an old saying springs to mind:

> Lord (Buddha, Allah, Ghost who walks, God ... insert the deity of your choice)
> Grant me the serenity to accept the things that I cannot change,
> The courage to change the things that I can
> And the wisdom to know the difference.

Which method is best for you? Let's first look at some common situations that cause stress. This will help you to decide if they are changeable. Some common causes of stress include the following internal and external factors:

(a) Your personality type
   Research has shown that certain personality types are likely to suffer from stress. These people, known to psychologists as Type A personalities, tend to push themselves hard, be rarely satisfied with their own performance, are hostile in traffic, and are intolerant of other people. Ring any bells?
(b) Repressed anger
   Are you carrying a deep grudge against someone who offended your self-esteem at some stage: a divorced partner, or an ex-boss, for example? Repressed anger has been shown to be a major stress agent, particularly in men.
(c) Guilt
   People develop guilt about a whole range of issues: eating too much, sexual guilt, guilt because of early childhood experiences, just to name a few. Women tend to be vulnerable to guilt-related stress.
(d) Negative self-talk
   Any time you rethink negative thoughts, your stress level will naturally rise. People who tend to brood, sulk or feel resentful are particularly prone to this type of stress. Cynical, mistrusting people are also very prone to high stress levels.
(e) Wrong job
   A job that you dislike, or that does not suit your natural strengths and weaknesses, can be a major cause of stress.
(f) Change
   A new job, a relationship separation, moving house, changing work

conditions ... anything that represents a change also represents a stress factor. Modern life and technology are not only changing more quickly than ever before, but the rate of change is accelerating. No wonder we're all so stressed.
(g) Anything else that you can think of
You're partner, co-workers, traffic, your children, your parents, money, that leaking tap, lack of time, too much time ... I could go on for pages. So far, I've barely scratched the surface.

Are you starting to see how many causes of stress may be in your life? Are you going to change them all?

Not likely.

Sure, you may be able to alter one or two obvious, major causes of stress in your life—your job, for example. Furthermore, working on your own attitudes—such as decreasing your resentment toward other people who have wronged you—can produce major benefits in stress reduction. However, it is extremely unlikely that the world is going to slow down for a couple of months, just so that little old you and I can take a breather.

Some people take this approach to an extreme: they resign from their jobs, and move to a self-sustaining farm in the hills, content to live out their days doing nothing but ambling through the woods, recording their thoughts in a journal. Sure, it's good work if you can get it, but I'd guess that this solution is not going to suit most people.

Commonsense will tell you that most of the stress agents in your life are outside your bounds of influence, and therefore you cannot change them.

So what do you do? Simply, you learn to accept those things that would formerly have distressed you, and to reduce the manifestations of any stress that you may experience.

In short, you have to do what Doc did in Graph Five: lower the dotted line that represents your stress level. The easiest way to do this is to learn *deep relaxation of your mind*. In the next chapter, we'll examine in detail how to achieve this peace of mind, and the benefits that come with it.

Let me end this chapter with a few statistics that I find not only surprising, but a bit silly. A study in the United Kingdom investigated the attitude of the public toward deep mental relaxation and hypnosis. The researchers put three questions to a large number of people with chronic pain, and tabulated their responses.

First, the subjects were asked a simple question: if their doctor recommended a tablet that would cure their pain, would they take it? One hundred per cent of respondents said 'yes', they would take the tablet.

The researchers then asked the subjects a second question: if your doctor recommended that surgery would cure your pain, would you have the operation? Here, 65 per cent of people said yes, 15 per cent were not sure, while 20 per cent said that they would refuse the surgery. Fair enough.

Finally, they were asked a third question: if your doctor recommended that hypnosis would cure your pain, would you undergo the treatment? Only 40 per cent of people said that they would agree to be hypnotised, while 20 per cent were unsure. Surprisingly, 40 per cent of people would flatly refuse such a treatment, even though they trusted their doctor and knew that it would cure their pain.

Think about it. Compare the dangerous and painful consequences of surgery with that of deep relaxation and hypnosis. Yet many more people would accept the dangers of anaesthetic, tolerate post-operative pain, and endure hospital food, rather than have a few sessions of deep relaxation!

From where does this irrational fear arise? Is it a deep-seated mistrust of allowing another person to manipulate our minds? Is it a fear that we will be exposed as unable to cope by ourselves? I don't know.

An Australian psychiatrist has written of the reticence of many of his patients to perform simple relaxation exercises. He cites cases in which he spent many treatment sessions not teaching or practising the exercises, but simply trying to convince the patient that they would work. Not only that, but even after the patient had reaped considerable benefits from the exercises performed in his surgery, many patients refused to continue them at home in front of their family or friends.

Again, I do not know why this attitude exists. However, this self-awareness is a very real problem for some people. My only advice is this: the sooner you start the relaxation exercises, the sooner this irrational feeling will go away.

I know that many joggers feel the same sense of self-awareness when they first start their exercise regime. Often, a runner will feel very embarrassed during his or her first few attempts, believing that people are staring or sniggering at them. Nothing could be further from the truth. Be honest and straightforward about your exercises, and the benefits that you receive from doing them, and you will soon discover how to relax your way to better health and a pain-free spine.

22

How to decrease stress

Drink more beer and eat more cake?

'I know how to relax. It's easy. I just grab a six pack out of the fridge, lie on the couch, and watch sport on television all day.'

'If I want to relax, I just drop the kids off at Mum's place, then call a girlfriend to go out for coffee and a huge slice of mud cake.'

Sorry. Relaxation is not that simple.

Sure, the alcohol or chocolate may temporarily make you feel better. Moreover, for many men, doing something simple like watching sport is a simple way to forget problems, while many women find that a good chat will help them resolve their difficulties. Although you may find these activities enjoyable, they unfortunately don't produce the deep mental relaxation that you need to rid yourself of stress and its associated pains and problems.

The colloquial use of the word 'relaxation' differs from the concept to which I am referring. Here, the term 'relaxation' does not mean eating, drinking and being merry, but rather refers to the practice of deeply calming your state of mind. From now on, if I use the term 'relaxed' I am referring to a state of *deep mental relaxation*, not to how you feel when you are having fun.

What exactly is a *deeply relaxed mind*, and how does it differ from your normal state of mind? A deeply relaxed mind is a floating, uncritical mind, which thinks its own thoughts. If your mind is deeply relaxed, you do not analyse, worry, or direct your mind in any way. Your thought patterns have no logic, and you do not attempt to understand, resolve or clarify any thoughts that enter your head.

You may be vaguely familiar with this state if you've ever found yourself daydreaming. When you daydream, your mind drifts along without obvious direction. You are oblivious to your surroundings, and uncritical of anything that occurs nearby. The moment of reverie just before you fall asleep provides another close approximation.

When you're doing the relaxation exercises, you must learn to let yourself go into this deeply relaxed, floating, drifting state of mind.

You will soon be learning how to perform relaxation exercises. The exercises have four main benefits:

1. You will learn how to relax your muscles, easing any tension or tightness.
2. Your relaxed state of mind will diminish your pain perception. (However, please be aware that deep mental relaxation should never be used to repress pain of unknown origin. The techniques can be so powerful that even very dangerous pain can be masked. Use your commonsense, and consult a spinal health practitioner or doctor if you are unsure.)
3. The calm and peaceful feeling will stay with you after you have finished the exercises, promoting general wellbeing.
4. When your mind is deeply relaxed, you can use various other techniques to alter your way of thinking about your back pain.

Let's now look at some simple hints on how to best perform these extremely useful relaxation exercises.

Some practical considerations for performing the relaxation exercises

DO NOT BE PUT OFF BY THEIR SIMPLICITY
Because of the deeply relaxed state of mind that the following exercises engender, the instructions that you give to yourself are, by nature, very simple. Your mind, in its current active state, will probably perceive the instructions as so straightforward as to be almost useless. Do not be put off by this simplicity!

Complicated sentences or detailed instructions would not be as readily accepted by your relaxed mind as simple, direct statements. As you progress through the exercises, your mind will gradually let go, and the simple statements will have a deep impact on your way of thinking.

PRACTICE MAKES PERFECT
Don't worry if at first you have difficulty in achieving a fully relaxed state. These mental routines are like any other skill: they take time, practice and persistence to learn properly. Very few people would expect to pick up a golf club for the first time and hit a perfect drive. Skills such as this take training and practice to master. Most of my mates have been playing golf for fifteen years and are still no closer to having a decent swing.

Similarly, deep mental relaxation is a skill that is not self-evident, but must be learned. Don't be surprised if your first few efforts are not a spectacular success. Frequently, beginners have trouble with random thoughts and worries interrupting the flow of the exercises. If this happens, simply 'let the thought go', and gently redirect your attention back to the exercise phrases. I'm sure with a little practice that you'll start to experience that calm, floating feeling, and will soon discover how natural and peaceful it is to relax.

IT GETS QUICKER
You will find that when you master the skills of relaxation, you will be able to achieve a calm, peaceful mind far more quickly than during your first attempts. During the first few weeks that you attempt these exercises, you may find that it takes half an hour or more to achieve a deeply relaxed state. After a few months of practice, most people can achieve deep relaxation within five or ten minutes.

I have seen experiments in which highly practised subjects were able to block out all pain signals after only twenty seconds of relaxation. They proved their immunity to pain by keeping their hands in a bath of icy water for two minutes, without any increase in pain level, heart rate or respiration. I wouldn't advise you to try that experiment at home, but if you've ever fished through the bottom of an ice-filled cooler, searching for the last cold beer can, then I'm sure you can appreciate how deeply relaxed these subjects must have been. And they could achieve this painless state of mind in just twenty seconds!

Not only that, but as you improve your mental relaxation skills, you will find that the feeling of calm stays with you for longer periods. Many people who are experienced in these techniques find that they require only a few minutes of relaxation exercises to maintain an all-day feeling of calm and peacefulness. Not a bad pay-off for five minutes' effort. Don't you agree?

BE ALERT AND AWAKE WHEN YOU PERFORM THE EXERCISES
Many people believe that when you sleep your mind is completely relaxed. This assumption is not necessarily true. Many people sleep fitfully, tossing and turning ideas through their mind all night. Others find that each time they awaken, a problem is churning away in their semi-conscious mind. Many people take drugs or alcohol in order to sleep, both of which can promote a false sense of relaxation. Compare these states to a floating, calm, peaceful mind as described above, and you will see that sleep does not necessarily provide deep relaxation.

For this reason, you should perform these exercises when you are alert and fully awake. Otherwise, you may nod off to sleep before you have achieved a fully relaxed state, and you won't achieve the benefits for your mind, body or spine that it can bring.

Later, when you have mastered the exercises and have reaped the benefits of a relaxed mind, you may wish to use the exercises to help you fall asleep at night. However, I suggest that you avoid this practice for at least six weeks, in order that you make the fastest possible progress with your new skill development.

USE A POSTURE THAT IS SLIGHTLY UNCOMFORTABLE

Most people naturally presume that a warm, cosy, comfortable position will assist with mental relaxation. In fact, the opposite is more likely to be true: a slightly uncomfortable posture will help you attain a more deeply relaxed mental state.

An overly comfortable posture can trick your brain into thinking that you are relaxed. By keeping your body slightly inconvenienced, your mind will realise that it has not yet achieved a fully relaxed state, and will continue to allow your muscles and mind to let go.

Picture a Buddhist monk, or a Himalayan yogi, deep in meditation. How do you think they would position themselves? On the couch? In a hammock? On a soft, feathery bed? Not likely. Most people who are adept at deep relaxation sit on a hard floor, often in a crossed-legged position. In this 'lotus' posture, the meditating person can pull their feet further underneath them as they reach progressively deeper states of relaxation. This action creates extra tension and mild discomfort in the legs, thus inviting the mind to relax even more deeply.

This principle is useful for you, too, although you may not wish to take it as far as the lotus position. Just make sure that you are not too comfortable, and you'll be fine.

WHAT POSTURE IS BEST FOR THE EXERCISES?

Your back pain type provides a guide as to which posture to adopt. Types A and C may wish to try sitting. Just ensure that your chair is supportive and not too heavily padded. Your feet should be resting flat on the floor, with your hands on the armrests or in your lap. Your head may drop forward onto your chest as you relax more deeply.

Types B and D will probably be more comfortable in a lying posture, possibly with a pillow under your knees. Here, I recommend that you lie on a firm surface such as the floor, rather than a soft, comfortable bed. You may use a small pillow or, preferably, a folded towel under your head, if necessary.

The ideal posture for you depends upon many factors, such as the time and place that you have put aside in which to perform your relaxation exercises. In general, any posture will do, so long as it is not too comfortable.

Some other general hints for posture are:

- Keep your limbs symmetrical.

HOW TO DECREASE STRESS

- Minimise or loosen your clothing.
- Keep your arms and legs uncrossed.

WHERE TO DO THE EXERCISES

In the beginning, you should choose a place in which you feel totally safe and secure. Have your back or head nearest to the wall, which will provide you with an extra feeling of safety. Take the telephone off the hook, and put up a physical or otherwise tangible 'do not disturb' sign. The light should be dim but not dark, and the room should be relatively quiet. These provisions will allow you to more easily slip into an unguarded, relaxed state of mind.

As you improve your relaxation skills, you should move out of your comfort zone. Progress through steps such as trying the exercises with the radio or television turned on. In this way, you will learn to tolerate and relax against background noise. You may wish to try the exercises in a more uncomfortable location—one expert used to lie on a rocky stone wall in his garden—or with your eyes open. By increasing the uncomfortableness of your surrounds, you will teach your mind to relax in a variety of circumstances.

After a few months' practice, you will be ready to attempt the exercises in real-life situations. People skilled in these techniques can attain a deeply relaxed state in almost any situation, from a crowded bus to walking down the city street. Athletes, such as swimmers and runners, may even wish to try the exercises when training. Many great athletes have even used them in the midst of competition!

Finally, you can use the techniques in known stress situations. Imagine how useful your relaxation skills would be in anxious situations, such as before your next big job interview or after-dinner speech. Of course, these techniques, once mastered, will prove invaluable when you are suffering from acute or chronic spinal pain.

A word of commonsense: don't try these exercises while driving home from work, or while operating the backhoe that you've hired for the weekend from the hardware store. Obviously, a floating, uncritical mind is not an appropriate state in which to attempt dangerous, reactive or mentally challenging tasks.

REALLY 'FEEL' THE INSTRUCTIONS

The relaxation exercises are represented by a series of phrases that you will say to yourself. However, just repeating the statements to yourself does not necessarily ensure that your mind will follow the instructions. You must really try to 'feel' the instructions, and allow your mind to follow as they suggest.

This practice of *allowing* your mind to feel the instructions—rather than forcing it to follow them—is one of the keys to obtaining a deeply relaxed mental state. Again, this method of thinking requires practice, but will come soon enough if you persist, relax, and keep gently reminding yourself of its importance.

LEARN HOW TO LET GO OF PHYSICAL TENSION
Some people find it very difficult to fully let go of physical tension in their muscles. To discover if you are one of these people, try this simple test.

Have someone else lift your arm into the air, and hold it for a few seconds. Then, without warning, they should suddenly release your arm. Observe what happens. If your arm naturally flops to your side without resistance—it should drop with a completely passive flop, not an active, pulling down movement—then you are probably fairly physically relaxed.

However, you may find that your arm hovers in the air for a few seconds, indicating moderately high stress levels. Some people are so physically tense that they are unable to let their arm fall at all, instead just deliberately lowering it to a resting position.

Letting go of muscle tension is a vital skill that you must learn. To be able to let go of muscle tone, you must first learn to identify it. In Chapter 14, you learned how to evaluate muscle tone in your biceps muscle. Following is a simple task that will revise your skills in identifying increased muscle tone.

Sit or lie comfortably. Now concentrate on your right thigh. Feel, and try to really experience, how much tone and tension are in the muscle. Next, pretend that you are going to lift up your right leg. Don't actually move it, but simply pretend that you are about to, so that its weight on the bed or chair is minimal. Do you sense the increased tension in the front thigh muscle?

The state in which you are now holding your right thigh muscle is one of increased muscle tone. Palpate your thigh with your fingers, and compare its suppleness to that of your left thigh. You will note that the right side feels much harder, while your left thigh muscle is softer, relaxed and more pliable.

Now relax the muscle, and experience the feeling of softening, and 'letting go'. This 'letting go' feeling is very important, and forms the basis for the following exercises. Try to develop a conscious awareness of muscle tone and the all-important feeling of letting go while you are performing the relaxation exercises.

DON'T WORRY IF YOU CANNOT REMEMBER THE INSTRUCTIONS WORD FOR WORD
As you perform the relaxation techniques for the first couple of times, you will probably have to read the phrases from this book. This method

is fine, and will help you to develop a sense of the exercises.

As you become more adept, you should close your eyes and mentally repeat the instructions to yourself. Do not worry if you cannot remember the instructions perfectly. As long as you remember the general stages of the whole process, you can virtually invent your own relaxation phrases as you go.

The phrases below are just examples, which will help to get you started. You may find that some ideas work for you, while others have no calming effect whatsoever. Fine. Stick with the instructions that work best for you, and disregard any that you don't find helpful.

As you create your own phrases, always use positive instructions such as 'I feel . . .' or 'I am . . .', rather than negative instructions such as 'I do not feel . . .' or 'I am not . . .'. For example, use a phrase such as 'I feel calm and relaxed' rather than telling yourself 'I don't feel stressed'. You will see later why this type of positive thinking is so important.

The relaxation exercises

The relaxation exercises below follow a natural, logical sequence of stages that will guide you from being alert and tense, through to being fully, deeply relaxed.

First, you will prepare your mind for the relaxation that is to follow. Then, you progressively relax each body part, using a technique known as *contract–relax*. To perform the contract–relax technique, follow these simple steps. Try it as you read, by squeezing your right hand into a fist.

1. Tighten the target muscle as firmly as you can, and hold for a few seconds as you experience the tension in the muscle.
2. Then, on your next outward breath, allow the muscle to suddenly and completely relax. Experience the feeling of letting go.
3. Allow yourself another inward breath. Then, as you exhale, relax the same muscle even more completely. Just aim for the same 'letting go' feeling that you used in Step 2. Try to really feel the relaxation.
4. When your next inward breath arrives, move on to the next muscle as described.

This routine may sound complicated, but it is very simple and logical when you're used to it. In short, you tightly contract a muscle, then spend your next two exhalations relaxing it, before moving on to the next muscle group.

After physically relaxing your major limbs and trunk, you move to your face, scalp and eyes. Then allow the relaxation to permeate through to your mind. You will start to feel as though you are floating, and your thoughts will wander as you gradually slip into deep relaxation.

Once in this state of mind, you have three options, which we'll discuss later. Finally, after having worked through all the stages, you slowly and gently bring yourself back to reality, feeling relaxed, calm, peaceful and pain-free.

Let's now examine these steps individually, and discover the simple exercises that can make such a difference to your physical and mental wellbeing.

By the way, the following sections won't make very interesting reading if you simply skim over them. I suggest that you try the techniques as you read. That's right ... try to feel and use the simple phrases as you go. In this way you will experience first-hand just how simple and effective these techniques can be. Do it!

(1) PREPARATION FOR RELAXATION

Take a slow, deep breath. Let your whole body relax as you allow yourself to exhale. Do not force the breath out; simply allow it to flow out of your body, like a long sigh.

Repeat this long, relaxed sigh two more times, aiming for a more relaxed, calm feeling during each exhalation.

Inwardly experience the following sentiments as you slowly and carefully repeat them to yourself. (Remember, their simplicity is a virtue that you will come to appreciate.)

I have nothing else to do for the next twenty minutes.
This is my time to relax.
I feel safe, I feel secure.
I deserve to feel relaxed.
It feels good to relax.
I feel calm.
Calm and relaxed.

Now take another deep, relaxing breath, and move to Stage 2.

(2) PROGRESSIVE PHYSICAL RELAXATION

Use the following movements and phrases to guide you through a cycle of contract–relax exercises.

Turn your attention to your feet.
Think about your feet.
As you breathe in, curl your toes up tightly.

Feel the tension in the arches of your feet.
Breathe out, and relax your feet.
Let go of your feet.
Allow yourself to take another inward breath.
As you exhale, relax your feet even further.
Feel the relaxation.
It feels good to relax your feet.

Turn your attention to your calf muscles.
Think about your calf muscles.
As you breathe in, push your toes away from you.
Feel the tension in your calf muscles.
Breathe out, and relax your calf muscles.
Let go of your calf muscles.
Allow yourself to take another inward breath.
As you exhale, relax your calf muscles even further.
Feel the relaxation.
It feels good to relax your calf muscles.

Get the picture? The process may sound repetitive, but as you try the exercises, you will see that a simple, repeatable formula is best.

As you have already relaxed your feet and calves, I suggest that you next move to your thighs. First, tighten and relax your quadriceps muscles. Then contract your hamstring muscles, which is most easily achieved by pressing your heel into the floor. Then move to your front hip muscles (pretend to lift your leg in the air) and then to your buttocks (squeeze your bottom cheeks together). Simply follow the same pattern as you did when you released your feet and calf muscles. After this, you may find it useful to let your *whole* legs go, and reaffirm your commitment to ease and calm. Try some phrases such as these:

My whole legs are relaxed.
Utterly relaxed.
Relaxed and loose.
It feels good to relax my legs.
My legs are so relaxed that they are heavy.
I can feel the weight of my legs
My legs feel dead and heavy.
My legs are so relaxed that I can hardly feel them.
My legs feel distant—almost as if they belong to someone else.
My legs are distant and heavy.
Utterly relaxed.

By now, you should be starting to experience an overall feeling of calmness and relaxation.

Now continue to use this technique on the other major muscle groups in your body. Most people find this technique is most effective if they follow a rough anatomical pattern through their body, from legs to trunk, then to your arms, and finally to your head. For example, perform a two-breath cycle of relaxation on each of the following areas, just as you did for your leg muscles:

Tighten your tummy muscles ... relax.
Arch your lower back slightly ... relax. (Spend some extra time on the area that generally hurts the most.)
Tighten your chest muscles ... relax.

Once you have completed a contract–relax cycle for each of the above areas, reaffirm the relaxation of your whole trunk, just as you did with your whole leg area. Try some phrases such as these:

Allow yourself to feel your torso and back.
Feel the weight, heaviness and warmth of your back and torso.
You feel so heavy that you are sinking into the floor or chair.
Your body is so relaxed that you can no longer feel it.

Now move on to contract–relax exercises for your arms.

Pull your shoulder muscles up toward your ears ... relax.
Tighten your upper arm muscles ... relax.
Bend your hand back tightly at the wrist ... relax.
Grip your fingers into a fist ... relax.

Now completely let go of your arms and shoulders.

Feel the weight, heaviness and warmth of your arms.
Your arms feel distant and unattached, like they belong to someone else.
Your arms are relaxed, heavy and warm.
They feel good to be so relaxed and calm.

Finally, move to your neck muscles.

Arch your neck slightly, then fully relax the back of your neck.
Then tense the muscles at the front of your neck (if you are lying, pretend to lift your head off the pillow) then let it grow heavy.
Concentrate on the heaviness of your head and neck.

HOW TO DECREASE STRESS

Slowly let your neck go loose, and feel the weight of your head.

At this stage you may wish to repeat a few deep relaxing breaths, and reaffirm your overall calmness and peacefulness. Next, move onto Stage 3, in which you will deepen your physical relaxation into mental relaxation.

(3) MENTAL RELAXATION

Turn your attention to your cheeks.
Feel the relaxation in your cheeks.
Your cheeks are so utterly relaxed that you can feel the skin smoothing out.
Your cheeks are heavy and smooth and relaxed.

Repeat the above sequence for your jaw, then your forehead, your temples, and finally your eyelids.

Now, you will use the relaxation of your facial area to induce a deep relaxation of your mind.

You can feel your eyelids resting gently on each other.
Your eyelids feel heavy.
Heavy and relaxed.
Your whole face is relaxed.
Relaxation right through your head.
Your whole head is relaxed.
Deeply relaxed.
Relaxed right through your mind.
Your mind is relaxed.
Your mind is heavy, warm and comfortable.

(4) DEEPENING YOUR LEVEL OF RELAXATION

You feel calm.
Calm and peaceful.
Utterly calm, all through your body.
Your whole body is relaxed.
Your mind and body are totally calm, relaxed and peaceful.
You are so peaceful that your mind feels light.
Your mind feels so light and relaxed that it is starting to float.
Your mind is lightly floating.
Floating.
Your mind is drifting.
Drifting.

BACK PAIN

Floating and drifting wherever it wishes to go.
With each outward breath you grow even more calm and peaceful.
Utterly peaceful.

At this point—if you're still reading—your mind should be fully calm and relaxed. Your thoughts will wander about of their own accord, as in a daydream. Do not attempt to control your thoughts, but instead just let them come and go as they wish. Don't try to pass judgements, or to solve any problems. Just relax, and enjoy the feeling of letting go.

If thoughts—especially worries or problems—enter your head, *just let them go*. It's as though your thoughts arrive on a bus, but do not get off. You simply let them pass through without evaluation, like passengers on a bus who do not alight.

This final stage of deep mental relaxation is sometimes difficult for people to master. Sometimes, problems and worries just keep popping into your head. Fine. Let them. *Just don't think about them.*

When you have mastered this art of letting go of thoughts, you will have truly arrived at a state of peace, calm and deep mental relaxation.

Now, you have one of three choices.

(1) Do nothing
You can simply stay in this state for a few minutes, gently experiencing the warm, comfortable feeling that comes with deep relaxation.

(2) Imagery or visualisation
You can use other techniques, such as imagery or visualisation, to help you achieve an even more deeply relaxed state.

For example, you may wish to visualise a passive scene from nature, such as a waterfall, a sunset, or gently rolling waves on a beach. Alternatively, you may wish to picture and experience yourself in a favourite imaginary place (it doesn't have to be a pub). Other people find that mental tricks, such as a cool wind blowing through their mind, can help to clear away feelings of tension or anxiety.

Some find that associating different colours—the colours of the rainbow, for example—with different calming emotions is useful. Then, when their mind is properly relaxed, they simply picture the colour, and automatically experience the relevant positive emotion.

All of these 'tricks' are very simple yet effective. Many cassette tapes are available that will talk you through them.

(3) You can use a technique known as autosuggestion.
As your brain is now wandering and relaxed, it is very receptive and uncritical of any ideas and thoughts that enter it. When in this accepting

state, your brain will simply absorb any information that you supply it, without attempting to justify or analyse any instructions. You can then use this very useful state to help to alter your deepest perceptions and attitudes.

This area of mental exercise has many other names, including positive thinking, affirmations and self-hypnosis, all of which are essentially the same thing. These strategies are so effective in achieving a wide range of results, including decreasing your back pain, that we'll examine them in detail in the next chapter.

(5) RETURN TO WAKEFULNESS

After either performing visualisation, autosuggestion or simply relaxing for a few minutes, you are now ready to awaken back to reality. There are no real secrets here. My only suggestion is to arise slowly and gradually, and try to keep the feeling of deep relaxation with you as you do.

Many people like to use an abbreviated, reversed form of the progressive muscular relaxation. This technique involves gently feeling and moving your eyes, then your face and neck. You then continue this pattern until you have gently activated your arms, trunk, legs and finally your feet.

Other people prefer a reverse counting method. Here, you start counting from a number such as twenty, subtracting one as you take each inward breath. You gradually awaken yourself as you count, so that when you hit zero you are fully awake, alert, refreshed and ready to go.

I hope that you now have a solid grounding in the skill of relaxation. Below is a summary of the main points of the last few chapters.

- Stress is at epidemic levels, and causes many problems including back pain.
- Most people, probably including you, do not realise that they are stressed.
- The fight-or-flight response, a vestigial reaction from our prehistoric days, causes inappropriate responses to modern-day stress agents. These responses include overactivation of the mobility muscles, which ultimately causes musculo-skeletal problems.
- The fight-or-flight response also heightens your perception of pain via the opening of 'gates' in your spinal cord.
- When your stress level rises above your physical tolerance to stress, something in your body—your lower back, for example—must break down.
- You can increase your tolerance to stress by remaining healthy.
- You can decrease your stress level by changing the things that stress

BACK PAIN

you, which may or may not be possible, or by performing the relaxation exercises as described above.

Let's now look at another vital part of your mental approach to lower back pain: your attitude.

23

Attitudes, the placebo effect, and the power of the mind

The spinal health practitioner who resides within

Your attitude toward your back pain has an enormous influence on your recovery. Many studies of back pain recuperation rates show that your attitude is one of the most important factors in determining how much pain and suffering you have to endure.

A widely accepted maxim in modern psychology states that 'where the mind goes, the body will follow'. If you understand and fully appreciate this idea, then you will have a huge advantage in your quest to get rid of your back pain forever.

This principle can be seen at work in many spheres of human behaviour, especially in sport, where its effects are very apparent. For example, imagine two golfers—we'll call them Damian and Greg—on the last hole of a tournament, tied for the lead. As Damian tees up his ball, he realises that 250 metres away, on the left edge of the fairway, is a large, ominous sand bunker. In the back of his mind, Damian implores himself with the following instructions: 'Don't hit the ball into the bunker ... don't hit the ball to the left ... whatever you do, don't hook the ball ...'.

Soon, Greg is faced with the same shot. However, he gives his mind a different set of commands: 'Hit the ball onto the fairway ... hit the ball straight down the middle ... swing your club straight and true ...'.

Guess who won the tournament? Almost for sure, Greg would have walked away with the winner's cheque that day. For Damian, having pictured the bunker in his mind so vividly, was very likely to have hit the ball straight into it. Greg peppered his mind with images of the middle of the fairway, which is probably where his ball landed. Why did these results occur with such predictability? Simple: where the mind goes, the body will follow.

This effect was illustrated even more lucidly in one research study. The researchers connected an EMG machine (a device that measures the amount of electrical activity in a muscle) to the legs and arms of some elite downhill ski racers. The racers then imagined that they were skiing down a particular mountain, even though in reality they were lying perfectly still on the researchers' table.

The EMG readings were then matched with the skiers' descriptions of their actions during the race. The results were uncannily accurate. Each time the skiers reported that they were visualising a jump, their leg muscles automatically increased their activity, i.e. they performed a tiny contraction that was undetectable to the naked eye. The skiers' arm muscles tightened as they imagined pushing with their stocks, while their leg muscles tightened appropriately during sharp turns.

The skiers' minds could not distinguish between a real experience and one that was vividly imagined. In short, the skiers' muscles automatically followed and performed what their mind was visualising.

This reaction is not confined only to the sporting world. 'Where the mind goes, the body will follow' forms an inseparable part of our everyday life. For example, picture in your mind a person who is downhearted and depressed. Really try to visualise this person. Now, picture the same person in a joyful, happy mood. Consider this question: what posture did your imaginary person adopt in each situation? Usually, a depressed mindset is associated with low muscle tone, a drooping head and a slumped back, while a happy, exuberant mind gives a decidedly more upright and buoyant posture. This difference illustrates that your muscles are influenced not only by your imagination, but by your mood as well!

Can you see that your state of mind has a huge effect on your physical body, not only during sporting events, but also in virtually every task that you attempt each day. In many different ways, your body reacts *automatically* to the images in your mind.

Guess what happens to your spine if you keep thinking about your sore back? Think about that question, and apply the principle of 'where the mind goes, the body will follow'. The answer should be obvious: *the more you think about how much your back hurts, the worse it will become.*

Unfortunately, this mindset is exactly what most people tend to do. We focus upon and worry about everything that is wrong, while ignoring the positive aspects of any situation.

Consider the following exercise. First, mentally list all the body parts with which you don't have any problems. For example, how are your elbows, your fingernails, the middle joint of your left little toe, your right kidney? What about diseases, such as polio, Paget's disease, paracoccidioidomycosis, or pachydermoperiostosis, just to name a few—count how many of those you *don't* have. Your lists, were they an exhaustive collection of all of your body parts and systems that work perfectly, would have millions of entries. Yet despite all of these wonderfully functioning, pain-free parts, you probably only concentrate on the parts that are sore, or don't work properly, such as your spine.

As you saw above, this preoccupation with your sore or stiff areas has one effect: it makes them worse. Are you starting to see why a positive attitude to your back pain is so important?

Back problems can be difficult to ignore, as the pain and dysfunction often cause reciprocal mental stress and tension. In more severe or prolonged cases, back pain can also precipitate other mental states, such as agitation, anger, frustration and depression. These feelings increase your stress level, which then worsens the original problem. A vicious cycle can develop, which can be very difficult to break.

Often in these situations, the worry, resentment or brooding that comes with back pain can cause more stress than does the physical injury. Not only that, but the *fear* of pain can be as debilitating, if not more so, than the pain itself. Some people live their lives never daring to do anything more challenging than watch television for fear of hurting their back. This irrational fear is, in itself, a huge problem, which seriously hinders recovery.

For all of the above reasons, a positive attitude to your back pain is a vital part of your rehabilitation.

Does this all sound like bad news, and yet another problem that must be overcome if you are to relieve yourself of your spinal troubles? Despair not, for this effect works just as well in the forward, positive direction as it does in the backward, negative direction. In other words, if you can get your mind to believe that your troubles are resolving, then your body will follow it to health and wellbeing. Your back pain will start to magically disappear.

If this theory sounds a bit airy-fairy to you, or if it sounds like a wishy-washy dream of some alternate hippy therapists, then consider this fact: this power of the mind to cure the body is not only real, but is the most conclusively proven effect in the history of medical science.

I'll repeat that last sentiment again, in case you weren't paying attention. *The healing power of the mind over the body is the most conclusively proven effect in all of medicine.* In medical and other health studies, it goes under the pseudonym of the *placebo effect*. Let's take a closer look at this interesting phenomenon, and see how you can use it to help cure your back pain.

Whenever a new drug—or any other treatment, for that matter—is introduced, it must be tested on a large number of patients to see what effects, beneficial or harmful, it produces. Every good study then compares the results of the drug trial to what is known as a *placebo group*. This group, which is matched as closely as possible for conditions and symptoms to the medicated group, does not receive any real treatment. Instead, they receive a placebo treatment, which is a pill that has no effect whatsoever.

Usually, the placebo drug is a capsule that looks identical to the real drug, but is filled with nothing but harmless sugar. Of course, neither the control group nor the real group knows of the placebo. All subjects believe that they are taking a real drug.

Why do researchers go to this huge amount of trouble when they test a new drug or treatment? The reason is that those who take the placebo treatment always show a remarkable improvement as well!

Despite the fact that they have only swallowed a harmless sugar pill, many subjects in the placebo group report an improvement, sometimes even a complete cure, of their symptoms. In general, about thirty to forty per cent of people report an instant, seemingly miraculous cure following treatment that consists of absolutely nothing.

For example, in a study investigating the efficacy of new anti-inflammatory medication in eighty-eight arthritis sufferers, the same number of subjects reported relief following ingestion of a placebo as did patients who took the drug. Those patients who received no relief from the tablets were then given a placebo injection. This theoretically useless injection cured sixty-four per cent of the remaining difficult-to-cure cases.

Another study investigated the ability of a placebo drug to reduce post-surgical pain. One group of subjects were given intravenous doses of morphine (a very powerful pain-relieving drug), while the other group were given an intravenous placebo drug. The results showed that 52 per cent of the patients on morphine experienced satisfactory pain relief, while the placebo group had satisfactory relief 40 per cent of the time. In other words, the placebo was 77 per cent as effective as morphine, one of the most powerful pain-relieving drugs available.

The placebo effect works in other ways. For example, a group of patients were given a placebo pill, but were told that it was a new antihistamine drug. Funnily enough, 77.4 per cent of these patients reported a side effect of drowsiness, a common and well-known reaction to antihistamine medication.

For a placebo to work effectively, the patient must really believe that it will work. This effect was demonstrated in a study in which two groups of patients with ulcers were administered drugs. The first group of subjects were told that the tablets contained a new drug that had been proven to drastically reduce the symptoms of stomach ulcers: 70 per cent reported significant relief from their symptoms. The members of the second group were told that their tablets contained a new experimental drug, whose effect on ulcers was largely unknown: only 25 per cent of these patients received adequate relief. But guess what? Both groups received identical tablets: a placebo!

I could continue to cite thousands of other studies that show the amazing ability of a placebo drug to cure an amazing array of illnesses.

As mentioned earlier, the placebo effect is by far the most well-proven theory in all of medical science.

How does a placebo create this wonderfully powerful healing effect? Possibly, some of the healing powers are due to *attribution*: the patient would have recovered anyway, but attributed their improvement to the drug. However, this concept can not explain why many chronic patients, who have suffered with an ailment for years, suddenly recover when treated with placebo medication.

Many people have studied the placebo effect, trying to discover how it produces such amazingly powerful results. When all the hype, science and hoopla are stripped away, the answer is simple: it makes you *think positively*. The placebo drug creates an expectation in your mind that you will improve. Naturally, these positive thoughts and expectations soon become reality.

The placebo effect provides a wonderful illustration of the maxim with which we started this chapter: *where the mind goes, the body will follow*.

So how does this information apply to back pain? Well, if you can learn to create this placebo effect in yourself, you can reap the considerable, powerful benefits of this health practitioner who resides within your mind.

You have already seen how negative thinking and stress can produce damaging effects on your health and your spine. You now know that positive thinking—which the placebo effect automatically creates—has overwhelmingly beneficial effects. Let's now learn how to turn damaging negative thoughts into positive expectations.

Getting rid of negative thinking

The first step to positive thinking is to rid yourself of negative, self-damaging thoughts and attitudes. This subject is obviously extremely complex; psychologists and psychiatrists spend years studying and treating this condition alone. However, you may find that the following information at least gets you thinking, as you may not even realise that you are carrying negative thoughts about your pain. For example, do any of the following situations ring true? Have you ever . . . .

- moped about the house, feeling sorry for yourself, grumbling that your painful back is ruining your day?
- made your problems known to your friends, family and acquaintances, telling them all about your insufferable pain?
- felt a sense of relief when your spinal health practitioner diagnosed you with a 'serious problem'?

- felt annoyed that no one else seems to care about your back pain?
- felt glad that your back pain was allowing you time off from work, or other unpleasant tasks?
- blamed someone else for causing your back pain?
- blamed a situation, such as a work task, or stressful situation, for your back pain?
- become frustrated that your back injury has no blood, swelling or bruising with which you could prove to people that you are suffering?
- tried some silly, medically unproven 'miracle' pill or treatment that was supposed to cure your condition?

Any of these thoughts familiar? If you sometimes think in any of these ways, then your mind, focusing on your problems, will soon start to drag your body down with it, causing even more pain, frustration and tension.

How do you avoid these negative thoughts? If you find yourself thinking this way, the first step is to ask yourself the following questions:

1. How do I feel at present?
We've already established that you feel frustrated, tense, fed-up and in pain.

2. How would I like to feel?
Naturally, most people would like to feel relaxed, calm, happy and pain-free.

3. Are my thought patterns helping me to feel relaxed, calm, happy and pain-free?
No, they are not. In fact, your negative attitude is clearly making your problem worse.

4. Then why am I doing something that makes me feel so bad?
This final question is by far the most important. Your honest answer will guide you to the best method in reversing your negative pattern of thought.

Note that you are not asking yourself why you have a sore back. This question has many answers, to which this entire book is devoted. You are asking yourself why your *attitude* to your pain and disability is one that is clearly making you worse.

You don't have to pry deep into your childhood experiences and inner psyche to discover the answer. Just consider the question honestly.

By asking yourself these simple questions, you will see, in clear form, the basis of much of your negative thinking. Now let's see how to turn this negative, destructive attitude into a positive, helpful frame of mind.

Techniques for positive thinking

Most of the following techniques can be used at any time. You can try them when you are in pain, in the car, on the toilet, or on the telephone while your Aunty Doris chatters unendingly about a dispute with her neighbours over the garbage bin. However, they are far more effective if you use them regularly, especially when performed in conjunction with the relaxation exercises that you learned in the last chapter.

As you know, a deeply relaxed mind does not criticise or analyse any new information that you present to it. Your mind simply accepts the thoughts as true, and automatically alters its attitudes and reactions. This effect is best seen during hypnosis, in which a hypnotist can convince a willing, hypnotised subject of the most absurd possibilities. Here, you will be using a similar technique known as *autosuggestion*.

For this reason, the instructions for these positive-thinking exercises are very simple. As with the relaxation exercises, your mind will respond more readily to simple, straightforward statements than to complicated, detailed, logical instructions. Please do not be discouraged by the seemingly simplistic nature of the following exercises. I urge you to try them, and you will soon see how effective they can be.

AFFIRMATIONS

Affirmations are simply positive phrases that you repeat to yourself, either mentally or verbally. These phrases have an enormous effect on your mind, for while it is true that 'where the mind goes, your body will follow', it is equally true that 'where your speech goes, your mind will follow'. Therefore, you can control the reactions of your body just by thinking, *or even saying*, the right sentiments.

You can clearly see the effect of affirmations in elite sporting situations. Phrases such as 'Come on, you can do it' are commonplace in virtually every sport, and represent the simplest, most basic form of an affirmation.

To apply this technique to your lower back pain, you simply use positive phrases to convince your mind that you are well. Just repeat the phrases for a few minutes, either silently to yourself, or audibly.

Remember, these phrases are far more powerful if you use them when your mind is in a deeply relaxed, receptive state.

Below are some examples of such phrases. You can pick a few of these that you feel will work for you, or you can create some of your own. However, ensure that the sentiments are positive, not a double-negative type of phrase. Remember Damian the golfer, who told himself not to hit the ball in the bunker, but unerringly shot directly into the middle of the sand.

EXAMPLES OF POSITIVE PHRASES	EXAMPLES OF PHRASES TO AVOID
• My back feels healthy and strong.	• My back does not hurt.
• My back is calm and relaxed.	• I cannot feel any back pain.
• My back feels wonderful.	• My back is not tense or tight.
• I am strong, healthy and relaxed.	• I am not sick.
• My back muscles are loose and relaxed.	• I do not feel any pain or tension.
• My spine is 100% comfortable.	• My back is pain-free.
• I feel confident and strong.	• My back will not retain any pain.
• My back will remain relaxed and healthy during any activity.	• My back will not hurt after lawn bowls today.

Why not say a few of the phrases now, aloud if you please. You may surprise yourself!

VISUALISATION

As mentioned previously, your mind cannot distinguish between a real situation and one that you vividly imagine, as demonstrated by the champion skiers in the EMG study. You can use the technique of visualisation to help practise your attitudes and responses to many different situations.

I'm sure you've heard the old adage that 'practice makes perfect'. One Australian football coach refined this saying to '*perfect* practice makes perfect'. Luckily, you have a place in which you can practise perfectly every time: in your mind.

You can use the visualisation techniques to perfectly practise perfect responses to any situation that would previously have disturbed you.

The technique is, again, remarkably simple. During your *first* visualisation session, picture the problem in your mind. Then, after you have fully examined and experienced every detail of the picture, you abruptly change its polarity so that the situation is now as you would like it to be. In other words, you change the image so that it now depicts you solving your problem.

You then visualise this new, perfect picture for the ensuing few minutes, and in subsequent sessions. Never again should you visualise

ATTITUDES, THE PLACEBO EFFECT, AND THE POWER OF THE MIND

the picture containing the problem. Remember, your mind will go where your thoughts take it, so make sure that your thoughts are always showing the ideal situation, the solution.

Let's look at a few examples to see how visualisation can work.

Suppose that you feel extremely angry and tense each time your partner leaves their dirty clothes on the bathroom floor. Just the sight of the dirty jocks, socks and shirts makes your blood boil, and the subsequent stress makes your back ache for the next few hours. You've tried, you've really tried, to change your partner's habits. But no amount of berating, bribery or begging has made a difference. Instead, you decide to change yourself, by altering the way that you respond to the same situation.

To use a visualisation technique to help you overcome your stressful reaction, you would first picture yourself walking into the bathroom when your partner has left the floor covered with dirty clothes. See yourself becoming angry, and really experience the feelings of tension and frustration that your response brings. Vividly imagine the slowly ebbing backache that grows with your tension levels.

Now, change the polarity of your vision. Again, picture yourself walking into the bathroom and seeing the filthy floor, but this time see yourself as calm and relaxed. Really experience this new response. Feel the relaxation. Imagine yourself responding exactly as you would like. See yourself as calm, relaxed and 100 per cent comfortable in your spine. Practise this response in your mind, and never again return to the old vision of a frustrated, aching, angry you.

After a few sessions, particularly if you combine this visualisation with your deep mental relaxation, you will find that this practised response becomes your natural reaction. This may take up to six weeks, but if you practise this response diligently in your mind, then it will definitely happen. Never again will you feel stressed or pained by dirty clothes on the bathroom floor. Note that you have not changed the external situation; you have simply changed how you respond to the same stimulus.

You can also use this technique to practise physical responses. Many athletes visualise themselves successfully performing their chosen sport. Next time you are watching an elite sportsperson just before a competition, take note of their behaviour. Sometimes you can actually see them visualising every nuance of their performance.

One athlete who won an Olympic Gold Medal in middle-distance running showed so little emotion after crossing the line in first place that friends later quizzed him on his lack of happiness. His reply was that he had already won the race thousands of times in his mind, and that this particular race was no different. He *knew* he was going to win. In fact, he was *bored* of winning that race. Visualisation can be very powerful.

Similarly, you can use visualisation to practise physical elements of your back pain prevention program. For example, let's say that your back aches if you repeatedly lift with a poor technique. Unfortunately, your job as a supermarket grocery handler requires you to perform hundreds of lifts every day. In the rush and hustle of your work, your lifting technique often falters, and you find that your back pain is increasing as a result.

To help you with this aspect of your management, first perform your mental relaxation exercises. Then imagine yourself working frantically, behind schedule, with dozens of awkward heavy lifts to complete before closing time. Visualise your lifting technique failing and your stability muscles flagging as you lose concentration. Feel your back pain increasing, and your stress level rising.

Now, change polarity. Imagine the same busy situation, but this time see yourself in control. Visualise your posture as perfect, and your lifting technique as infallible. Your stability muscles are firm, and your spine feels flexible and strong. Imagine that you easily complete all of your required lifts with ease, with no pain and no stress. Well done!

If you practised and rehearsed this scene in your mind for a few weeks, the next time it arose you would respond exactly as you had 'practised'. Remember, your mind cannot tell the difference between a real and a vividly imagined situation. Perfect practice makes perfect.

Note that in all these situations, you practised and visualised your response in advance. You cannot relax and visualise a perfect response if you have already triggered frustrated emotions. It's no use cleaning your teeth if they've already developed a cavity! For visualisation to be effective, you must train your mind *in advance* to replace the negative reactions with more favourable, automatic responses. In this way, you won't have to subdue any feelings of tension, because *they won't even occur*.

FIVE STEPS TO PREVENT THE ONSET OF BACK PAIN
The following technique was popularised as a treatment for migraine headaches. Here, I have adapted it for use with back pain, where it should work equally well. In fact, you could apply this exercise to any stress-related illness at all. The idea of the technique is to use relaxation, visualisation and affirmation techniques to banish any back pain before it gets started.

Step One: As soon as you feel the first twinge of a pain, immediately stop what you are doing. Do not wait five minutes, for if you do a pain-tension-spasm-pain cycle may come into effect.

ATTITUDES, THE PLACEBO EFFECT, AND THE POWER OF THE MIND

Step Two: Perform your relaxation exercises. In the beginning, this may take you up to half an hour. However, with practice you should be able to achieved a suitably relaxed mind within five minutes.

Step Three: Slowly work through the following positive phrases:
I can feel back pain coming on.
I do not want back pain.
I do not deserve back pain.
I want my back to remain relaxed, comfortable and healthy.
My back is relaxed, comfortable and healthy.

Step Four: Come out of your relaxation phase, and undertake a different activity from what you were doing when the pain started. At the very least, you should assume a different posture.

Step Five: If the twinge of pain returns, then immediately repeat the whole process.

In this chapter, you have seen how your mind has remarkable subconscious control over your body. The well-proven placebo effect illustrates the powerful positive effect that the mind can have on the body. You have learned some simple techniques to turn your negative thought processes into positive feelings, and so generate healing and health in your spine.

24

The effects of drugs

No, I'm not talking about marijuana

Drugs and back pain

Don't let the title of this chapter mislead you. We will not be discussing whether that marijuana joint you smoked at a party back in the '70s caused your present bout of back pain. Instead, we will examine the effects of medically prescribed drugs, not only with regard to your spinal injury, but to the rest of you as well.

First, here's the standard disclaimer, just so that some irresponsible idiot doesn't try to sue me. The following information is intended as a guide only. In *all cases* you should check with your doctor and pharmacist before commencing, or stopping, any drug treatment.

Four main groups of drugs are sometimes used to alleviate the symptoms of back pain.

(1) Non-Steroidal Anti-Inflammatory Drugs. These drugs are usually referred to by the acronym NSAID. They are referred to colloquially as 'anti-inflammatories'.
(2) Over-the-counter medication. This group includes simple analgesics such as paracetamol and aspirin, as well as preparations that combine these drugs with codeine.
(3) Muscle relaxants and sedatives.
(4) Spinal injections of cortico-steroids (see Chapter 34).

Note: A list of common NSAID medications is listed in the 'Appendices'.

As NSAIDs are the most commonly prescribed drugs for low back pain, the following discussion will centre on this group. We will look at NSAID use in three situations: first, for chronic back pain that has been ongoing for longer than one month; second, for recently injured, acutely painful backs; and third, when they are used in a cream or gel.

Following the discussion on these three aspects of NSAIDs, we'll briefly look at the other classes of medication.

NSAIDs for chronic, ongoing back pain

Although NSAIDs are frequently prescribed, I feel that regular NSAID use is sometimes overused in the treatment of chronic, ongoing back pain. The risk–benefit ratio of NSAIDs is too high to justify their continued daily use to treat this condition. The reasons that the risks outweigh the benefits are fourfold:

1. NSAIDS often do not work very well for specific, localised conditions such as back pain.
2. NSAIDS have side effects, some of which can be severe.
3. You may unknowingly injure yourself while taking NSAIDs.
4. Long-term NSAID use encourages drug reliance, rather than encouraging you to accept the responsibility for curing your back pain.

Let's now look at these reasons individually.

(1) NSAIDs often do not work very well for specific, localised conditions, such as back pain
Simply, many patients do not receive much relief from chronic back pain after taking NSAIDs. Studies suggest that fifty to sixty per cent of patients experience a satisfactory response to the first NSAID that they are prescribed. However, if you compare this percentage to that of placebo drugs (often about forty per cent) you can see that little difference exists.

NSAIDs have also been used in an attempt to hasten recovery following sporting injuries, such as ligament sprains. Studies have shown that these injuries heal at the same rate whether anti-inflammatory medication is taken or not. So if the medication does not help an ankle sprain heal any more rapidly, why would it help a lower back sprain?

Furthermore, you may be able to obtain similar pain relief from other less harmful tablets. One study tabulated the responses of arthritis sufferers to an anti-inflammatory drug, and then compared them to a matched group who took simple paracetamol. There was no significant difference between the responses to either drug.

Why don't anti-inflammatory drugs always decrease the pain associated with an inflamed spine? Two explanations spring to mind. First, and this is a really simple reason, the tablet doesn't know where to go. The drug does not know that you have a painful back. The agents that decrease the joint inflammation effect your little toe just as strongly as

BACK PAIN

your lower back. So any effect on a damaged disc or joint is very *non-specific*, and therefore close to useless for such localised injuries.

Second, NSAIDs do not address the cause of inflammation. Even if you had a perfect drug that could completely halt the inflammatory process, your joints would retain their inherent problems. No tablet, no matter how potent, can loosen a stiff joint, support an unstable one, or loosen a caught nerve.

Using drugs to treat chronic back pain is like putting a bucket under a leaking roof, rather than fixing the broken tile.

(2) NSAIDs frequently have side effects, some of which may be severe
Most people who take NSAIDs realise that these drugs can irritate your stomach. Your doctor and pharmacist should have warned you about this possibility before prescribing this medication to you. Below are some further facts to ensure that you are fully aware of the dangers of these drugs. These statistics are from the pharmacy industry itself; they are not trumped-up figures from anti-drug fanatics. After reading this list, you will realise that NSAIDs have side effects that are sometimes more damaging than the original problem they were supposed to help.

- In the UK, NSAIDs constitute 25% of 'Adverse Response to Drug' reports, even though they account for only 5% of the prescriptions.
- Roughly 30% of all peptic ulcer complications are attributable to NSAIDs, with the rate rising to 50% for elderly women.
- Patients taking regular NSAIDs have four times the chance of developing gastric ulcers, three times the risk of stomach bleeding, and six times the risk of developing a hole in their stomach wall, as compared to an average population.
- Here's one that should really worry you: approximately 30% of patients on NSAIDs who had a *life-threatening* haemorrhage *did not have any prior symptoms of gastric problems.*

NSAIDs can also affect many other bodily systems. In particular, they can cause or exacerbate the following conditions:

- Long-term use can cause kidney damage.
- The NSAIDs thin your blood, meaning that any cuts will bleed more profusely.
- They can precipitate asthma attacks in susceptible people.
- They can elevate your blood pressure.
- If you are pregnant, they can cause problems for your foetus.

The side-effect rollcall does not end there. Even if you escape without serious problems, you may end up with either nausea, vomiting or diarrhoea, all of which are common side effects. A whopping sixty per cent of patients will experience dyspepsia—a burning, irritable stomach—in response to prolonged NSAID use.

How long does it take before these symptoms become clinically relevant? Obviously, the answer varies significantly from one person to the next. However, one study, which used a small scope to look at the stomach lining of NSAID users, noted changes in some patients after a week. Most subjects had obvious damage after one month. A general rule of thumb is that the higher your dose, and the longer you take it, the more side effects you will suffer.

After reading the above series of complications and side effects from NSAIDs, you should now compare them with the possible benefits. Is it worth the extra risk?

(3) You may inadvertently injure yourself while under the influence of pain-killing drugs

This statement should be interpreted with normal commonsense. Pain is a warning from your body that you are doing something wrong. Particularly when this signal is chronic, you should not simply paper over the problem by gulping down handfuls of pills. Why not use some of the other techniques in this book (go for a walk, perform some relaxation exercises, apply a heat pack, or do some exercises, for example) which not only provide pain relief, but also will help to repair and rehabilitate the source of your pain?

In some sporting circles, some athletes take this mistake one step further: they *knowingly* injure themselves—by overtraining—while under the influence of NSAIDs. They promote their constant use of pain-killing and anti-inflammatory drugs as 'proof' that they are dedicated, persistent, and will train through anything to achieve their goals. These obsessive personalities wear their NSAID 'addiction' like a badge of honour.

If this group includes you, then you have a problem. See a psychiatrist, and then take up knitting instead.

(4) NSAIDs encourage drug reliance

Drug reliance is a rapidly escalating problem. The trend of high-volume pill popping has itself become a disease. Perhaps someone should invent a pill to treat the obsessive disease of excessive pill popping!

With back pain, drug reliance makes even less sense than it does in many other illnesses. Normal back pain is not due to an evil disease that is taking over your body, it's not contagious, and you can't contract it like AIDS or hepatitis. Even with very chronic normal back pain, your blood tests will be normal, and the condition will not spread around your body like a cancer.

In contrast with many other diseases, back pain is a localised, specific, benign condition. Spinal problems have nothing to do with identifiable external invaders such as germs, which can be sensibly attacked with drugs like antibiotics. Back pain arises from your movements, your muscles or your mind, not from somewhere 'out there'. As such, the cure must come from *within*, not from a bottle.

If your doctor prescribes you long repeat courses of anti-inflammatory medication, he or she is unfortunately reinforcing the notion that something else will cure your pain for you, handily diminishing responsibility and effort on your part.

In short, drug prescriptions encourage you to take the easy way. Trust me, this strategy doesn't work. If drugs really could cure back problems then the world wouldn't be losing 50,000,000 (or whatever) work days per year due to back pain, and spinal health practitioners would long ago have been out of a job.

In summary, I feel that most people should not regularly be taking NSAIDs for long-term lower back pain. The lack of major proven benefits, the possible complications, and other more complete solutions all combine to make a sensible argument against the prolonged use of such medication. In my opinion, chronic back pain sufferers would be best served by using these drugs sparingly, or, better still, flushing them down the toilet.

NSAIDs for acute, severe pain

OK, now that I've finished bagging the long-term, regular use of NSAID medication, I'd better have a look at another question: what *is* the place for anti-inflammatory drugs in the treatment of spinal pain?

In some circumstances, the short-term use of NSAIDs is beneficial. For example, if you are in acute severe pain, or have suffered with recent traumatic back pain—kicked off a horse, for example—then NSAIDs should be your drug of choice, provided you have no history of gastro-intestinal disturbances or asthma. If you are in severe pain, then the temporary relief and relaxation that the drugs provide will, in many cases, outweigh the potential risks.

Although the bucket-under-a-leaking-roof analogy remains relevant, sometimes this strategy is best, particularly if the storm is still raging outside.

If you have acute, severe lower back pain and you wish to take NSAIDs, then the following guidelines will help to ensure that you have minimal trouble.

- Ensure that you eat before taking the tablets. By the way, I mean eat a proper meal, not a teaspoon full of cottage cheese on a water cracker biscuit.

- Do not take any other drugs, such as aspirin.
- Discontinue taking the NSAIDs as soon as your severe pain has started to subside. You do not have to complete a full course, as is the case with antibiotics.
- Do not exceed a week of continuous use if possible.
- Inform your doctor and pharmacist if you have previously suffered from gastric problems, high blood pressure, kidney disease, haemophilia or asthma, or if you are currently pregnant.

If you limit your NSAID use to the above circumstances, then you have a low risk of developing complications.

Topical NSAIDs—creams, gels and liniments

After realising the significant side effects of oral anti-inflammatory medication, the drug companies sensibly decided to change their approach. They decided that patients would be better served not by swallowing tablets, but by rubbing NSAID cream into their painful areas, and so hopefully lessening the dose needed to affect the target area.

This thinking is obviously a step in the right direction. Certainly, these creams and gels do not have nearly as many side effects as the oral preparations. However, we now come to another question: do they work? Unfortunately, in many cases, the answer is 'not really'.

One obvious difficulty with using NSAID creams for back pain is that most people will inadvertently apply the cream to the wrong area. Recall Chapter 9 on nerve injuries and referred pain, in which you learned that the painful area is often far removed from the true injury site. Many back structures refer pain long distances, to seemingly unrelated areas. Believe me, locating the exact source of diffuse back pain is no easy task.

If you rub the anti-inflammatory cream into the area of referred pain, rather than into the real injury site, then you will not obtain effective results. This would be like trying to extinguish a fire by spraying water through the tips of the flames, rather than onto the base of the fire.

Secondly, doubt exists as to whether the active ingredients in the cream can penetrate deeply enough into the joint to effect real benefits. Lumbar structures such as discs are very deep within the body, and are covered by layers of muscles, bones and ligaments. I find it very difficult to believe that the active ingredients in the drug could penetrate halfway through your body, neatly sidestepping the skin, the connective tissues, the muscles and the joint capsule, before depositing themselves neatly onto the problem area.

One recent study indicated that the drugs do not directly penetrate into the local joint tissues, but rather are absorbed by the blood stream, then transported around the body and into the joints in the usual way. This theory was supported by the finding that the concentration of the drug was the same in both knees, despite the cream only having been applied to one knee. If this theory is true, then we run into the same problems that oral NSAIDs had: the anti-inflammatory medication does not have enough concentration at the injury site to be of much use.

Various studies have compared the efficacy of anti-inflammatory preparations to ordinary moisturising cream—a placebo, in other words. These studies found that there was very little difference in the pain-relieving properties of the two substances. The NSAID cream was only *slightly* more effective at relieving pain and inflammation than was ordinary hand cream.

With this finding in mind, allow me to indulge in some simple mathematics, which will illustrate why I hesitate to recommend anti-inflammatory creams. At present, a 75 gram tube of a well-known anti-inflammatory cream has an active ingredient with a very long, unpronounceable name, at a concentration of three per cent. By my calculations, this tube therefore contains about 2.25 grams of the drug, while the rest of the tube is essentially hand cream.

Now let's look at the cost. An equal-sized tube of moisturising cream retails for about one-eighth the cost. The anti-inflammatory cream, by virtue of the 2.25 grams of medication, is seven times more expensive. Given this substantial mark-up I'd be wanting impressive, instant results. I certainly wouldn't be happy with 'slightly better than placebo'.

OK, I admit that this argument doesn't hold up under intense scrutiny of economic and market forces. But I hope it at least makes you stop and think before you spend your hard-earned money on something that is unlikely to help relieve your pain very much, and will not help the underlying cause at all.

Other commercial preparations such as liniments contain chemicals that create a feeling of warmth. These preparations are essentially harmless, and contain no active ingredients that directly affect your spinal injury. Nor do they actually create warmth in your joints. Liniments simply react with your skin to create a feeling of warmth.

If liniments or anti-inflammatory creams make you feel better for a while, then fine, use them. You won't die. Just be aware that all of the above arguments—particularly those that relate to treating the cause and not the symptoms, and cost-effectiveness—apply.

Over-the-counter analgesics

The most common over-the-counter pain-killers are aspirin and paracetamol, both of which are sometimes combined with codeine. While you may have so far gathered that I am fundamentally against the ongoing or frequent use of drugs to treat back pain, on occasion you may simply feel the need for temporary pain relief. Fair enough. If you ever find yourself suffering a temporary escalation of your pain, then you may wonder which over-the-counter analgesic is best for your problem.

Obviously, different people will respond in different ways. However, the general guidelines for using over-the-counter medications for low back pain are as follows:

- If your stomach and airways are in perfect condition, then aspirin should be your medication of choice. The mild anti-inflammatory effect of aspirin gives it an advantage over other drugs.
- If you have ever experienced tummy problems or asthma, then avoid aspirin. Aspirin is very similar in nature to the NSAID group, and hence has similar effects and problems. Use it wisely and prefer paracetamol.
- If you have suffered an acute, traumatic, violent injury to your back, then you should avoid aspirin for the first 24 hours. Aspirin, like other NSAIDs, tends to thin your blood, and so may worsen any internal bleeding or bruising if you use it too early.
- Do not exceed the recommended dose. This rule sounds like commonsense, but many people ignore it.
- Keep all over-the-counter drug use to a minimum and remember that there are many other ways to deal with your problem.
- Finally, many new drugs are being released onto the over-the-counter market which are, or contain, NSAIDs. These preparations should be approached with the same guidelines as for the prescription-only tablets: they are fine in small, infrequent doses, but potentially harmful when taken over a prolonged period.

Muscle relaxants and sedatives

This group includes drugs such as Valium, as well as some other commercial pain-killers (Mersyndol) that have a small amount of muscle relaxant. These medications are occasionally prescribed by some doctors for acute lower back pain.

If your doctor has prescribed these drugs so that you, who would otherwise be in agony, have a decent night's sleep, then fair enough ... for one or two nights, three at the most. However, if the prescription is to promote relaxation, decrease muscle spasm or to mask pain in a chronic condition, the reasoning is very questionable.

First, muscle relaxants don't affect the underlying cause of the problem. As you read way back in Chapter 7, muscle spasms are almost never the primary cause of lower back pain. Muscle relaxants have no effect on other more likely pain-producing structures, such as the joints, discs and ligaments, nor do they effect the inflammatory process.

Furthermore, muscle relaxants may worsen the injury. If your back is unstable (a type A or B) then it requires muscular support, not drug-induced relaxation. Muscle relaxants further decrease the already inhibited support that your stability muscles are providing for your spine.

Third, as you will read later, rest is a very poor option for even very painful lower back sufferers. Movement and activity provide a far quicker and more effective means of pain relief than does rest. Yet these tablets, with their effects of drowsiness, weakness and lethargy, encourage, and even compel you to lie in bed all day. Why take a drug that creates a harmful effect?

Finally, these drugs not only encourage reliance, but some of them are physically addictive. Some people who start on a course of muscle relaxants find the habit very difficult to cease, and end up with other psychological and physiological problems.

In summary, I believe that these types of medications are generally over-prescribed, and that they have a limited place in the management of lower back pain. These types of drugs should be restricted to a couple of nights, and used only if you are suffering severe physical or emotional stress from acute lower back pain, with due reference to the stability of your injury.

Summary

If your back pain is severe, then temporary use of NSAIDs or other analgesics is fine. However, please don't use them repetitively, or over a prolonged period, as the benefits do not outweigh the concerns. By the end of this book you will have many safer, more beneficial techniques for back pain relief at your disposal that I suggest you try instead.

25

Diet, nutritional supplements and natural remedies

How I plan to make a fortune

You are probably aware of the basic rules for sensible, healthy eating. Maybe you even follow them. Millions, if not billions, of books and magazines are available on the subject of diet, so I will not bore you with a rehash of old information that you have no doubt read a thousand times. Instead, we will examine how your ordinary, everyday diet can affect your spine, and investigate the actions of natural remedies, vitamins, minerals and other supplements.

Your daily diet and its relationship to back pain

You may be asking yourself why anyone would include a section on diet in a book about back pain? However, three good reasons exist to examine and/or modify your diet with regard to lower back pain.

(1) YOUR DIET IS IMPORTANT FOR YOUR OVERALL HEALTH
Commonsense will tell you that a healthy person will recover from injury more quickly than will someone whose diet consists of chewing gum, coffee, and cola.

A balanced intake of vitamins and minerals will assist your body to optimally perform its natural healing responses. Simply, I am talking about the basic strategies of healthy eating with which I am sure you are familiar, with emphasis on freshness and variety.

Good eating habits improve your body's capacity to cope with the normal difficulties of everyday life. By eating healthily, and thereby raising your physical tolerance to stress, you can help to decrease the impact of anxiety and tension upon your body. Often, the result is less back pain.

(2) BEING OVERWEIGHT CAN AFFECT YOUR SPINE
To find your ideal weight, simply take your height in centimetres, multiply it by sixty-seven, and divide by the year of your birth. Then add

fifteen if you own a dog, and add the digits together if you've ever owned a cat, divide by pi, then add ... oh, forget it. Most of you probably know whether you're grossly overweight or not.

Seriously, if you're not sure, or if, like me, you're prone to kidding yourself about such matters, then you can use the following simple method to check. To calculate your *body mass index*, simply divide your weight in kilograms by your height in metres, then divide by your height again.

If your answer is below twenty, then you're too skinny; if its above twenty-five, then you're on the porky side. If your body mass index is higher than 30, then you're *waaaaay* over.

For example, suppose that Harry is 1.78 metres tall, and weighs 88 kilograms. His body mass index is 88 divided by 1.78, then divided by 1.78 again, giving a total of 27.7—definitely on the high side. Or consider Kate, whose height of 1.65 metres and weight of 42 kilograms give her a reading of 15.4, which is far too low to be healthy.

Note that heavily-muscled, highly trained people may have a body mass index of over twenty-five without being overweight. Use your commonsense in deciding if you belong in this category.

Any surplus body fat has a detrimental effect on your spine. Logically, the lower vertebrae bear more of your body weight than do the higher levels. As your lower back is the most frequently injured area, commonsense will tell you that any extra kilograms are a huge extra burden for these susceptible joints to bear.

Excessive body weight can be particularly troublesome if you gain it in a short space of time, as your joints will not have a chance to adaptively strengthen to the higher demands. Furthermore, you learned in Chapter 16 of the huge effects of leverage when you bend or lift. In this case, the negative effects of each extra kilogram are multiplied, making them an even greater liability.

And, by the way, spinal health practitioners find it easier to diagnose and treat thinner people, as the joints and muscles are far easier to feel.

In short, a trim you is more likely to avoid back pain than would be a heavy, obese you.

(3) YOUR DIET CAN HELP TO DIMINISH THE EFFECTS OF OSTEOPOROSIS

Most people are now well aware of the damaging effects of osteoporosis. In this condition, your bones lose their calcium, meaning that they become less dense and more brittle. Osteoporotic bones are therefore very liable to fracture.

In the spine, this bone weakness is most commonly represented by crush fractures of the vertebral bodies (refer to Chapter 6). Elderly

DIET, NUTRITIONAL SUPPLEMENTS AND NATURAL REMEDIES

women are most at risk of this condition, but elderly men should not be complacent.

Diet, particularly your calcium intake, has a role to play in the prevention of osteoporosis. Please consult the first section of the 'Appendices' if you are interested in learning more about this condition.

A FEW MORE POINTS ABOUT DIET

Some recent studies have shown that a diet high in oily fish (mackerel, salmon and sardines, for example) may help to decrease the inflammation levels in patients with rheumatoid arthritis. However, directly attributing less low back pain to a fish diet is taking a lot of liberties with the results, rather like asserting that the outcome of a cricket game is obvious after only one ball has been bowled.

As you will see later in the chapter, almost every claim that certain foods or supplements decrease pain or inflammation has been ultimately unproven. However, I feel on morally higher ground in suggesting that you add some fish to your diet for one simple reason: seafood is good for your general health anyway.

Many studies have linked high-fish diets to improved general health and wellbeing. Furthermore, fish is relatively low in kilojoules, has 'good' fats for healthy arteries, and, most importantly, tastes great on the barbeque. One Australian doctor says that only four healthy things do not have side effects: laughter, sex, vegetables and fish. By including more of the latter two in your weekly diet, and more of the other two in your daily life, you will not only become healthier, but also gain a few percentage points head start on your back pain.

I don't wish to bore you with rules and regulations for healthy eating. I'm sure that you know them as well as I do. If you need extra attention in this area, then consult a dietician about how to make basic, simple changes to your eating habits.

Don't be afraid to try the positive thinking techniques and affirmations that we discussed in Chapter 23. These techniques can be a very useful adjunct to your willpower when you are making the difficult change from pie-scoffing, cola-quaffing porker to a healthy, energetic, trimmer you.

So you can see that there are many good reasons to include a healthy, fresh, varied diet to your armament of strategies with which to attack your lower back pain. But what about nutritional supplements? Aren't there dozens of products—vitamins, minerals, food supplements and natural remedies—that can ease inflammation, reduce pain and swelling, or otherwise cure back pain? Let's now look at these products to see if they have any value in your quest for a pain-free life.

Vitamins, minerals, nutritional supplements and natural remedies

I've already figured out the sequel to this book. It's going to be called *The NEW MIRACLE DIET that will get rid of your back pain forever!* This book will be an international bestseller, and my publishers, bless their souls, will make a well-deserved fortune.

The miracle-cure diet book would not discuss any causes of back pain, nor would it contain any advice on strengthening or stretching. It wouldn't mention lifting techniques, posture or stress management, and would have no information whatsoever on chairs, beds, sports, fitness or drugs. The book would simply provide a few theories about diet and back pain, which it would prove by citing testimonials and case studies about how the new wonder supplement has cured others of their ailments.

I'll also promote and sell a wonder herb that has been 'proven' to cure all types of bodily aches and pains, as well as arthritis, the flu, tinnitus, lethargy, hay fever, ingrown toenails, headaches, and, why not, impotence as well. Millions of people around the world will swallow these expensive but miraculous herbal pills by the dozen. Daytime talk show audiences will hear about how I discovered the secret recipe on an ancient clay tablet in the Sahara desert. No one else would know about the magical combination of mystery ingredients, except for the ancient Egyptians and, of course, me. I'll become rich and famous.

This whole miracle-diet-book-herb-pills-cure concept would be wonderful, but for one minor problem. It wouldn't work.

Simply, no vitamin, mineral or natural remedy has been shown to cure back pain. However, this simple fact obviously doesn't bother those who promote health supplements as miracle cures. The Arthritis Foundation spend a great deal of their time and resources in educating the public to be wary of such claims. I'm about to do the same thing.

About a decade ago, an anti-inflammatory fad diet swept throughout the world that relied on green-lipped mussels. Shops sold out of mussels for months, and their price went through the roof. Similarly, celery tablets had their day in the sun, as did zinc supplements, copper bracelets, evening primrose oil, and additives such as willow bark and devil's claw. Some practitioners promoted an anti-acidic diet formula as the basis for curing all bodily ills, while almost every month a cure-all herb is promoted on a current affairs show. Noni juice, now also sold in concentrated capsules, is the latest cure-all food supplement on the scene.

Another craze occurred about two decades ago that relied on eating nothing but grapes for a few days. Someone even made money by publishing a book on the subject. Sure, I like grapes, especially when they've been juiced, fermented for a few weeks in barrels and then stored in a bottle. But how anyone, *anyone*, would believe that a grape-only diet could cure all of the problems that lead to back pain and arthritis, I'll never understand. Besides, I reckon that you'd end up with an awful case of the runs . . .

Other fallacies include alfalfa tea, megadoses of vitamin C, extracts of animal hormones or other strange secretions, periodic fasting, yeast, and even, believe it or not, yeast elimination. A further rollcall of back pain quackery includes protein supplements, garlic (sorry grandma), honey, kelp, watercress and aloe vera. Proponents of such products have made claims for their anti-arthritic and pain-relieving powers. Not surprisingly, all of these remedies have now fallen into obscurity, just as will the next lot of miracle additives.

Think about it. Imagine that you have a stiff, scarred disc in your back that is pressing on a spinal nerve. Your muscles are weak and unsupportive, and the surrounding area has accumulated so much microtrauma that you should really call it megatrauma. Your posture is poor, your work chair is a bar stool, and you are so tense that your muscles have more knots than a crocheted coat-hanger cover.

Do you *really* think that just by downing a few vitamin pills or eating some natural remedy that all of these problems will suddenly vanish? Will something that goes into your stomach have the power to fix your posture, reverse the accumulation of microtrauma, decrease your stress levels, increase your strength, and return all of your joints to a normal, healthy and flexible state?

You're not that silly, are you? Yet thousands of people still try fad diets, expensive supplements and strange-sounding health foods that are supposed to cure them of their back pain, decrease the inflammation, or perform a host of other amazing functions. Please, for your own sake, don't waste your time and money.

Most health supplements that are supposed to improve back pain profess to have natural anti-inflammatory properties. This may be true—after all, aspirin is a derivative of tree bark. Furthermore, I don't mean to imply that natural medicine does not have any use at all, or that it has no place in the health-care field. Alternative medicine is now making genuine inroads into the treatment of many conditions. However, before you rush out and buy a shopping trolley full of desiccated zebra's hoof (or whatever) to help cure your *back pain*, compare the anti-inflammatory potency of the supplement to that of a specifically developed NSAID tablet.

You have already learned how even the concentrated power of strong NSAID drugs has only a minor overall effect on lower back pain. Even *if* the herb or foodstuff has some anti-inflammatory properties, the active ingredient will be present in such relatively low amounts that it would be effectively useless. If even the highly concentrated, specifically developed drugs have only a minor influence on your pain, then what hope does a trace amount of natural anti-inflammatory agent in a foodstuff have? Close to nil, I suggest.

Other remedies make a variety of claims, such as 'anti-oxidant effect', 'increases collagen formation' or, my personal favourite 'flushes toxins from your body'. Those evil toxins! All of these 'effects' have no proven action on lower back pain.

Let's have a quick look at how vitamins and other food supplements affect your body. Understanding their function will enable you to competently assess the claims made by any remedy. This knowledge will also illustrate why megadoses of vitamins or other supplements are simply a waste of money.

Vitamins and food supplements do not have any *active* effect on your body whatsoever. This statement may surprise some people, so I'll repeat it: vitamins and food supplements have *no active effect* on your body. Nor does your body use them for fuel. Instead, their job is to assist other normal reactions to proceed with greater ease.

Vitamins work via a process that chemists call *catalysis* (cat-TAL-ee-sis). Catalysis means that you accelerate a chemical process by adding another substance, which is labelled a *catalyst*. It is important to understand that the reaction already occurs naturally, but the catalyst makes it much faster and more efficient. Furthermore, the catalyst is not permanently affected by the reaction, and nor is it 'burned up' or used as fuel.

In your body, vitamins act as catalysts. In other words, they accelerate or facilitate processes in your body that are already occurring. As such, vitamins do not have any *direct* action on your body. Furthermore, they are not expended or destroyed by the reaction.

Chemistry tells us that if a catalyst is present in a sufficient quantity, adding more of it will not make the reaction any quicker or more powerful. In short, enough is enough. This simple fact has obvious implications for your intake of vitamins and minerals. The warning on the label spells this message out very clearly: 'Vitamin supplements can be of assistance only if dietary intake is inadequate'. Yet many people choose to ignore this truth, and think that if taking one vitamin pill is beneficial, then taking two, ten or 100 must be better. Sorry, it doesn't work this way. If enough of the catalyst is present, taking extra will provide NO benefits whatsoever. Nil. None. Zilch. Zip. Zippo. Squat. Diddly-squat. Zero.

Let's look at a simple analogy to illustrate how a catalyst works, which will illustrate more clearly the catalysing action of vitamins.

DIET, NUTRITIONAL SUPPLEMENTS AND NATURAL REMEDIES

Imagine a big, fat, jolly man, who we will call Christopher, who loves to eat pizza. Every evening, Christopher sends his young daughter Louise to Giovanni's Italian Food Emporium to pick up a large pizza. Louise dutifully walks to the shop, collects the pizza, and then walks home, which takes her about an hour. This routine occurs every night in their household.

After a while, Christopher decides that he does not like waiting so long for his nightly pizza, as it is cold by the time his daughter arrives home. He buys Louise a bicycle, which allows her to complete the journey to and from the pizza shop in only ten minutes.

Christopher then acts a bit foolishly. He reasons that as buying one bicycle for his daughter made the trip faster, then two bicycles would make it quicker still. Just to make sure, he purchases Louise five new bicycles, which he hopes will have his pizza delivered piping hot, only seconds after Giovanni bakes it.

Of course, Christopher's strategy fails miserably, for Louise can ride only one bicycle at a time. The other bicycles stay in the garage, until Louise graduates from high school ten years later when they are donated to charity.

The bicycle is a perfect example of a catalyst: it speeds up a natural occurrence, and makes the routine task far more efficient. However, note that the bicycle *cannot do anything by itself*. Furthermore, the bicycle—the catalyst—is not permanently affected or used up by this process.

Vitamins work in exactly the same way as the bicycle: they assist and accelerate normal bodily reactions, but *do not do anything by themselves*. Nor are they used up, or permanently changed, by the process.

Just as extra bicycles did not further shorten Louise's trip time, taking higher doses of vitamins and minerals doesn't produce any additional improvement in your bodily function. As soon as you have enough of these substances in your body, extra supplements are of no benefit whatsoever. They are strained out by your liver, and end up down the toilet.

The health food industry argues that, due to our hectic modern lifestyle and excessive food processing, most of us do not naturally obtain the nutrition that our bodies require. Here they have a fair argument. Commonsense will tell you that an occasional pick-me-up like a multivitamin pill will do neither your body nor your wallet any harm. I am not protesting against commonsense nutritional augmentation. However, I hope to convince you to interpret with a good dose of scepticism the specific and sometimes extravagant claims made by many so-called health foods, particularly those that relate to back pain.

It's an interesting exercise to compare the claims of natural remedies with those of medical drugs. For any drug company to make a claim about what a particular medication will cure, government regulations insist that they repeatedly and rigorously test it. They must compare the test results with a control group who take nothing but a placebo, and must check and recheck for effects and side effects. Only when the drug has been thoroughly proven to work are the manufacturers permitted to release it for general prescription.

Here's the silly bit. Because food supplements, vitamins and minerals are not drugs, the government does not require them to undergo any testing procedures. Nor are the manufacturers of natural remedies limited in how they advertise or promote their products, and they do not have to scientifically justify any claims that they make about the product's effects. The manufacturers of natural or food-based products can make virtually whatever claim they like, without having to provide any hard evidence that it is true.

Does this policy sound ridiculous to you? If so, then you should seriously question the value of the supposed claims on the label or marketing brochure of any such product. *Buyer beware!*

When evaluating the claims of any health product, ask yourself the following questions. The answers will help you to decide how rigorously its assertions would hold under proper evaluation.

(1) HOW WERE THE CLAIMS PROVEN?
In most cases, a natural supplement will have no proof whatsoever that it does what it claims. To be accepted as a reliable, genuine treatment option, the product must have been repeatedly tested by reputable, *unbiased* research groups on a large sample of people. Furthermore, at least one study must have compared the product's effects to a placebo. Very few natural products have been submitted to this level of scrutiny.

Many products use testimonials as 'proof' of their healing powers. The marketing material provides pages of quotes, case histories and glowing letters from grateful devotees, each assuring you of the wondrous benefits of the product. These testimonials, even if they are true, are not worth the paper on which they are printed.

Vested interests, bias, outright fibs, and, of course, the placebo effect, make such advertising an insult to your intelligence. Please, do not ever be coerced into buying a product by testimonials alone.

(2) WHAT ARE THE SIDE EFFECTS IF I TAKE TOO MUCH?
Every action has a reaction, so any substance that has an active effect on your body will probably have side effects. If a product professes to have wonderful healing powers yet no side effects, even if you swallow the whole bottleful, then a red light of doubt should immediately flash in your mind.

(3) DOES IT CLAIM TO CURE A WIDE RANGE OF PROBLEMS OR ILLNESSES?

Commonsense dictates that the more generalised a treatment, the less specific it can be to a particular condition. If an additive or supplement is supposed to help a range of unrelated conditions, from period pain to impotence to insomnia to acne, then you can be assured that its effect on something as local and identifiable as a back injury will be negligible.

(4) WHERE DOES THE PRODUCT COME FROM?

You should immediately be suspicious of any product that is only available by mail order, or from only one location. Similarly, you should doubt any health product that is sold door-to-door, via pyramid sales schemes, or over the Internet. In short, you should question the validity of any product that is promoted directly to the public, rather than through registered health professionals.

Immediately forget any product that is made from a 'secret formula' or one for which the manufacturer claims to have rediscovered an ancient 'Chinese/Japanese/Indian/insert-your-favourite-exotic-minority' remedy.

Generally, you may find it useful to think about this question: if you were trying to sell a product of dubious therapeutic benefit, how would you market it? Would you sell this product through educated professionals who will ask you lots of tough questions, or would you advertise direct to the public in a magazine?

Do I sound like a hardened sceptic? I hope so. And I hope that I have convinced you to use some healthy scepticism when evaluating any back pain treatment from a bottle, whether it be a natural or medicinal product. Please demand proof, hard proof, of their efficacy. And I don't mean an advertising brochure in a chemist or health food shop, either.

I realise that the proposition is tempting. Simply change your diet for a few weeks, swallow a few tablets, or add a sprinkling of some magic herb to your tea each morning, and two weeks later you're pain-free forever. Sorry, it just doesn't happen. Spinal problems are far too complex and varied to be cured by such a simple solution. As with drugs, the easy way out just does not work.

A good healthy diet—sure. Occasional generalised augmentation with a multivitamin or other food supplement for overall good health—why not? But to anyone considering a natural remedy that claims to cure your back pain or arthritis, I have only one thing to say: Why give yourself expensive urine?

26
Fitness and exercise
How sweat can cure your back pain

Hippocrates, 2400 years ago, said the following wise words:

All parts of the body which have a function, if used in moderation and exercised in labours to which each is accustomed, become thereby healthy and well developed and age slowly; but if unused and left idle, they become liable to disease, defective in growth, and age quickly. This is especially the case with joints and ligaments if one does not use them.

Hippocrates would have made a great spinal health practitioner.

Being generally fit and healthy brings many advantages to your back pain management program. Recent studies have shown that regular exercise is one of the simplest yet most effective ways of improving your spinal pain. Not only that, but exercise has many positive 'side effects'.

In this chapter, we'll firstly look at the benefits that regular cardiovascular exercise bestows upon your spine, which I hope will provide you with some additional motivation to start an exercise program. Then we'll look at the specifics: the how-when-which-where-what of making aerobic exercise part of your daily routine.

Advantages that regular cardiovascular exercise confers upon your spine

1. YOU WILL LOSE WEIGHT
As you read in Chapter 25, extra body weight increases the risk of your spine accumulating microtrauma. This risk is multiplied when you bend or lift, meaning that any extra kilograms can be an even greater liability than you might assume.

Regular, prolonged cardiovascular exercise is an excellent way of reducing weight, and so directly benefits your spine not just while you are exercising, but virtually every other waking minute of your life.

2. YOU WILL INCREASE YOUR PHYSICAL TOLERANCE TO STRESS

Regular exercise is great for just about every bodily system. Your heart, lungs and circulatory system were all designed with regular movement in mind. Even your bowels need regular exercise to work efficiently; if you're ever feeling a bit clogged up, go for a jog and see what happens!

When your major bodily organs are working efficiently, the health benefits flow through to the rest of your body. If you are generally healthy, then your body and mind—and that weak link at the bottom of your spine called your lower back—can cope with the normal stresses and strains of everyday life without capitulating.

3. YOUR STRESS LEVEL WILL DECREASE

Not only will exercise help to increase your tolerance to stress, but it can decrease your overall stress level. There are many mechanisms by which exercise helps you to feel more relaxed.

First, prolonged gentle exercise encourages the brain to release chemicals called *endorphins*. Endorphins, which are chemically similar to morphine, are a natural pain-killer and relaxant. Long-distance athletes such as 100-kilometre ultra-marathon runners sometimes enter a state called a 'runner's high' in which the level of endorphins in their bloodstream is so high that they literally feel no pain. You may not achieve quite this level of euphoria with your undoubtedly more modest exercise regime, but you will hopefully experience the natural relaxing and pain-relieving effects of endorphins in a more subtle way.

There are also psychological reasons that exercise helps to decrease stress. On a most basic level, physical exercise helps you to work out your aggression in a non-violent way. In Japan, some companies have a room in which pictures of the boss are taped onto a dummy. Disgruntled employees can punch, kick, thump, or otherwise attack the dummy-boss in any way they please. In this way, the worker can dissipate his or her frustrations before they accrue to a dangerous, health-affecting level. The physical demands of sport and exercise serve a similar function, although obviously in a less conspicuous way.

Furthermore, many people find that the regular, soothing rhythm of a steady jog, swim or ride has a calming, hypnotic effect.

Others find exercise relaxing because it allows them some uninterrupted time to themselves. In this fast-paced, 24-hour-a-day, rapidly changing world, some quiet, private time should be considered not only a privilege, but a necessity.

A friend of mine, when asked why he liked a sport as repetitive and boring as swimming laps up and down the pool, replied that anyone who dislikes the peaceful solitude of swimming laps obviously doesn't work hard enough at their job. His reply overstates the case, but makes the point that while exercising, you can leave your busy work life, hectic schedules and constant interruptions behind for half an hour.

Please do not doubt the stress-relieving properties of regular exercise. They are very real, and a more-than-useful partner in your fight against back pain.

4. YOU WILL STRENGTHEN YOUR BONES
Before you continue, answer this simple multiple-choice question.

Q. At approximately what age do your bones stop regenerating and growing?
(a) At puberty—between the ages of ten and fourteen.
(b) When you stop growing—between the ages of sixteen and twenty-one.
(c) For women, at menopause, and for men, at about forty years of age.
(d) Never. Even the bones of a 100-year-old are constantly growing and regenerating.

If you answered a, b, or c, then you may be surprised to know that your bones never stop growing. They are not, as you may imagine, dead and stagnant, but constantly update and replace themselves.

Furthermore, your bones are very reactive to outside forces, and grow stronger in response to exercise, just like muscles. Bones not only increase their density when you exercise, but cleverly manage to lay the new bone in the areas of greatest need. So regular weight-bearing exercise will not only strengthen your bones, and so prevent stress fractures, but will guard against osteoporosis.

5. YOU WILL KEEP YOUR JOINTS MOVING
Your spine, like most joints in the body, requires regular movement to maintain its extensibility and suppleness. The smooth linings of cartilage that cover your joint surfaces do not have a blood supply. If they did, then the blood vessels would soon be squashed as the bones rubbed together.

Instead, the joints rely on a special fluid for their nutrition, called *synovial fluid*. Each time you move a joint, the fluid washes over the joint surfaces, lubricating and feeding them, just as polish nourishes leather. Of course, if you don't move your joints, the cartilage is not fed, and it soon becomes brittle and weak, just like a piece of leather left out in the sun.

Because cardiovascular exercise generally requires large movements of all body parts, it is useful for maintaining general joint function.

Sport provides an added benefit of repetitive movement, without the dreariness of thousands of repetitions of a stretching exercise.

6. YOU WILL MAINTAIN MUSCLE TONE
General exercises will also increase your basic level of spinal muscle tone. Particularly if you are unfit or normally sedentary, this extra tone and strength will benefit your spine enormously.

However, be aware that increased strength from sports or gym is likely to be accrued by the mobilising muscles, rather than the injury-preventing stabilising muscles. To lessen the risk of your exercise program causing a muscle imbalance, you should add some stability exercises, as outlined in Chapter 14, to your warm-up or cool-down phases.

Guidelines and frequently asked questions about exercise

WHAT ACTIVITY IS BEST FOR MY BACK PAIN TYPE?
The most important factor in choosing an exercise activity is that you should enjoy it. As *regular* exercise over a *long period* is the key to accruing benefits, you will benefit from choosing a fun and relaxing activity. If you keenly anticipate your exercise sessions, then you will find it far easier to form a long-lasting habit.

Furthermore, you must have the facilities handy. There is little point in choosing swimming if your nearest pool is an hour's drive away, or in commencing a cycling program if you don't own a decent bicycle.

Of course, your chosen activity must fulfil three qualifying criteria. First, it must get you moving: big, whole body movements, using your arms, legs and spine. Second, the activity should increase your heart rate and make you puff. Third, you should be capable of sustaining the activity over a long period, making it an *aerobic* activity.

Sorry, but bridge, poker, canasta, 500, chess, Doom, tic-tac-toe and pinball do not count as aerobic exercises. Nor does watching sport on television, not even if you watch an entire iron-man triathlon from start to finish. Instead, you should choose an activity that makes you puff— not so much that you can't carry on a conversation, but not so little that your respiration rate barely deepens. Walking, running, swimming, cycling and rowing are the most obvious examples. Other common choices include rollerblading, surfing, kayaking and bushwalking.

Your back pain type serves as a useful indicator as to which of the major aerobic sports is likely to be of most benefit to your spinal problem. As a rule, type A spines will be best suited to activities in which your spine is held in flexion, such as rowing. The opposite holds true for type B spines, for whom activities such as walking will be the least likely to cause any exacerbation. Conversely, stiff spines such as types C and D may benefit from activities that encourage their spine to move into the stiffest direction, particularly if the initial sessions are controlled and gentle.

The table below provides a guide in this regard. These suggestions are very general, and while many exceptions will exist, they should at least increase your chances of choosing an activity that suits your back problem.

Table 26.1
Suitability of common sports for each back type

Key to symbols

?	This activity may make your problem worse, so proceed with caution.
+	Your spine will probably tolerate this activity.
++	Your spine should tolerate this activity, and will probably improve if you begin gently, then gradually increase your workload.
+++	Your spine should improve with this activity, if you gradually increase your workload.

	Swim	Walk	Run	Bicycle*	Row
Type A	+	?/+	?	++	++
Type B	++	++	+	?/+	?
Type C	+++	+++	++	++	++
Type D	++	++	++	++	+++

* The data for bicycling assumes that you are riding in a 'race' position—leaning forward with your weight on the handlebars. If you intend to use an exercise bike in an upright sitting position, then the data for walking is more appropriate.

If after three weeks you find that your problem is worsening, then substitute the suggestions for type A with type C, or type B with type D, and vice versa. Of course, you should not expect that one or two exercise sessions will instantly or permanently cure your pain. But if you persist at your program for a month or two, I'll *virtually guarantee* you that you will feel better. Persistence *will* pay off!

WHAT PRECAUTIONS SHOULD I TAKE BEFORE EXERCISE?

If you are over forty or grossly unfit, then you should consult your doctor for a general health check before commencing any exercise program. A *stress ECG*, in which your doctor can study your heart's reaction to exercise, is a useful screening device for cardiac problems.

FITNESS AND EXERCISE

Furthermore, you should warm up your spine before playing any vigorous sport or activity. The stretching and stability exercises that you learned in Chapter 14 provide an excellent guide.

Please remember—this point is very important, and frequently overlooked—unstable spines need muscular activation, not just stretching, during your warm-up. The exercises to reactivate and awaken your stability muscles are just as important in any good warm-up routine as are the stretching routines, particularly if you have an unstable spine.

The stability exercises are not taxing, and will not induce fatigue. In contrast, the stability exercises awaken and facilitate the muscles, and prepare them for the very important job of protecting your spine.

Many sporting teams, even those with professional coaches and conditioners, often fail to observe this simple principle, and then wonder why so many of their players constantly injure themselves. To avoid the disappointment of re-injuring your spine, you should perform some simple, low-key stability exercises as outlined in Chapter 14 before you next attempt a vigorous or different sport or activity. Your back will thank you for it.

HOW OFTEN SHOULD I EXERCISE?

Aerobic exercise is most effective when performed four to six times per week. If you exercise less frequently, the benefits will be so slow to arrive that you may become frustrated. On the other hand, you should allow at least one day of rest each week for your body and spine to recover. Even Olympic athletes schedule rest days into their training regimes.

When you start your exercise program, I suggest that you perform an easy session *every* day, with just one rest day per week. This regularity will help you to develop the habit of exercising, and will keep you motivated. After three weeks you can then exercise with the frequency and intensity that your lifestyle and commitment suggest—perhaps four or five times per week.

HOW LONG AND HOW HARD SHOULD I EXERCISE?

Below is a concise summary of generally accepted exercise guidelines. By using a stopwatch and your heart rate as a guide, you can easily gauge the correct intensity and distance for each session. Don't worry about measuring distances, performing time trials, working high repetition speed sets, or any other such techniques. You can add these elements into your program later if you wish. Simply use gentle, sustained, regular exercise along the following guidelines, and you will progress just dandily.

The first column of Table 26.2 indicates your average fitness level, which you will have to estimate. If you have not performed any regular exercise over the last six months then you are probably a beginner. If you usually play sport once or twice per week then you may be at the intermediate level, while those of you who qualify for the advanced group will already be training regularly. You should also consider the physical demands of your occupation when making this estimate.

The second and third columns show the period, in minutes, for which you should sustain your exercise session. As a hard day of training should always be followed by an easier effort, two figures are provided—one for more intense days, and another for lighter 'recovery' sessions. If you are training six days of the week, then I suggest that you alternate between these two figures. If you are exercising four times per week, then you should use the higher figure for most sessions, as your body will have ample time for recovery on your rest days.

The fourth column shows the percentage of your maximum heart rate at which you should aim to train. These figures—60%, 70% and 80%—are generally accepted exercise guidelines for each fitness level.

Your maximum heart rate, which you can estimate by deducting your age from 220, is shown in brackets at the top of the next five columns, along with your age group. The figures in these columns provide a ready reckoner to indicate your target heart rate, which you should aim to sustain during your entire exercise session.

Table 26.2
Exercise guidelines: Duration and heart rate

Level	Mins on Hard Day	Mins on Easy Day	Heart Rate % of max	Target Heart Rate by Age Group				
				25–35 (190)	35–45 (180)	45–55 (170)	55–65 (160)	65–75+ (150)
Beginner	20	15	60%	114	108	102	96	90
Intermediate	25	20	70%	133	126	119	112	105
Advanced	35	25	80%	152	144	136	128	120

Let's consider two examples.

Lolita is a fifty-six-year-old teacher who has rarely exercised. She decides to embark upon a walking program four days per week. She rates herself as a beginner, and, by reading the above chart, knows that she should walk for 20 minutes each day, and should keep her pulse rate at about 96 beats per minute.

Jock is a thirty-one-year-old labourer, who finished his football career only two years previously due to ongoing back and hamstring problems. He embarks upon a swimming program that he hopes will decrease his pain and stiffness, as well as burn off a few extra kilograms. As he is still reasonably fit, Jock rates himself in the intermediate category. By consulting the above table, Jock sees that he should swim for about 25 minutes, at a pace such that his pulse rate stays at about 133 beats per minute. The following day he should swim a recovery session of about 20 minutes.

HOW SHOULD I PROGRESS MY PROGRAM?
The most important rule of exercise progression is to proceed slowly. Many people drop out of exercise programs because they pushed themselves too hard, too early, and became tired, injured or, most likely, disenchanted.

By contrast, very few people quit self-paced exercise programs because they found it too easy.

The most objective way to steadily improve your fitness level is to increase the *duration* of each session by 10% every two weeks. Keep adding to the time by these small increments every two weeks, without increasing your intensity.

When you have reached the recommended time limit for the next level, keep your session duration the same, and instead progress your program by increasing your intensity.

To do this, simply increase your target heart rate by 10% every two weeks, until it, too, reaches the next stage. Then you should slowly increase your session time again until you reach the next level, whereupon you should again incrementally raise your target heart rate.

By gradually incrementing your distance and then your target heart rate, you will steadily progress through the fitness levels without the all-too-common side effects of excessive early enthusiasm.

For example, suppose that Lolita, from our example above, dutifully completes her first two weeks of walking. She has been exercising for 20 minutes per day, four times per week, and has kept a slow but steady pace so that her heart rate hovered around 96 beats per minute. She now must add 10% to the time of her daily walk.

To simplify calculations, Lolita simply adds six seconds per minute. For example, she adds $20 \times 6 = 120$ seconds, meaning her new session time is 22 minutes. After a further two weeks she adds a further 10%, increasing her walk time to 24 minutes and 12 seconds. (For simplicity, you can round the figures to the nearest minute, but I'll keep them precise for this example.) After her next progression, Lolita finds that her new time of 26.36 minutes is now in the intermediate range.

Two weeks later, Lolita is ready for another step up. This time, she keeps her exercise time period the same, but increases her target heart rate by 10%. She finds that by walking more quickly she can raise her heart rate to 105 beats per minutes, which is about 10% above her old target rate of 96 beats. After two further weeks, Lolita raises her target heart rate by a further ten, bringing it to 116 beats per minute—also in the intermediate range.

In less than three months, Lolita has safely and slowly improved her fitness from an unfit novice to a healthy intermediate-level performer. The increments were so carefully controlled that at no stage did she feel distressed or overly tired. What a simple way to make yourself feel better!

WHAT HAPPENS IF I MISS SOME TRAINING SESSIONS?

Never try to make up a lost session by cramming it in the next day, particularly if you are training hard. Simply put the missed session out of your mind, and continue the next day as if nothing happened.

If you miss up to two weeks of training, you should return to your previous level. However, if you have missed more than two weeks, then I suggest you drop back by 10%, and then gradually move forward again.

WHAT ABOUT HYDROTHERAPY AND AQUA-AEROBICS?

Because hydrotherapy and aqua-aerobics are performed in water, the spinal stresses and strains are minimised while exercising. You can take advantage of this buoyancy by stretching your joints and working your body more safely and/or vigorously than you could on land. Furthermore, some custom-designed hydrotherapy pools are heated, and so provide extra loosening for tight spinal muscles and joints.

Hydrotherapy is an excellent exercise choice for many people, including elderly people, those with easily exacerbated pain, overweight people, and injured athletes who must maintain cardiovascular fitness while waiting for an injury to heal.

When exercising in water, the speed of your movement will affect its outcome. If you perform a movement slowly, then the water will provide buoyancy, making these actions ideal for stretching. Conversely, if you move quickly, then the water will provide resistance, and so can be used for muscle strengthening and toning. Water also provides a medium for a hard, yet safe, cardiovascular work-out, from which your body will recover rapidly.

Hydrotherapy classes are available at most public pools, most of which now have either spinal health practitioners or registered instructors to guide you through the movements. Alternatively, you can choreograph your own session.

A good hydrotherapy session should begin with slow stretching movements, progress to cardiovascular routines, and then add faster power-building exercises, before finishing with a warm-down. The content can be as wide and varied as your imagination itself.

You will probably achieve the best results if you establish an aim for your sessions, and incorporate each element around that goal. For example, suppose your aim is to stretch your spine and to increase flexibility. Here, the stretching exercises in Chapter 14 provide an excellent starting point, as you can readily adjust most of the movements so that you can perform them in water. Conversely, if your aim is to increase your muscle tone, then you should intersperse stability exercises with fast-paced twisting, moving and kicking activities.

Other activities such as cycling and running lend themselves to hydrotherapy. No, I'm not suggesting that you ride your old rusty Malvern Star along the bottom of the pool. Heavens, the streamers on the handlebars would get soggy! Rather, you can imitate the actions of other sports in the water, using buoyancy vests if appropriate. For example, you may wish to run or ride 'on the spot' for a few minutes. Or perhaps you could try some short 'sprints' of, say, ten or twenty seconds, followed by timed recovery breaks. Don't be afraid to throw in a few laps of swimming as part of your hydrotherapy session.

ARE THOSE EXERCISE MACHINES THAT I SEE ADVERTISED ON TELEVISION ANY GOOD?

Every year the fitness industry markets yet another whiz-bang exercise machine that will 'firm and tone your muscles, and burn away fat and kilojoules, without causing any stress to your joints'. These contraptions utilise a variety of mechanisms, with early models resembling exercise bicycles with arm levers, while later developments have included all manner of sliding, gliding, riding, skiing or pumping gizmos. They always seem to have names such as 'Ezi Glider 4000' or 'Trim Toner 2000'. I'm not sure what the numbers mean, but there you go.

In theory, most of these machines seem generally sound. Their actions fulfil the criteria of any good cardiovascular exercise program in that they use large body movements, raise your pulse rate, and can be sustained for the required length of time. Furthermore, most of these machines really *are* kind to your joints, with a minimum of jarring.

My only concern is born from years of observation: if you purchase one of these machines, it will probably end up in the cupboard under the stairs, along with the exercise bike, the mini-trampoline and all of the other failed attempts at starting a fitness program. In my experience, very few people manage to maintain an ongoing habit of exercising on a stationary machine. Be honest, do you really think you'll still be exercising on one of these machines in two year's time?

Yet thousands of people walk, jog, swim or ride their way to health and fitness every day, and many make it a lifelong habit. If I were you I'd ignore the hype surrounding latest gizmo machines, take up walking, save yourself $300, and use it to visit the coast for the weekend instead.

Other sports and activities

Obviously, sports such as football, tennis, squash and basketball also demand a high level of aerobic fitness. However, the high-velocity, uncontrolled nature of these sports means that they are less likely to cure your back pain. I do not mean to imply that if you have a sore back then you should not play these sports. If you play them for fun, fitness and competition, fine. However, I would not start playing one of these sports if your only motivation is to help your back problem.

Nevertheless, certain spine types are more suited to particular sports and activities than others. The following lists provide a rough guide. As before, there will be many exceptions.

The first column shows pastimes that generally require lots of spinal extension. They should be approached with caution by those of you with type A spines. Type C backs may find these choices OK, so long as you begin slowly, and allow your spine plenty of time to adapt to the extra demand. Most people with type B or D spines should be able to cope with these activities without too much trouble.

Conversely, the second column gives examples of sports that tend to be more flexion orientated. Hence, you type Bs out there should appoach these activities with caution, while type D spines should ensure that they start slowly. If you are a type A or C, then your spine will probably cope just fine with the activites in the second list.

Type A: Approach with caution **Type C: Begin slowly** **Types B & D: Less likely to have trouble**	**Type B: Approach with caution** **Type D: Begin slowly** **Types A & C: Less likely to have trouble**
Athletics	Billiards & snooker
Basketball	Canoeing
Cricket (bowling)	Cricket (batting)
Diving	Croquet
Football (all codes)	Cycling
Gymnastics	Golf
Surfing	Kayaking
Tennis	Lawn bowls
Volleyball	Motor racing
Water skiing	Hockey
Weightlifting (Olympic)	Rowing
Wrestling	Squash

If you play a sport that you think might hurt your spine, or you are unsure about a certain activity, then use the following guidelines to evaluate its suitability.

GUIDELINES FOR ASSESSING THE SUITABILITY OF A SPORT OR ACTIVITY FOR YOUR SPINE

If your back

(a) does not hurt while you are performing the activity
(b) does not ache when you have cooled down, and
(c) is no stiffer the following morning

then this activity is a good choice for your spine. Please continue with this activity, even if your well-meaning neighbour insists that it will ruin your back.

However, if you feel pain during or after exercise, then your decision is not as simple. When you first feel your pain increasing, continue your activity at a reduced intensity for about ten or fifteen minutes. Observe the response of your back pain, then work through the following guidelines.

- Your pain became worse as the session progressed
  If your pain continued to worsen as the session progressed, then this activity was probably not suitable for your spine at this time. I suggest that you avoid this activity for awhile—say three weeks— and retest yourself when your spine has improved. In the meanwhile, you can try other forms of exercise.

- Your pain stayed the same as the session progressed
  If your pain did not change as you continued to exercise through the session, then it *may* be alright for your spine. However, if your spine ached for more than two hours after you cooled down, or was noticeably stiffer the following morning than it was the previous morning, then the activity probably inflamed your spine.
  Here, I suggest that you choose a different activity for a while. Alternatively, you could try decreasing the time, intensity or distance by a quarter and retesting yourself two days later. If the stiffness and pain return, then try a different activity for awhile.

- Your pain gradually dissipated as the session progressed
  After your spine warmed up, you may have found that your pain gradually decreased. In this case, the activity is probably alright for your spine, and you should find that the aches lessen as you become

fitter. However, if you find that your spine aches for more than two hours after the activity, or is noticeably stiffer the next morning, then you should consider reducing the intensity or distance for a few weeks.

You can use these guidelines to evaluate any sport or activity. From lawn bowls to lacrosse, wrestling to rock-climbing and croquet to karate, the above guidelines will help you to evaluate whether your passion is helping or hurting your back. You may be pleasantly surprised to discover the tremendous spinal benefits of a long-forgotten favourite pastime.

These guidelines are also useful to evaluate work duties, or other home tasks, such as gardening. In general, you can use them to analyse the effect of any prolonged or repetitive task on your spinal condition.

Summary of how to organise your exercise program

1. Consult Table 26.1, and select an activity that suits your back pain. Make sure that you choose an exercise that you enjoy, and one for which you have the facilities readily available.
2. Have a medical check up, if necessary.
3. Consult Table 26.2 to determine your exercise duration and pulse rate targets.
4. Warm up your spine, using stretches *and* stability exercises as outlined in Chapter 14.
5. Start. *Today!*
6. Do not miss a day for three weeks. Establish a habit of exercising.
7. Progress slowly and steadily, by no more than 10% every two weeks, as described above.
8. If you feel back pain while exercising, then evaluate the activity using the guidelines above. Reduce or change your activity, if necessary.
9. Enjoy your new healthier lifestyle. You will soon be trimmer, healthier, more relaxed, more flexible and stronger. Your back pain will decrease as well. What are you waiting for? Get sweaty—it's good for your spine!

27
X-rays and scans

*The diagnosis you have when you're
not having a diagnosis*

This chapter has an interesting format. First, I am going to tell you about the various types of X-rays and scans that spinal health practitioners sometimes use to help diagnose your back pain. We'll discuss which type of test is best for each condition, and tell you all of the clever things that these complex, sophisticated machines can do. Then, to round off our discussion, I'll explain why everything that I've told you about radiology with regard to back pain is wrong.

Radiology for back pain uses four main modalities:

(1) X-rays
(2) CT scans, also called CAT scans (computerised axial tomography)
(3) MRI (magnetic resonance imaging)
(4) nuclear bone scans.

Let's briefly examine these modalities individually, and see what they can tell you about the source of your back pain.

X-rays

Most people are familiar with a standard X-ray. These machines work by shooting a beam of radiation through your spine, which is picked up on the other side on a film, or plate. Because your bones do not allow the radioactive beam to pass through as readily as the other tissues, your bones show up as white on the X-ray. Hence, the developed prints depict a 'shadow' of the bones.

X-rays are very limited in what they can detect—far more limited than most people realise. They show a shadow of the bones, and virtually nothing else. Nevertheless, X-rays may be useful in the following situations:

- Plain X-rays are a useful screening device following trauma (such as a motor vehicle or sporting accident), as they readily show serious injuries such as fractures.

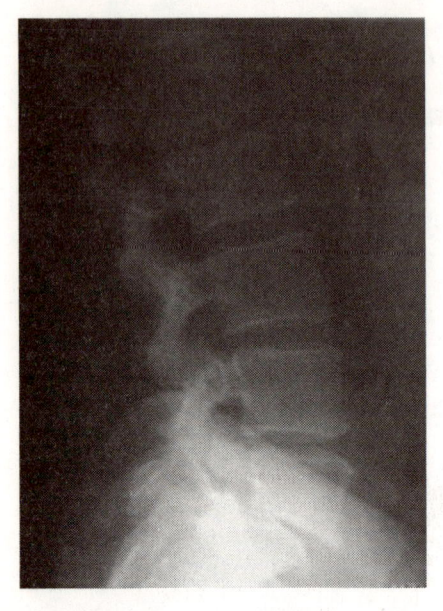

A standard X-ray of your lumbar spine—a 'shadow' of the bones. (N.B. If you look carefully you may see that the bottom vertebra has slipped forward a bit on the sacrum.)

- Although X-rays do not show the disc tissue, the height of the disc can be estimated by looking at the distance between the vertebrae. A decrease in disc height may indicate deterioration or spondylosis.
- A displaced vertebrae or large stress fractures can also be detected. However, small stress fractures are often undetectable on normal X-ray pictures.
- The surfaces of the facet and sacro-iliac joints can be seen, showing if any major degenerative changes are present.
- The general alignment of the vertebrae is displayed, which some practitioners interpret to help realign your spine.

As X-rays are quick, easy and cheap, they are ordered more frequently than any other screening test. Unfortunately, X-rays do not show disc tissue, ligaments, nerves, tendons or muscles, and so miss a huge proportion of the causes of low back pain.

CT scans

CT scans (computerised axial tomography—also known as CAT scans) are more complex than X-rays. They work by firing a pattern of multiple X-rays through your back, and detecting the amount of energy that passes through. A computer then analyses the data, and forms a cross-sectional picture of your spine. A series of these cross-sectional pictures is taken, which provides a far more accurate picture of the internal workings of the spine than does a plain X-ray film.

As such, CT scans supersede all of the uses for plain X-rays as discussed above, as well as being useful in the following areas:

- They can demonstrate the intervertebral disc, and so can show major bulges and herniations.
- They provide a more accurate assessment of any degenerative changes.

- Smaller injuries, such as stress fractures, can be detected with greater accuracy.
- CT scans also show muscles, and so can provide an estimate of their size, which can be used to spot long-term weakness.
- The intervertebral canal and spinal cord tunnels can be examined to see if the nerves have enough room to pass through them unimpeded.
- CT scans can also 'see inside' your back, and so can detect nasty causes of lower back pain, such as tumours.

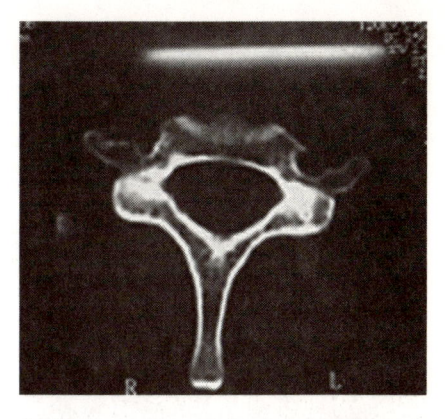

A CT scan of a vertebra, viewed from the top. The vertebra appears in cross-section, which can provide additional insights. (N.B. Just in case any radiologists are reading, I should confess that this is a thoracic vertebra, not a lumbar vertebra. A slight difference in shape is the clue.)

While CT scans provide far more information than plain X-rays, they are still limited by a fairly low resolution. As such, they cannot accurately detect injuries to finer structures such as ligaments, tendons or nerves.

MRI

MRI (Magnetic Resonance Imaging) uses magnetic fields and radio waves to create cross-sectional pictures of the spine. The images are created by analysing the response of the molecules to radiation, so the images are finely detailed. These state-of-the-art scanners can accurately depict almost any lower back structure in two or even three dimensions. MRI scans can detect subtle ligament and nerve injuries, as well as minor fractures that are invisible to all other forms of radiology. Tiny tumours can be detected, as well as pockets of inflammation or infection.

In short, MRI scanning provides a wonderfully detailed picture of your spine. The major disadvantages of this modality are its high cost, and its time-consuming nature. If you're claustrophobic, then you'd hate the MRI experience, as it demands that you lie very still in a small tunnel for half an hour or so. MRI scanning has another significant advantage in that it does not, like X-rays and CT scans, expose you to any electromagnetic radiation, thus lessening the chance of side effects, such as cancer.

BACK PAIN

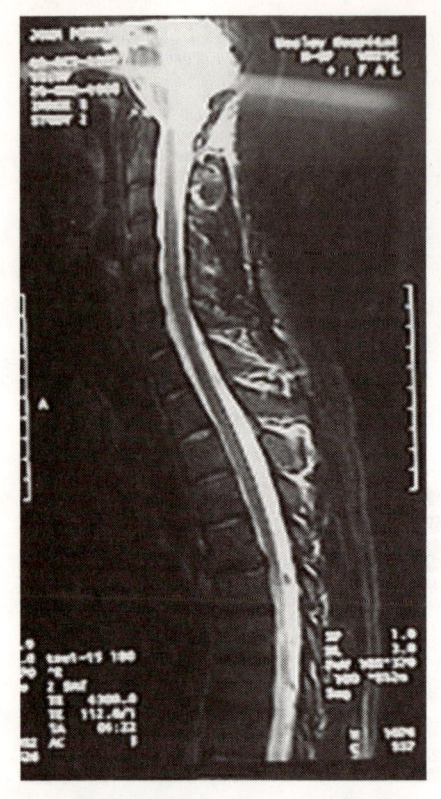

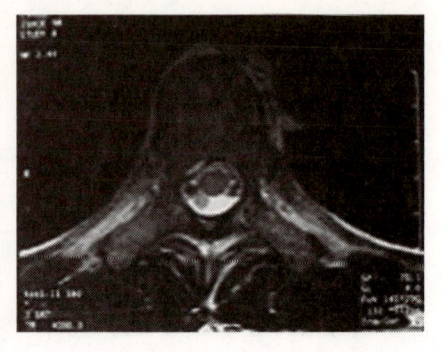

Two MRI scans. The picture on the left depicts a cross-sectional side-on view of the whole spinal column. That bright thing down the middle is the spinal cord. The block-like structures to the left of it are the vertebral bodies.

The right picture shows a cross-sectional view of a single vertebra. By comparing it to the previous CT image, you can appreciate the extra detail revealed by an MRI scan. Those squiggly little lines and blobs all have great meaning to a trained eye. By referring to pictures in the first section of this book, you should easily be able to spot the spinal cord, the vertebral body, and the transverse processes.

Bone scans

Before you have a bone scan, a doctor injects radioactive chemicals into your blood stream. After a couple of hours or so, the radiologist uses a camera to detect the radioactivity that your body is emitting. As an inflamed site attracts more blood, and hence more radioactivity, than does normal tissue, the injury will show up as a 'hot spot' on the developed print.

Bone scans are useful for detecting sensitive injuries, as the changes in an injured cell may occur before any structural changes are evident. However, bone scans have the disadvantage that they cannot accurately localise the source of pain. A hot spot only shows a general area of concern, rather than a specific structure.

How effective is radiology in diagnosing the source of back pain?

Any doctor will verify that radiology is an inherent and important part of the investigation of many medical conditions. However, despite this fact, and the information above, you will soon see why radiology has a limited place in the investigation of most cases of low back pain.

As mentioned above, recent advances in radiology, such as MRI scanning, can now provide a very accurate, detailed picture of your spine. So does this mean that the source of your pain can now be accurately diagnosed in almost every case? Unfortunately, no, it doesn't.

Even perfect, finely localised scanners such as MRI play a minor role in the diagnosis of lower back pain for two main reasons:

(1) They often show major problems in people with healthy, pain-free spines, i.e. false positive findings.
(2) They often show that nothing is wrong at all, even in patients with severe pain, i.e. false negative findings.

Let's look at these two related areas to discover the limitations of radiology in diagnosing your lower back pain.

FALSE POSITIVE FINDINGS

The hope that improved scans such as MRI would diagnose lower back pain with greater accuracy turned out to be forlorn, as unfortunately these scans frequently detect alarming abnormalities in normal, asymptomatic people.

One study performed MRI scans on a large group of people who had never experienced any lower back or leg pain, and whose spines were clinically in perfect condition. The results showed that about fifty per cent of these completely healthy people had at least one bulging intervertebral disc. Furthermore, about twenty per cent had a herniated disc, which is usually cited as a cause of severe lower back pain.

In the older population, the statistics were even more revealing. Nearly eighty per cent of pain-free subjects over the age of 60 had a bulging disc evident on their MRI scan, while more than a third had a herniated disc. Just about every subject had signs of arthritis, while about twenty per cent had spinal stenosis. Remember, these subjects were people who were experiencing no back pain or stiffness whatsoever.

Other studies have shown that roughly half of all people who have a displaced vertebra, spina bifida, or an extra vertebra have absolutely no pain at all. About forty per cent of patients whose MRI scan shows that they have Scheuermann's disease, a condition that is often blamed for severe thoracic stiffness and pain, have no history of back trouble.

These studies, as well as many other recent investigations, suggest that X-rays, CT or MRI scans often provide false positive results. The 'abnormalities' that they detect are in fact normal occurrences, and probably have nothing to do with the patient's current problem. Detailed scanning technology has taught us that problems such as degenerative changes and bulging discs in the lower back are so common as to be considered normal, and are clearly not necessarily painful or debilitating.

FALSE NEGATIVES

In contrast to the above findings, many patients with disabling pain have X-rays or scans that show nothing abnormal at all. Even people with extremely severe, chronic pain may have an MRI scan that shows everything is 100% okay. This lack of an identifiable pathology disturbs many people, and often creates consternation if the case is part of a legal claim.

A clear scan or X-ray does *not* indicate that there is nothing wrong with your spine, and it definitely does not imply that your symptoms are all in your head. The reason that scans often show up as 'nothing abnormal detected' is that they cannot detect the *real* cause of lower back problems.

Can you remember our discussion in Chapter 10, in which you learned that most spinal pain is caused by movement abnormalities, such as *stiffness* or *instability*. These factors cannot be reliably detected by even very accurate scans, no matter how powerful their resolution. This simple fact explains why even a severe back problem may not show up on a scan.

To further explain this concept, take a close look at the picture below. Study it carefully, and try to spot any variations between the three jars.

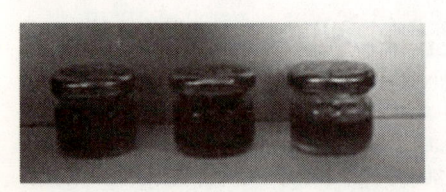

Spot the difference!

X-RAYS AND SCANS

You probably cannot see any obvious differences between these three jars. The differences are even more difficult to spot in the second picture, which is an X-ray-like 'shadow' of the jars.

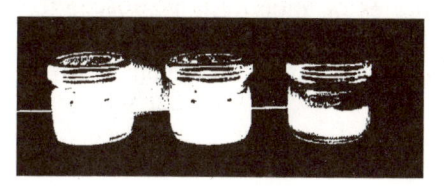

If you can spot the difference here, then you have a huge future as a radiologist!

So would it surprise you to know that the lid on the first jar is screwed on very tightly, the second sealed with normal tension, while the third jar's lid has been screwed down loosely.

Obviously, it would be very difficult to reach this conclusion based on the pictures alone. A far easier, reliable and more accurate method would be to simply twist the lids. You could tell in an instant exactly which jar had a stiff lid, which was normal, and which was loose.

Your back joints are the same. Even a highly detailed picture from a scan cannot tell you whether your joints are stiff, normal or unstable. An X-ray has virtually no hope of providing this vital information. An easier and far more reliable method is the one employed by every good spinal health practitioner: to observe, test and feel the movements of the spine.

I hope you can now see the limited place that radiology has in the diagnosis of your lower back pain. Intrinsic, unavoidable limitations mean that healthy spines often show up as badly damaged, while spines that are causing agonising pain can show up as clear.

A recent study showed that of every 10,000 X-rays taken for lower back pain, the pictures provided unexpected and useful information on only four occasions. The rest of the cases could have been diagnosed just as effectively by a clinical examination alone. That means that about 2499 out of every 2500 X-rays are a waste of time and money.

Your spinal health practitioner should not rely on radiography to diagnose your lower back pain. If your spinal health practitioner relies on radiography alone to evaluate your condition, then I advise you to seek another opinion. Any practitioner who relies solely on radiology to form a diagnosis is clearly out-of-date, or cannot be bothered to properly examine your spine. Save your money and time, and go somewhere else.

SO DOES RADIOLOGY HAVE ANY PLACE IN DIAGNOSING LOWER BACK PAIN?

In the initial stages of lower back pain, radiology is relatively useless. Usually, the cause of the pain can be identified by a thorough clinical examination. X-rays and scans add very little information, and sometimes create red herrings through false positive findings.

However, if the problem is not improving as expected, or if the symptoms are unusual, radiology becomes far more important. The following list shows situations in which radiology is very useful:
- Scans can help exclude certain causes of lower back pain, such as cancer.
- In difficult-to-localise conditions such as arthritis or generalised spondylosis, an X-ray or scan can add clues as to which level is the most likely source of the pain.
- They can reassure both patient and practitioner that chronic, hard-to-treat back pain is not due to a serious or unexpected problem. A sound general rule is that any spinal pain that has not responded to treatment within three months should be investigated by either CT scan, or, preferably, an MRI scan. This simple rule ensures that the spinal health practitioner is not inadvertently missing a more sinister problem.

In summary, while radiology is very useful in many branches of medicine, it is not very helpful in diagnosing the source of ordinary, acute lower back pain for a few reasons.

X-rays show only bony detail, and thus miss a huge proportion of the structures that often cause spinal pain. CT scans, while far better, are still inherently limited by their technology. Even with very clear, accurate pictures as obtained from an MRI, radiological diagnosis remains elusive. False positives are commonplace, with many otherwise healthy subjects showing 'serious' spinal problems. Conversely, even the most sensitive scanners cannot detect stiffness or instability, which are often the most significant underlying cause of back trouble.

As such, practitioners should not rely on radiology alone to determine the cause of your problem. Any practitioner who uses radiology for this purpose is incompetent, or at least inadequate, in their duties. While scans can be reassuring—particularly if the problem is tricky or slow to respond to treatment—they will never take the place of a thorough clinical examination.

28
Pregnant women and children
Extra concerns for vital times

Pregnancy

Pregnancy and the first year after your baby's birth are very dangerous times for a young woman's spine. The reasons and precautions for pregnancy-related spinal pain are many ... as if labour wasn't painful enough already!

(1) THE PREGNANCY HORMONES AFFECT YOUR LIGAMENTS AND DISCS

When you become pregnant, your body releases a hormone called *relaxin*. This hormone, as its name suggests, helps to loosen and relax the ligaments and other soft tissues in your body. This effect allows the pelvic and spinal joints to stretch so that they can accommodate the developing baby, and allow it passage during delivery. Unfortunately, this very useful process has the side effect of decreasing the stability of your spinal discs and ligaments.

Women who suffer most with pregnancy-related lower back pain are likely to be those with type A or type B spines. As these spinal types are inherently unstable, they will probably be worsened by the effect of the relaxin. It follows that if you feel pain for the first time during your pregnancy, then your spinal type is likely to be A or B.

Conversely, those people with type C or D spines may find that their pain improves during their pregnant months. As the hormones loosen the ligaments and discs, previously stiff and painful joints will relax, temporarily alleviating the cause of the problem.

(2) THE GROWING BABY WILL STRETCH YOUR ABDOMINAL MUSCLES

As the foetus develops and grows, it gradually expands toward your abdominal cavity. The first muscle with which it makes contact is the transverse abdominal muscle, which is not only the lowest abdominal muscle, but also the deepest.

As you know, the transverse abdominal is one of the most important muscles for stabilising and supporting your lower back. So when the growing baby squashes against this muscle, your lower back receives considerably less support, and therefore has a higher risk of developing problems.

Any instability in your lower back is hit with a double whammy. Not only do the hormones loosen your ligaments and discs, but also your major supporting muscle is severely disadvantaged. If you have an unstable spine and fall pregnant, then you will require plenty of extra diligence to avoid aggravating your problem.

(3) YOUR GROWING ABDOMEN WILL CREATE POSTURAL PROBLEMS

As your pregnant tummy becomes larger, its sheer bulk will create postural problems. For example, your centre of gravity will move forward, meaning that you will have to compensate by leaning slightly backward. Spine types A and C may find that this posture aggravates their condition. You type A's are really copping it here, aren't you?

Your larger tummy also limits your options for finding a comfortable lying or sleeping position. For example, women with type B or D spines may have previously found that lying prone on your stomach helped relieve their pain. However, this position is rarely comfortable if your tummy is the size of a watermelon.

(4) YOUR LOWER BACK MUST SUPPORT EXTRA WEIGHT

The extra weight of the baby, the placenta and the amniotic fluid (usually about ten to fifteen kilos) adds to the pressure on your lower back. This weight will obviously disappear in one sudden rush during labour, but during those last few months the extra kilograms can, for reasons already outlined, be a real burden on your spine.

(5) YOU WILL BE REQUIRED TO LIFT FAR MORE FREQUENTLY

In the first few months (make that years) after the baby is born, most new mothers (and fathers) find that they must lift far more frequently than ever before. Furthermore, the lifting is often very awkward, such as hoisting a baby capsule into the car, or carefully lowering a sleeping baby (finally, after four hours, she's asleep) into a cot.

Or, for example, carrying the baby on one hip, a toddler on the other, a portable cot over your shoulders, a baby nappy bag in your hands, while simultaneously trying to open the boot, pat the crying baby, and prevent the toddler from sticking her lollipop into your ear.

Yes, those early child-rearing days require not only lots of patience, but also an excellent lifting technique. If you have recently been blessed with a baby of your own, then you may benefit from re-reading the chapter on lifting, keeping in mind your difficult baby-related lifts as you go.

(6) YOUR STRESS LEVELS MIGHT SKYROCKET

In Chapter 20, you learned how stress can inflame or cause back pain. You also learned how change is one factor that readily induces anxiety and stress. As any new parent will tell you, there are few, if any, greater changes in life than the leap from carefree, socialising, movie-going young couple to becoming the sleep deprived, dirty-nappy-inundated guardians of a dependent, crying, tiny human being.

Don't be surprised if your stress meter goes a little berserk during this period. As you know, high stress levels are often coupled with elevated pain perception and increased muscle tension, which makes this period an even greater hazard for your lower back.

I'm sure you can now see the pregnant and post-natal months are a perilous time for your lower back, especially if it is inherently unstable. The relaxing effect of the hormones, weakened abdominal muscles, awkward postures, increased body weight, frequent lifting and higher stress levels all combine to attack your spinal integrity during your pregnancy and soon thereafter. It's a wonder that any women survive pregnancy at all!

So what do you do to avoid pregnancy-related lower back pain? Let's look at the above situations, and examine a few commonsense ways to lessen the impact of each problem.

First, the relaxing effect of your hormones can be countered with a pelvic stabilising brace. These braces, which resemble a wide, soft belt, simply loop around the outside of your pelvis. By pulling the belt tight, you externally bind your pelvic bones together. This extra stability helps to prevent the problems associated with an unstable sacro-iliac joint, which is a major cause of pregnancy-related back pain.

Second, you should commence stability exercises *now*, before you become pregnant. I hope you're not too late! By exercising your transverse abdominal muscle in the early days, you will develop and maintain its tone throughout your entire pregnancy. It will be too late to start exercising in the eighth month when your tummy muscles are stretched further than a fisherman's story.

Of course, you can work on your other stability muscles, such as your multifidus and hip muscles, right up until your labour. In the early months following baby's birth, you can re-introduce the transverse abdominal contractions. You can easily combine your spinal stability exercises with pelvic floor tightening, which is a mainstay of post-natal therapy. In short, strong stability muscles are a key to preventing pregnancy-related pain.

Third, you should follow all of the general principles of care in this book, with emphasis on the information for type A or type B spines. When putting your back-care theory into practice, concentrate on known pregnancy problem areas, such as lifting and lying posture. Frequent sitting for long feeding sessions also deserves special attention.

One last hint: find yourself a good man. Apparently they're hard to come by, however if your husband/partner/de facto/boyfriend/friend/whatever can help—not only with the heavy jobs, but with the frustrating, stress-inducing tasks—then your pregnancy and post-partum year will pass with minimal emotional and physical stress. Good luck. You'll need it.

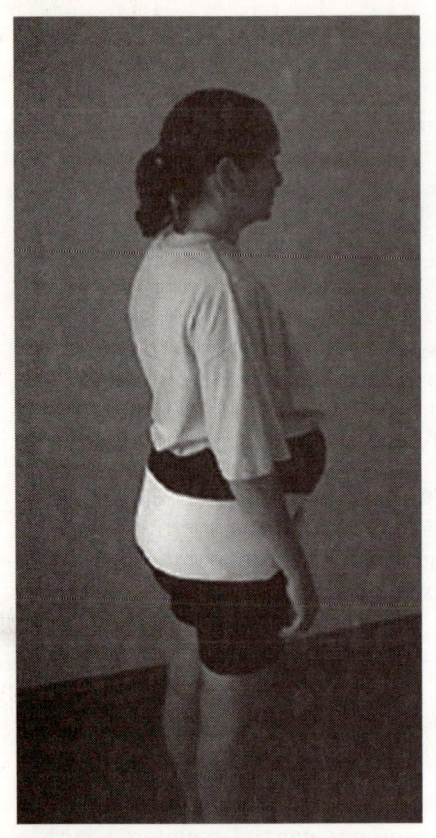

My friend Clare, modelling a pregnancy support belt. In her tummy is Edward, now a bouncing baby boy.

Children and adolescents with lower back pain

The most frequent comment that I hear about children with back pain is 'Ah, they'll be alright. Kids heal their injuries pretty quickly, don't they?'

Not only is this idea about adolescent back pain false, but the opposite is far more likely to be true. Back pain in children is usually more serious, and requires more intervention, than does an equivalent problem in an adult.

This contradiction occurs because of the nature of lower back pain. Recall from Chapter 3 that most cases of back pain are due to accumulated microtrauma. If a fifteen-year-old has developed back pain, then this implies that he or she has accumulated as much microtrauma in their short life as most people do in forty years. Commonsense will tell you that this child has significant problems with either posture, habits, muscle balance, stress, or whatever—to cause their back to degenerate at such an alarming rate.

This theory is supported, rather than denied, by the assumption that children heal more quickly than do their adult counterparts. For if a child's naturally rapid healing rate cannot repair the microtrauma, then the damage must be significant.

Young people with back pain have one other problem with which adults do not have to deal: their disc centres are very liquid. Recall that the nucleus of the disc dries as we age. The gooey, jelly-like nucleus of our youth hardens to a wizened crabmeat consistency by retirement age. The more liquid-like the nucleus, the greater chance that it will completely prolapse if the outer disc fibres are torn. This serious injury is therefore more likely during the younger ages.

If your child has back pain, then treat it with respect. If his or her problem persists, even if the pain is minor, then the injury warrants attention. The habits, postures and muscle imbalances that they correct in their adolescence will provide a platform for a healthy, active life, rather than gradual deterioration toward a pain-racked middle age.

29
A few other things that had nowhere else to go
The variety pack of back pain options

Orthotics

Some spinal health practitioners feel that orthotics—padded insoles that you slip into your shoe, which help to correct foot problems such as fallen arches—are a mainstay of back therapy. I concede that there is a loose association between foot position and back pain. (*Viz*: The foot bone's connected to the: leg bone ... the leg bone's connected to the: thigh bone ... the thigh bone's connected to the: hip bone ... the hip bone's connected to the—you guessed it—back bone. No prizes for the anatomical accuracy of this ditty, but you get the point.) I feel that the relationship is so distant that orthotics are unlikely to be of major or immediate benefit.

However, if you have very flat or stiff feet, then you will probably benefit by having them examined by a podiatrist. This advice doubles in value if you also have knee or hip pain. In these cases, the orthotics may provide other benefits to your musculo-skeletal system, so why not give them a go? Although I can't see how orthotics qualify as front-line artillery in your fight against back pain, they may form a useful ally to your other efforts.

Supports and braces

Back supports, corsets and other types of braces have a debatable place in the overall management of low back pain. Consider the important and recognised principles of back rehabilitation, such as exercise, strengthening and stretching. Furthermore, you will soon learn that rest is a poor, outdated option for the management of even very acute pain, and how those people who exercise fare better than those who don't. All of these factors indicate that braces are unlikely to be of much benefit, and may in fact hinder your improvement. As a rule, I suggest that you do not wear a brace.

However, there are, as usual, a few good exceptions to this rule. First, if you are about to perform a short-term activity that normally hurts your back but is unavoidable, then by all means temporarily use a brace. For example, suppose that you have to mow the lawn, and the last time you performed this chore your back pain increased dramatically. In this case, I would consider that wearing a brace for half an hour or so was the lesser of two evils.

Second, wearing a brace may temporarily allow you to mobilise (i.e. walk or otherwise exercise) sooner after an acute episode of low back pain. If you find that you can walk around the house with relative comfort while using a brace, but your pain forces you back to bed if you try to walk without it, then I would consider the extra support a good option.

Third, certain back types will respond more favourably to bracing and supporting than others. Generally, unstable spines like types A and B are more likely to benefit from temporary bracing than the stiffer types C and D.

Your back pain type will also guide you as to which type of brace is best. Type A spines, which detest bending backward, are best suited by a brace that is wide at the back, preferably with some reinforcing struts for added support.

Conversely, type B spines will benefit most from braces that stop the spine from flexing forward. Here, a brace that is wider at the front is more useful, while any posterior reinforcing will probably just get in the way.

In summary, braces prevent movement, and therefore do more harm than good for many back pain sufferers. However, some people, particularly those with unstable spines, may temporarily benefit from wearing a brace. You should not wear a brace continually; use it only during high-risk occasions or when your back is acutely painful.

Taping

Taping can provide temporary pain relief, and can assist with postural retraining or habit breaking. Like bracing, it may be occasionally useful, such as during acute pain, or before a difficult activity.

People with type B spines will probably gain the most benefit from taping, while some type D spines may also find that it helps. Type A might find that taping helps to contain any rotary instability, although they may find that it makes their pain worse. Type C shouldn't bother, as the position in which the tape holds your spine will probably worsen your pain.

There are two approaches for spinal taping. The first is a rigid style, which prevents most forward movement of the lumbar spine. The second is a more flexible method that allows some movement, and serves as a gentle reminder that you are losing the lordotic curve in your spine.

The rigid, stabilising technique is best used if your pain is severe or acute. This style is also useful if you are returning to work or other physically demanding tasks after a back-pain-induced rest, since it affords your back extra protection and stability during these vulnerable times. In short, rigid taping can be considered in the same class as back braces.

The flexible, reminder-type style is better suited to most other situations, as it allows some movement and muscle control, while helping to retrain better posture and habits.

You may wish to experiment with spinal taping to see if it improves your posture and/or pain. You'll have to convince someone else to apply the tape for you, as trying to accurately position the strips yourself is a waste of time. The method for applying these two techniques is as follows.

METHOD ONE
Flexible method
For postural retraining, and to remind you if you lose your lumbar lordosis

(1) The subject lies on his or her tummy. (If this position is painful, then this taping technique will probably not help very much.)
(2) Find the top of the subject's pelvic bones, and connect them with an imaginary line across their back. This line will intersect the vertebral column at about the L4 or L5 level. We will use this point as the centre of our tape application.

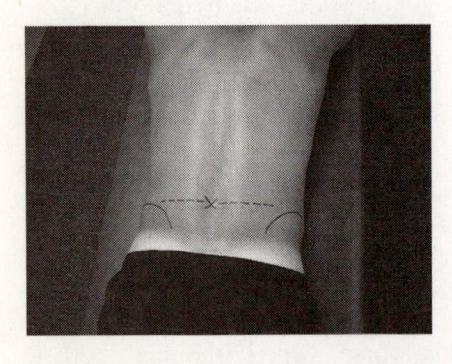

By using the top of the hip bones as landmarks, you can easily locate the approximate level of the L4 and L5 vertebrae.

(3) Cut two strips of semi-flexible tape about twenty centimetres (eight inches) long. The tape should be about five centimetres (two inches) wide.

If you do not have semi-flexible strapping tape (*Fixomull stretch* by Beiersdorf, is a good example) then ordinary rigid sports tape will do. Completely forget about using boxing tape, Sellotape or masking tape.
(4) Place the tape strips on the skin so that they form an elongated 'X', with its centre over the L4 and L5 area.
(5) Secure the tape top and bottom with anchor strips. You're finished.

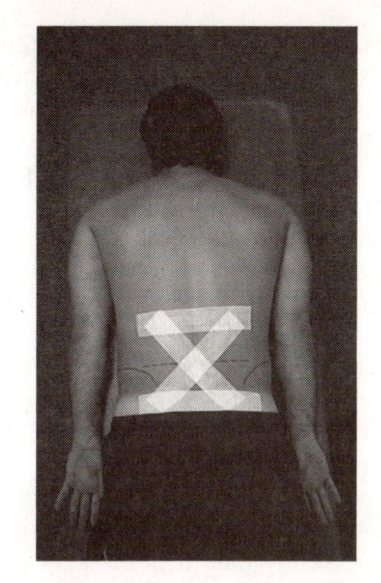

A completed 'flexible' tape job. Note that the centre of the 'X' is over the most affected level—often the L4 or L5 region.

Remember that the idea of this taping technique is to provide a reminder that you are losing your lordotic curve. So if you feel the tape tightening, you should immediately readjust your posture, or find a more efficient way of performing the task.

METHOD TWO
Rigid method
To prevent flexion of the lumbar spine and provide extra support during difficult tasks

(1) Proceed through Steps 1 to 4 as above, except you should use rigid sports strapping tape rather than semi-flexible tape.
(2) Apply a strip of tape between each corner of the 'X' so that you form a box.
(3) Working from one side, and overlapping the tape strips by about half of their width, add more vertical strips of tape to fill the box. After each vertical strip of tape, apply a horizontal strip so that you form a basket-weaving pattern. Continue layering the tape until the box is filled with overlapping strips.

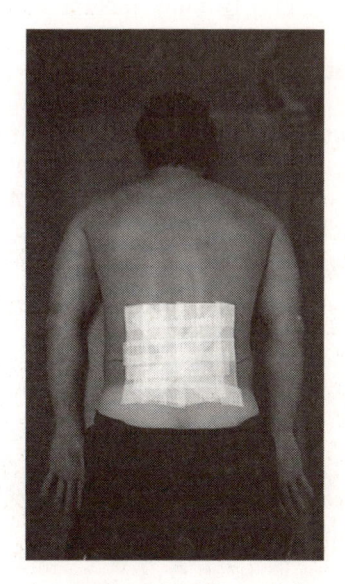

A completed 'rigid' tape job.

OTHER ADVICE REGARDING SPINAL TAPING

Some people are allergic to strapping tape. If your skin itches or burns under the tape then remove it immediately.

Generally, you can allow the tape to become wet in the shower, as its porosity allows it to dry. If you are concerned that the moisture will ruin your best silk shirt, then a few minutes under a hair dryer will solve your problem.

Leave the tape in place for about 24 hours. If you feel that the tape is particularly helpful, then you may leave it on for up to 48 hours. Beyond this period the tape becomes too loose to have any real functional effect, and will only irritate your skin. Therefore, two days is a sensible maximum time to leave the tape in place.

You may find that the tape is annoying, particularly if you use the rigid method. Try to be patient, and work with the tape, not against it. However, if you feel that the tape is worsening your original pain, then remove it. The tape has no long-term benefit, so if it is not helping immediately then it is unlikely to help at all.

Oh, by the way fellas, body hair really hurts when ripped off by tape. I mean *really* hurts. A thousand simultaneous exfoliations are not much fun. I've witnessed tears welling in the eyes of big burly footballers who would be loathe to admit that even being gored through the stomach by a rampaging buffalo was painful. Don't be brave—shave. You'll thank me for that advice, trust me.

Traction

Traction, affectionately known in my practices as 'the rack', uses a longitudinal stretching force to pull your spinal joints slightly apart.

To achieve this affect, traction uses two corset-like belts, one of which fits around your pelvis, while the other binds around your ribs. By applying a force—either mechanically with a machine, or passively with weights—the lower belt pulls on your pelvis, which in turn stretches your spine.

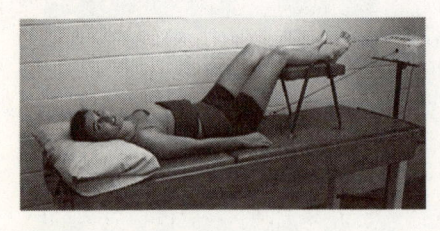

Debbie on 'the rack'.

Traction is used chiefly in two circumstances. First, many spinal health practitioners use traction in their consulting rooms, to help with the immediate treatment of back problems. Second, traction can be applied on a continuous basis in hospital for a few days, or even weeks, at a time.

Does traction help lower back pain? Sometimes. But not very often.

In-rooms traction is occasionally useful. I have witnessed some patients experience sudden, dramatic relief following just ten minutes of stretching. However, I have also seen some people's pain made considerably worse, while for the vast majority it does nothing at all. Unfortunately, I know of no clear way of predicting which types of spine will benefit from in-rooms traction, and which will not.

Furthermore, if your practitioner chooses to use traction, it should form only a part of your overall treatment plan. Traction does not replace the need for strengthening, stretching and mobilising techniques, which will do more to improve your overall condition than will any amount of 'the rack'.

Prolonged hospital traction is, I believe, a poor way of treating spinal pain. This practice completely ignores the principle that movement and strengthening are the keys to spinal rehabilitation. Any benefit could have been achieved by bed rest alone, and the results would have been even better with gentle exercise and movement.

Electrotherapy

Electrotherapy covers the broad range of modalities that many spinal health practitioners use to assist with the treatment of back pain. Some of these devices are very useful, while others provide little more than a glorified placebo effect.

I won't go into too much detail on each different modality. However, you may find the following list will help your appreciation of these commonly used treatments.

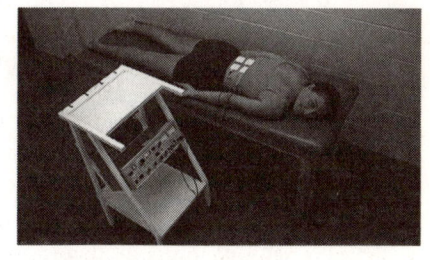

Debbie being zapped by an electrotherapy device.

- Ultrasound. This treatment works by bombarding the injury site with a high-frequency vibration, in much the same way that a radio speaker will vibrate if the music is amplified. This produces a microscopic massage-like effect, which is thought not only to break down the by-products of inflammation, but to control chemicals that regulate the inflammatory process.

- TENS. This form of treatment, known formally as Transcutaneous Electrical Nerve Stimulation, uses a modified electric current to produce a mild tingling sensation. This decreases the perception of pain via the 'gate control' theory as discussed in Chapter 21.

- Short Wave Diathermy. This treatment uses high-frequency electromagnetic waves to gently and deeply heat your injury site. It works in much the same way as does a microwave oven, so you'll know what a chook feels like as you defrost it in preparation for Sunday dinner.

- Infra-red lamps. Old-fashioned and out-dated method of heating. A hot water bottle is just as effective, but much simpler, cheaper and safer. I'd be worried if your spinal health practitioner is still using one.

- Magnetic Field Therapy. Each cell in your body has a minor electric charge, which makes it like a tiny magnet. When this therapy is applied, an oscillating magnetic field causes the cells to flip back and forth about fifty times per second. This effect may encourage healing, and loosen up cross-linked molecules within scar tissue.

- Laser. By applying a high-intensity light source of a single frequency, it is hoped that more energy can be supplied to the healing cells.

- Biofeedback. This device measures the activity in your muscles by measuring the electrical charge that is passing through them. As such, biofeedback is extremely useful for retraining weak muscles, or for relaxing overactive muscles.

As the preceding discussion shows, spinal health practitioners have access to a wide variety of technology to help you achieve your rehabilitation goals. However, a few general points require consideration.

First, electrotherapy is only the 'icing on the cake' of any good treatment. It is far more effective when combined with other measures such as soft tissue therapy, joint mobilisation and muscle imbalance correction. While the electrotherapy may help diminish pain, spasm and inflammation, the 'hands-on' therapy helps remove the underlying cause of the problem.

Second, many untrained practitioners now use electrotherapy. In particular, ultrasound is widely available, and TENS units can be purchased from department stores or mail-order catalogues. There are a few dangers to these increasingly common developments:

- Each modality has specific contraindications to its use. In other words, certain conditions may be worsened by inappropriate use of electrotherapy. It takes a trained therapist to fully understand the implications of every injury.

- Pain is a signal to your body that something is wrong. Covering the pain and inflammation by constant application of electrotherapy may cause an unwarranted delay in seeking more appropriate treatment.

- A practitioner who is not highly trained in injury diagnosis may inadvertently apply the electrotherapy to the wrong area, giving an ineffective treatment. For example, I once had a patient whose previous practitioner had applied ultrasound for two months to a 'torn hamstring muscle' without success. Subsequent examination showed that the problem was due to a disc problem in his lower spine.

In short, electrotherapy is a useful treatment adjunct in many cases of lower back pain. However, any practitioner who relies on electrotherapy alone is wasting your time. Similarly, do not let a glossy brochure tempt you into buying an electrotherapy device, as the results will probably be inadequate, and may be potentially harmful.

A few final words on electrotherapy. These types of treatments do not help you to lose any weight whatsoever. Not even one gram. If anyone ever tries to tell you that electro-stimulation will 'break up cellulite' or 'effortlessly burn away calories', then beware, for they probably have vials of snake oil, or potions of newt's ear, ready for your next treatment. Save your dollars and go elsewhere. Trust me on this one.

Nor will electrotherapy strengthen normal muscle. Yes, I realise that Bruce Lee once used electro stimulation for muscle strengthening. But that was in the '60s—right where that idea belongs.

Trigger point therapy

As you read in Chapter 7, muscular knots, known as trigger points, can sometimes contribute to lower back pain. Many different treatments have been developed to deal with these problem areas.

For example, some doctors perform a procedure known, technically, as a *percutaneous neurotomy*. It is sometimes called *Nesfield's treatment*. The technique consists of making a small incision—just a nick, really—underneath the spinal trigger points. This treatment bobs up on current affairs programs every few years.

Other trigger point therapies include anaesthetic injections, dry needling, and deep finger pressure. Apart from the fact that they don't cure the underlying cause of the trigger point, I can't see anything inherently wrong with trying these techniques as part of your program. They have almost no severe side effects, and are relatively inexpensive.

However, you'll probably find that the relief is only temporary, as the imbalance, posture or habit that caused the trigger point in the first place has not changed. You'd probably find that you improved permanently if you addressed the primary causes of your problem, rather then attacking the trigger points.

30

Heat or ice?

A frequently confused topic

Much confusion exists, not only among the general public, but also among health practitioners, as to which modality, either heat or ice, is best for treating back pain. Some practitioners always recommend ice, while others stick religiously to heat. Others recommend ice for 48 hours after an injury, then heat, while some practitioners have a dollar each way by recommending an alternating 'contrast application'. Furthermore, the recommended time and frequency of application seem to vary alarmingly from one practitioner to the next. Many patients justifiably feel confused after receiving such contradictory information.

Let's introduce some rational thought to the debate. Below are some guidelines that will help you to decide for yourself which treatment is best for your problem.

While ice and heat have many physiological effects on the body, one effect predominates for each modality. The main effect of ice is that it decreases the inflammatory response. The main function of gentle heat is to relax and loosen the muscles and other soft tissues. By considering these effects, we can decide when to apply each treatment.

In forming our guidelines, we must consider three situations. First, acute injuries, in which the pain commenced within the last two days. Then, we'll look at chronic injuries, which have been hanging around for one month or more. Finally, we'll look at the in-between group of sub-acute pain, in which the pain first appeared between two and thirty days ago.

If your pain is of recent origin *and* has been precipitated by violent trauma, then you have a true acute injury. Here, ice is best.

However, if your pain began recently, but due to only minor provocation, or if it just started by itself, then the pain is probably due to the accumulation of microtrauma. In other words, the current problem is an *acute exacerbation of a chronic condition*. Here, the decision is not as simple, so you must ask yourself two questions:

(1) Have you experienced this type of pain before? If so, then your injury is probably due to accumulated degeneration. In this case, heat is probably best.
(2) Is your injury site exquisitely tender, or very painful when you move only a small degree? If so, then your injury is probably very inflamed. In this case, ice is the treatment of choice.

If you are in doubt with any pain of recent origin, then try ice first, as it has fewer side effects.

If your injury is *chronic*, then heat is probably best. This advice doubles in strength if your spine is type C or D, as stiff spines usually feel better after heat application.

Now we come to a few areas in which the decision is not so black-and-white. For example, if your injury is *sub-acute*—i.e. it began between two and thirty days ago, then your decision may be tricky.

Another situation in which the general rules become blurred is if you have chronic pain from a type A or B spine. Because stiffness is not underlying your problem, you may not feel relief from heat, which is usually recommended for chronic pain.

The best strategy in these indeterminate situations is to follow the evaluation procedure of any good spinal treatment, which is known as *objective assessment*. To do this assessment, you should first perform a movement or task that makes your spine hurt: for example, bending forward, or walking around the block. Then apply the treatment—in this case ice or heat—then retest the same movement or task. The results of the second test, when compared to that of the first, will guide your next move:

- If your back moved more freely, or you felt less pain, then the treatment was probably the correct choice. Repeat the same dose again later.
- If your back was stiffer during the retesting movement, or if the task exacerbated your pain more easily, then the treatment was probably wrong. Test the alternative treatments, and see what happens.
- If the treatment seemed to have no effect, then it was either too mild, or was unsuitable. In this case, increase the time or intensity of application, and retest again. If the treatment still has no effect, then test an alternative in the same way.

Let's look at an example to see how to best choose between heat and ice:

Alison is a computer programmer who has never previously injured her back. One day, as she rises from her office chair to fetch a cuppa and a doughnut, she feels a twang in her spine. Her symptoms deteriorate over the next few hours. That night, when she arrives home, she can barely move without pain. Alison must decide whether to apply heat or ice to her injury.

First, she analyses her problem, and sees that she does not have a truly acute injury, as the pain started after only minor provocation. However, as her movements are very limited, she decides to try ice first, which she also knows is the safest option. To double-check her decision, she uses an objective assessment.

Before applying the ice, she tests her injury by bending forward, and finds that her hands only reach her knees before her pain increases. After applying ice to her spine, she re-tests the movement. Alas! This time, Alison can barely bend forward at all. Her hands reach only her mid-thigh area before her pain increases. Ice was probably the wrong treatment.

Soon thereafter she applies a heat pack, and repeats the testing procedure. This time her bending movement is far looser, and she is able to reach to mid-shin level. Alison now knows that heat is the correct choice for her current condition, and continues to apply heat with confidence until her spine has recovered.

Frequently asked questions about heat and ice application

HOW LONG AND HOW OFTEN SHOULD YOU APPLY ICE OR HEAT?
The duration of the ice or heat application depends upon the depth and size of the structure that you are treating. As lumbar discs and joints are very deep, and fairly large, a prolonged application is the best. As a rough guide, I suggest at least half an hour, which you can extend up to an hour if you wish.

The frequency of application depends upon so many factors that it is almost arbitrary. An acute injury will generally require frequent applications, as will a severe problem. Generally, aim for two to four applications per day.

IF I FIND THAT ICE IS BENEFICIAL FOR THE FIRST FEW DAYS AFTER MY INJURY, SHOULD I CONTINUE TO USE IT UNTIL MY BACK HAS RECOVERED?
Not necessarily. The above guidelines don't imply that your condition will not change. If you find that ice treatment is providing diminishing benefits, then test yourself objectively with heat. If the heat pack helps more than the ice, then change treatments.

Nor does this imply that you should automatically change from ice to heat after a few days. Many conditions create new inflammation every day, and will continue to respond favourably to ice until they are fully cured.

HOW SHOULD I APPLY ICE?
Real ice is best. There are many commercial ice packs on the market, but many of them don't seem to maintain their coldness as well as real ice.

On the other hand, commercial ice packs are more convenient. You may find it useful to keep two large commercial packs in the freezer, and change them after 15 or 20 minutes when the first pack loses its coolth (the opposite of warmth).

If you have a back injury that requires frequent icing, then consider purchasing a large bag of party ice (it doesn't cost much) and storing it in the freezer. (You can use the leftovers to keep your drinks cold when you recover.) Make a cold pack by heaping some ice into a plastic bag, sealing it, and wrapping it in a wet tea towel or dishcloth. Keep a bath towel handy to soak up any drips and spills.

The wet cloth around the ice bag is important to prevent the ice from freezing your skin, thus causing an ice burn. If you ever suffered from that most embarrassing primary school mishap of having your tongue stuck on an iceblock, you'll know what I mean. If you have sensitive skin or anticipate that you will require frequent ice sessions, then a thin layer of oil rubbed over your skin will also help to prevent ice irritation.

HOW SHOULD I APPLY HEAT?
There are many different ways to apply heat. The best method will depend entirely upon your budget, your posture and your preferences.

One reliable option is the good old hot-water bottle. Hot-water bottles are simple to use and hold their heat well. They are readily available, and inexpensive. Not only that, but hot-water bottles can double as a lumbar support device when you sit.

Of similar potential are the ranges of wheat-filled cushions, which you either soak in hot water or zap in a microwave. These items are also simple, cheap and effective. While the flattened shape of the wheat cushions devalues their potential as a lumbar support device, it makes them easier to use in positions such as lying in bed. Just be sure that you don't overheat them in your microwave. Oh, by the way, check that the product is mould-resistant before you purchase it, as I have heard of a few of these cushions going rotten.

Are you one of those people who has an infra-red ray lamp tucked in the top cupboard of your wardrobe, gathering dust? My advice would be to leave it there. Infra-red lamps, once a trendy item of home therapy, are now more out-of-date than safari suits.

The problem with ray lamps is that they do not provide any benefits that cannot be obtained far more cheaply and easily with, say, a hot-water bottle. The ray lamp only heats your skin, and does a poor job of penetrating to deeper structures. They have a high risk of burning if not used with care. Furthermore, you may have to adopt an awkward posture to effectively position your spine under the lamp. If I were you I'd sell your ray lamp in the weekend papers, buy a hot-water bottle instead, and treat yourself to a night out on the town with the change.

Electric-heat pads, which resemble small, wool-covered electric blankets, provide a useful addition to your heating options. The advantage of these commercially available products is that they can maintain their temperature indefinitely. Most brands have only a very low output, and so have very little chance of burning you, even with prolonged use. They are flat enough to be used in bed, although the manufacturers recommend that you do not sleep while using one, as this increases the chances of an accident.

If you have the type of back that is very stiff and achey in the mornings, then you may wish to connect your heat pad to a timer switch, as recommended in Chapter 18. By activating the heat pad an hour or two before you are due to awaken, your back will be warm and flexible when you arise.

Of course, hot showers and baths also provide heat for your spine. Many people find that their stretching exercises are most effective when performed immediately after, or even during, a hot shower or bath. The bath has the added benefit of providing buoyancy and support for your spine. However, be careful with baths if your pain is acute, especially if you have a type B or type D spine, or if you have tight nerves as revealed by Part Three of the quiz in Chapter 11. In these cases, the difficult postures and transitions to and from the bath may do you more harm than good.

In summary, the decision to use heat or ice is not always clear. However, by using the above guidelines, and choosing different applications to suit your situations, you can gain great relief from either modality.

31
Myth busting
What **doesn't** cause or cure back pain

What *doesn't* cause low back pain

OLD AGE
If your spinal health practitioner tells you that your spine is sore because you are getting old, and that you'll just have to learn to live with it, then I have one piece of advice for you: go somewhere else. The spinal health practitioner obviously does not know what he or she is talking about, and cannot be bothered to properly analyse your problem.

Old age does not cause low back pain any more than it causes headaches or sprained ankles. In fact, the peak period for the most severe forms of low back pain is between the ages of 35 and 50 years—a long way from the seniors bracket.

While signs of degeneration are very common on X-ray in the older population, this finding does not, as you read in Chapter 27, mean that back pain is more likely. For the same reasons, severe degenerative changes on X-ray do not mean that your spinal problem is necessarily more difficult to cure than someone with a clear X-ray.

In short, the principles of back pain management during later life are no different from any other age. Your age is not, I repeat not, causing your pain, and do not believe anyone who tries to imply that this is the case.

THE WEATHER
Some academics have postulated that decreasing air pressure is responsible for a minor increase in joint swelling. This would explain some arthritics' suggestion that they can tell when it is about to rain because their back aches. However, this theory does not explain why the same people suffer from the cold in winter, the winds in autumn, and the humidity in summer. Wouldn't have anything to do with the condition of your spine, by any chance?

Studies have shown no correlation between weather patterns and the average pain level of a large group of arthritis sufferers—although my grandfather would disagree ...

SCOLIOSIS

Scoliosis means a sideways-curving spine. When viewed from the back, a spine with a scoliosis will resemble an elongated 'S', rather than a straight line. The cause of true scoliosis is usually idiopathic, meaning that it just happens for no particular reason.

Would you be shocked if I told you that about eighty-five per cent of people with mild scoliosis suffer from back pain? I hope not, because you should already know that about eighty-five per cent of the general population also suffer from back pain, although their spines are straight. In other words, mild scoliosis itself is not a painful condition, and does not necessarily cause other conditions that lead to back pain.

Some spinal health practitioners go to extreme lengths to correct scoliosis. They suggest shoe raises or orthotics, electronic muscle stimulation, curve-correcting exercises, sometimes even rigid braces, all of which are designed to reverse this dreaded affliction.

I have reservations about the value of such attempts, and feel that they probably do more harm than good. Your spine is no doubt used to being held in its curved position, and any attempts to straighten it may simply provoke further problems.

In growing adolescents, a mild scoliosis often corrects itself. Conversely, if you've stopped growing, then the shape of your spine is fixed, and no amount of coaxing will convince it to straighten. In either case, you have very little to gain by trying to correct the 'abnormal' curves.

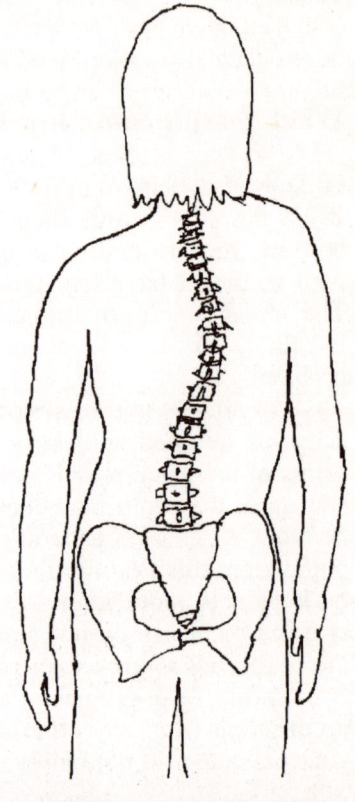

A typical case of scoliosis. Note the different hip angles and altered shoulder heights.

If you have scoliosis, then my advice is to simply let your curves stay as they are, and use all of the normal techniques, exercises, stretches and advice in the rest of this book.

However, before closing this section on scoliosis, I must mention two cases where important exceptions exist to the above guidelines.

First, if your scoliosis is *severe*, then it may lead to spinal problems that are potentially disabling. The medical method of classifying

MYTH BUSTING

scoliosis is to X-ray the spine, and then to measure the maximum difference in tilt between any two vertebrae. If this angle exceeds 35 degrees, then your scoliosis is classified as severe. In this case, gravity will tend to pull your spine into an even greater curve. Thirty-five degrees is a crucial point, and once the curve reaches this level, it will probably worsen.

If you have moderately severe scoliosis—say twenty degrees or more—then you should be under the care of a specialist who will monitor your spine each year, and intervene with rigid bracing or surgery if the curve worsens.

The second area of concern with scoliosis is if you acquire it suddenly. If your spine is normally straight, but develops a sudden sideways tilt or twist, then you probably have an identifiable back problem, such as an unstable disc. Health practitioners sometimes call this condition a 'list'. In this case, correction of your sideways curve

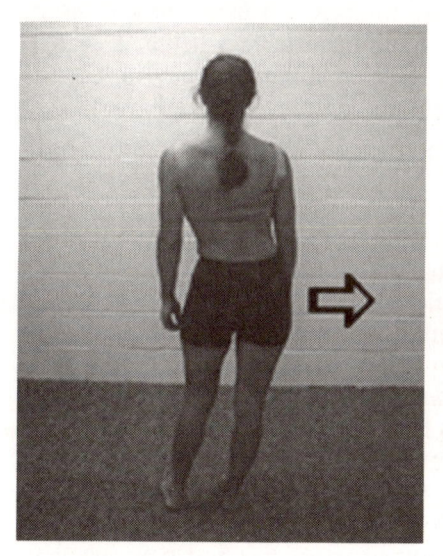

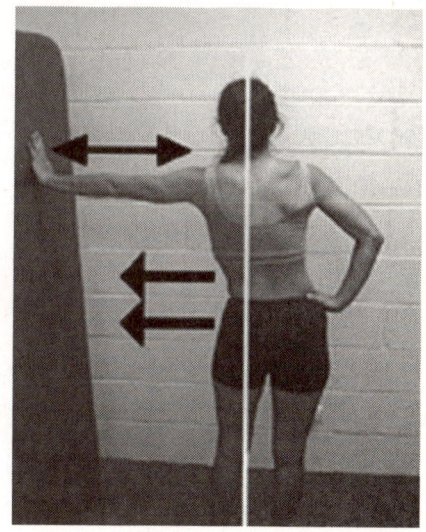

The left photograph above shows Debbie with a 'list', i.e. an acquired twist in her spine due to a lumbar injury. Note that her hips have moved sideways, as indicated by the open arrow.

The photograph on the right shows a technique that may help you to self-correct this problem should it ever occur. Start by ensuring that your feet are directly under your head, as indicated by the white line. Use a mirror if necessary. Then, after stabilising one arm against a wall, use the other hand to gently glide your pelvis across. Ensure that you keep your pelvis level. Hold this new position for five seconds, and then relax. Repeat about half a dozen times. If this exercise helps to relieve your pain or increase your range of movement, then repeat it three to five times per day until you are straight.

is an important part of your treatment, so you should see a spinal health practitioner as soon as is reasonably possible. You may also find that self-correction of the twist, as shown in the picture at right on the previous page, will help to relieve your pain and stiffness.

LEG LENGTH DIFFERENCES

Leg length differences are a commonly cited cause of back pain. As with scoliosis, I feel that if your legs have been different lengths for your entire life, then trying to equalise them will create more problems than it will potentially help.

One study evaluated a large group of industry workers and found no correlation between a two-centimetre limb-length inequality and back pain. A follow-up one year later showed that there was still no difference, indicating that minor leg length differences do not cause lower back pain.

However, if your leg length difference is acquired—after a broken leg, for example—then it makes sense to correct it using a shoe insert. Another situation where an insert may be beneficial is if you are often standing still for prolonged periods—say, as a bank teller. But for the vast majority of people, a natural, minor leg length difference is best ignored.

FIBROMYALGIA

Fibromyalgia means 'pain everywhere'. The rules for diagnosing fibromyalgia are simple: the patient has lots of tender spots and painful areas, but you can't find anything else wrong with them. There are no blood tests, X-rays or any other tests to confirm that you have this dreadful 'disease'.

In my opinion, 'fibromyalgia' does not really exist. There are many causes for widespread pain, of which you are no doubt already aware. For example, neural tension can cause multiple sites of pain, as can longstanding muscle imbalances. Mental tension and anxiety are obvious possibilities, while even a prolonged poor posture can create many tender and painful points. Many types of referred pain, particularly those from the nerve's connective tissue, can give rise to fibromyalgic-type symptoms. Often, a combination of the above factors creates the widespread pain associated with this diagnosis. I feel that spinal health practitioners who diagnose fibromyalgia are simply missing another condition.

If you have been diagnosed with fibromyalgia, then fear not. You are a prime candidate for a cure, simply by following the principles outlined in this book. Sure, it will take some hard work, but your chances of success are very high. Once you have fixed yourself, you can boast that you've discovered a 'miracle cure for fibromyalgia'.

What *won't* cure low back pain

REST

Except during a very severe, acute episode of low back pain, rest is a poor treatment option. The idea that rest will help to cure your low back pain is as outdated as is using leeches to purify the blood.

One recent study of a large group of patients, each of whom suffered an acute attack of back pain, showed that four days of bed rest was no more effective to reduce rehabilitation time than two days of rest. Even more significantly, no bed rest at all was just as good.

Other studies have shown that people who remain normally active, even during acute phases of low back pain, do better than those people who rest. Those people who keep moving following a back injury have been shown to require less treatment from health professionals, and have less chance of developing long-term back pain, than those who rested.

Bed rest has side effects. For a start, your stability muscles weaken very quickly when disused. Consider space astronauts, who, after only a few weeks in space, are so weak that they cannot even walk. Your spinal support muscles suffer a similar fate when you rest in bed, with predictably disastrous consequences for the stability of your joints.

Did you know that your bones lose their strength at the rate of about 1.5 per cent for each day of bed rest? Resting in bed is a sure-fire way to give yourself a case of osteoporosis.

As you read in Chapter 26, your joint cartilage quickly becomes sick if it is not regularly moved, as the synovial fluid that nourishes it is not circulated properly. Not only that, but bed rest causes your muscles and tendons to stiffen, further heightening any muscle imbalances.

Early mobilising and exercising encourages the scar tissue to form in the right places. If you move and exercise while your spine is healing, the cells that repair the damaged tissue construct the new fibres in the areas of highest demand. However, if you rest while your injury is healing, the scar tissue forms in aimless clumps. This weak, restricting, scar tissue is next-to-useless, and is a frequent cause of ongoing joint stiffness or instability.

If you have chronic, long-term back pain, then you should already know after reading this far that stretching, strengthening and exercising are the keys to recovery, not rest. If your spinal health practitioner advises you to rest for your low back pain, then run for your life—he or she probably has a bucket of leeches in the corner, ready to purify your blood.

ANY TREATMENT THAT HAS NO SIDE EFFECTS

One inescapable law of the universe is that everything that has an action also has a reaction. So any treatment with absolutely no side effects probably has no effects either, and most likely is doing nothing at all. You should be sceptical of any treatment that claims to help back pain, but promotes itself as having no side effects whatsoever.

ANY TREATMENT THAT IS THE SAME FOR EVERY PATIENT
Every few months, another so-called miracle cure for back pain pops up on current affairs shows on television. Often the promoter has a gadget, exercise device or new technique that they claim will help almost everyone with back pain. These gadgets vary widely, from those cheaply available to the public, to other more elaborate devices that are the possession of a spinal health practitioner who no doubt paid handsomely to import this 'state-of-the-art' technology. In all of these cases, ask yourself one simple question: is the treatment from this machine/gadget/device the same for every patient?

If the answer to this question is 'yes', then be assured that the device is probably a waste of time and money. As you know, all spines are different, and respond in vastly different ways. To claim that one single exercise, routine or device can cure vastly different problems—for example, the unstable spine of a young gymnast, and the stiff, aching spine of an eighty-year-old lawn bowls player—is stretching the bounds of probability.

Proper spinal treatment requires individual assessment of the nature and behaviour of the problem. Any therapy, device or treatment that ignores this inescapable fact is doomed to failure.

INVERSION MACHINES
You know the ones: those machines into which you strap your feet, then swing upside down and hang like a bat for five minutes. These machines are supposed to reverse 'postural drag' on your spine, and to stretch it with a traction-like effect. Do they work?

Usually, no. Inversion machines are unlikely to help your spine for several reasons. First, these machines offer the same treatment for every problem. As you read above, this approach automatically invalidates the likelihood of success for any device.

Second, the only place you hear about 'postural drag' is from the makers of the inversion machines. I do not know of any study that correlates this mystery condition with low back pain. Strengthening your stability muscles is surely a far more effective way to counteract a poor posture than is hanging upside down for five minutes, and then being upright the other 955 waking minutes each day.

Third, the traction effect provided by these machines to your lower back is very limited, as your legs receive most of the stretch. Most of the traction effect of an inversion machine occurs in your ankles, with your knees receiving the next strongest dose, and your hip joints after that. Your sacro-iliac joints are next in line, while the traction effect of your remaining body weight is spread over your next thirty or so spinal joints. Obviously, any localised effect on the pain-producing structure in your lower back will be non-localised and extremely minimal.

Furthermore, hanging upside down can injure your leg joints, or cause problems with high blood pressure, and sometimes headaches. In short, don't bother with inversion machines.

VIBRATING HEAT PILLOWS AND CHAIRS

While vibrating heat pillows have no intrinsic faults, they achieve very little that you could not obtain with a hot-water bottle or a small electric-heat pad. The vibration has no real therapeutic value, but probably adds significantly to the cost of the device.

If you have a vibrating heat pillow or chair, then by all means use it, as it will help in a small way toward your overall rehabilitation. However, please don't buy one on the promise that your troubles will be cured forever, or on the testimonials of other back pain sufferers on the brochure.

HYPERBARIC CHAMBERS

Hyperbaric chambers were originally developed to help errant scuba divers recover from the 'bends'. Their combined oxygen and pressure therapy enables your blood to carry a higher concentration of oxygen to the tissues, supposedly hastening your healing rate.

Hyperbaric chambers allegedly help a vast range of conditions, including burns, skin wounds, strokes, headaches, gangrene, plastic surgery and sports injuries. While the extra oxygen may help to slightly accelerate the healing process in some of these conditions, I doubt very much whether it would help your back pain. Furthermore, this type of therapy can be dangerous, and so must be performed under the active supervision of a medical doctor.

These chambers generally require that you sit in them for two hours per day, several days per week, in order to reap any supposed benefits. I'll guarantee that if you spent this time exercising, deeply relaxing, or even taking a walk, that your back pain would progress at a far quicker rate. With the added expense, dangers and side effects of hyperbaric chambers, I advise you not to waste your time.

MAGNETS

Yet another attempt to provide a miracle cure with an overly simplistic yet marketable solution. Magnets have no proven therapeutic benefit for lower back pain. Don't bother.

32

What to do if you are in acute, severe pain

I hope that you never need this advice

By acute, severe pain, I am referring to pain that has just started within the last day, and is so severe that you are unable to bend, sit or even walk without searing agony. If you ever find yourself in this situation, then observe the following rules.

- THE FIRST AND MOST IMPORTANT RULE IS TO *RELAX*.

Calm your body and mind. Tension and anxiety will make your problem worse, so at all costs you should try to remain calm, peaceful and relaxed. If necessary, review the relaxation exercises in Chapter 22, which you have, I trust, already practised for many months.

- BE *REASSURED* THAT YOU HAVE A NORMAL, ALBEIT SEVERE, CASE OF BACK PAIN.

Sudden onset lower back pain, except after violent trauma, is almost never due to a serious, evil cause. If you presently have severe acute lower back pain, then you probably have a disc or joint injury, possibly with some nerve damage. Although your pain is excruciating, let me assure you that the cause is not life-threatening or serious, nor will it lead to paraplegia or permanent disability. Now is an excellent time to try some positive thinking, affirmations or visualisation.

- *REALISE* THAT THE PAIN WILL PASS.

Even the most severe lower back pain usually settles to a bearable level of its own accord within a few hours, and nearly always within a day or two.

- *RELATIVE REST* IS ALSO IMPORTANT.

I use the term 'relative' because, as you know after reading Chapter 31, complete, stationary bed rest is not good. Instead, try some very gentle, easy movements within your pain tolerance.

Exercises 1, 2, 5 and 6, as described in Chapter 14, are useful for acute back injuries. Make sure that you use only the lowest level exercises, and move just to the onset of your pain. Gentle pelvic tilting is also helpful. Here, simply lie on your back with your knees bent, and softly arch and relax your spine. Perform about half a dozen repetitions

WHAT TO DO IF YOU ARE IN ACUTE, SEVERE PAIN

of each exercise about five or six times per day. The best time to exercise is immediately following ice or heat application.

In between your exercise sessions, find a comfortable lying posture. Experiment with yourself, or consult Chapter 18 for guidelines in this regard. However, avoid long periods of rest. Instead, you should start activities such as gently walking about the house as soon as you are able. Use a back brace and/or crutches if necessary. Remember that gentle early mobilisation is a key to the correct management of your problem.

Keep this thought in mind: normal daily activities such as walking and gentle mobility exercises will *not* hurt your back. If these activities cause pain, then they are simply pointing out to you that your spine has previously been injured. Therefore, you should continue to set goals for your own mobility and ignore any minor pain.

However, I suggest that you avoid prolonged sitting, repetitive bending and heavy lifting for a few days after your injury. In general, you should aim for a combination of gentle walking and light mobility exercises, occasionally supplemented by relaxed comfortable lying when necessary.

- *RESIST* THE TEMPTATION TO SEEK A MIRACLE CURE FROM A SPINAL HEALTH PRACTITIONER.

Treatments such as manipulation will probably only worsen your pain at this stage. There are no miracle cures for acute lower back pain, and your spine cannot be 'clicked back into place'.

Consider this question: if you sprained your ankle, would you expect that a practitioner would be able to magically 'click' your ankle to make it function perfectly, just a few hours after you injured it? Of course you wouldn't. Your spinal injury is like any other injury, and takes time and patience to settle. You will only disappoint yourself and probably exacerbate your pain if you search for a miracle cure.

- ORGANISE A *REVIEW* WITH YOUR DOCTOR IF YOU ARE ANXIOUS.

During this acute phase, your doctor is unlikely to be able to offer much more treatment than reassurance and perhaps a drug prescription. If this advice will help you to relax, then fine, make an appointment. However, be aware that travel to and from the practitioner's room may do more harm than good for an acutely injured back, so try to organise a house call if possible.

Anti-inflammatory medication, which is now available over the counter, is usually most useful in this situation. Follow the guidelines in Chapter 24, and check with your doctor and pharmacist.

BACK PAIN

- USE *ICE* OR *HEAT*. (SORRY, I'VE RUN OUT OF 'R' WORDS.)
Consult Chapter 30 for guidelines. If you are unsure, then try the ice first, as it is less likely to exacerbate any inflammation. Generally, the easiest way to apply ice or heat when your back is acutely painful is to lie on your side with a pillow between your knees. Then fold a towel in half lengthwise and tuck one end under your waist. You can then use the towel as a binder to keep the ice or heat pack in place.

- *DON'T BOTHER* GOING TO HOSPITAL.
Lower back pain is not a condition that requires or benefits from hospitalisation, unless it was precipitated by severe, violent trauma. Another exception might be if you are alone, infirm or elderly, and cannot care for yourself due to your immobility.

Most people who arrive at hospital with back pain are simply X-rayed, told that they have 'done a disc', and sent home to bed. The whole episode, including the travel, the examination, the radiology and, not least of all, the waiting, usually makes the pain considerably worse. My advice is to use your commonsense, but in most cases save yourself the trouble.

- *RETURN* TO YOUR NORMAL ACTIVITIES OF DAILY LIVING AS SOON AS POSSIBLE.
Many studies have shown that people who quickly return to their normal activities fare much better than those who avoid exertion. As mentioned earlier, the presence of pain does not necessarily mean that you are doing the wrong thing. Commonsense, combined with the principles outlined in this book, will guide you in this regard.

In summary, just remember to stay relaxed, trust that the acute phase of your pain will soon pass, think positively, and move gently. Return to your normal activities as soon as you are reasonably able. If you follow these simple tips, then you will take giant (metaphorical) leaps along the path toward getting rid of your acute back pain as quickly as possible.

33

Choosing a spinal health practitioner

The choice is yours

So you've got a sore back. I'm sure that you're already aware that advice from friends and relatives flows freely.

Your aunt recommends that you see her chiropractor who is 'just wonderful', while your best friend has been prescribed a new wonder drug by her doctor. A lady in a shopping centre whom you've never met gives you fifteen minutes of free advice about the merits of naturopathy, while your father encourages you to visit a physiotherapist who cured his problem. Your brother recommends acupuncture, an acquaintance from the sports club swears by deep tissue massage, while someone you met at a party drunkenly insisted that colonic irrigation was the only proven cure for back pain. What do you do?

The number and variety of spinal health practitioners seems to be growing every year. The approach taken by the disciplines sometimes seem so diverse as to be incompatible, while at other times they have so much overlap as to be almost indistinguishable. The competency standards of spinal health practitioners varies widely, not just between professions, but within them as well. No wonder the back pain 'consumer'—you—is so confused.

During this chapter, you will learn some guidelines about how to choose a good practitioner. In the next chapter, we will discuss the basic similarities and differences between various types of spinal treatment.

What makes a good spinal health practitioner?

As you are no doubt aware, the approaches to treatment of spinal pain are wide and varied. Nevertheless, you can apply some consistent standards across the whole range of disciplines, and from one practitioner to the next, to help you to decide who is best qualified to help you to get rid of your back pain.

Of course, you want someone whom you trust, and with whom you feel confident. The treatment should be cost effective, and should be in harmony with your way of thinking. These points are self-evident, and require no further explanation. Below are some further questions and standards that you should consider when choosing someone to help you with your spinal health care.

(1) YOUR PRACTITIONER SHOULD HAVE A HIGH LEVEL OF TRAINING AND EDUCATION

A high level of education and training is your single best insurance policy when choosing a spinal health practitioner. Education standards among various professions vary widely, and sometimes vary within individual professions.

As you have no doubt gathered, back pain is a very complex area. The skills required to competently assess and treat your spine do not come easily. I suggest that three years of focused training is a *minimum* period required to learn the basics of human anatomy, physiology, kinesiology, and a whole lot of other 'ology' words that constitute a rounded, thorough understanding of back pain. Any practitioner without this basic level of education will probably miss vital elements of your problem, leading to any ineffective, negligent or possibly even dangerous treatment.

A trusting patient—you, for example—has no simple way of knowing the true level of training and competence of a practitioner. Sure, you could ask, but this is, for most people, an ungainly way of establishing trust. And I'm sure the answer would be biased!

One method of ensuring that your spinal health practitioner has a basic level of competence is to stick with professions that have adequate prerequisite training. Following is a summary of typical training levels for many spinal health practitioners.

Medical doctors must complete a Bachelor of Medicine degree, and one year of compulsory internship upon graduation. Many universities are now making Medicine a post-graduate degree, meaning that any aspiring doctors must complete another degree of their choice before they even start. Furthermore, general practitioners must have further experience and training. Obviously, most of a doctor's study will be in areas other than lower back pain.

Manual therapists such as *physiotherapists, chiropractors* and *osteopaths* must all complete a Bachelor degree from a university or college, and sometimes a Masters degree as well. This study generally takes about four or five years, and is dedicated, in the main, to musculoskeletal medicine.

Acupuncturists vary widely in their training standards. Some practitioners have passed a four-year university-accredited Bachelor degree in acupuncture and Chinese medicine, while others have studied a six-week course.

Other health professionals such as medical doctors are now learning acupuncture. Again, the standards of education vary widely, with some practitioners doing extended study, while others complete brief weekend training courses before poking needles into unsuspecting patients.

Naturopathy and *homoeopathy* are generally completed as part of a two- or three-year diploma from a college. Some university-aligned colleges are now offering expanded courses as a four-year Bachelor degree. However, like acupuncture, the educational standards vary widely, with some practitioners having completed only minimal certificate or correspondence courses of a few weeks' or months' duration.

Massage can be studied independently as a certificate course, usually of a few months' duration. There are many variations of massage, each of which can be learned through additional short courses. Some colleges also have a two-year diploma in remedial massage, which doubtless covers most of these areas. Reflexology, a form of foot massage, is also usually learned through a certificate course. Elements of massage are often taught as part of other disciplines.

Other types of therapies have varying educational requirements. For example, *Feldenkrais* practitioners generally complete an eight-month course, spread over four years. Other alternative choices, such as *aromatherapy* and *iridology*, can be completed either via short certificate courses, or as part of other disciplines like naturopathy.

Of course, all good practitioners will continue to study and update their knowledge and skills throughout their entire career.

(2) YOUR PRACTITIONER SHOULD BE GOVERNMENT-REGISTERED IF POSSIBLE

Government registration provides a guarantee that the professional has completed the minimum required study for his or her profession. Registration also ensures that those practitioners who act in a criminal or negligent way can be struck off the register or suspended, offering you a basic level of protection.

All doctors, physiotherapists, chiropractors and osteopaths must be government-registered. No one can claim to be a member of these professions unless they are registered; to do so is an offence punishable by law.

Unfortunately, other professions—including acupuncture, naturopathy, homoeopathy, massage and all other alternative therapies—do not require any government registration.

If you choose a therapist who is a member of a non-registered profession, then you have no guarantee that the practitioner has completed adequate training. In fact, the practitioner may have simply read a book on the subject, liked the idea, and opened a business. This is perfectly legal for unregistered professions, and something of which you should be very aware.

I do not mean to imply that non-registered health-care professionals are incompetent, or that they would be unable to help you with your problem. I know of many non-registered practitioners who have not only honed their manual treatment skills to a fine level, but have continued to study and research their chosen field. I am sure that there are thousands of non-registered practitioners who are dedicated, hard-working and caring people. However, in their midst lurk a few quacks, and unfortunately there is no current legislation to help protect you from encountering one of them.

I was recently sent an information brochure from a natural therapy school, which demonstrated the potential for underqualified people to enter the health-care market. The brochure advertised a variety of courses ranging from astrology to tasseography (tea cup reading, for all you uneducated souls out there) that were proudly marketed under the banner of *'Just imagine being able to set up your own business, backed up by a diploma in the subject of your choice'*. One such course was remedial massage, which contained units of study such as anatomy, physiology, shiatsu and—I shudder—manipulation. This course consisted of twelve lessons *by correspondence*. This in-depth study could be completed in (and I quote) 'just a few hours each week . . . in as little as (6) six months'.

Hmm.

I don't know about you, but I would certainly not be clever enough to master the intricacies of spinal anatomy, physiology, massage and manipulation in a few hours a week over six months. After four years at university I was still confused! Moreover, a correspondence course is hardly an ideal way to learn practical, hands-on treatment skills. Yet a person with this minimal, inadequate level of education could quite legally open his or her own business as a 'remedial massage therapist and manipulation expert'. Scary.

Many health associations are lobbying the government to introduce compulsory registration for their professions. This step is an excellent move, and one can only wonder why it has not already been implemented. I feel genuine sympathy for those dedicated, educated members of non-registered professions who have no way of controlling the standards of their 'colleagues'.

However, until the laws are changed, you have no assurance that a non-registered practitioner has achieved adequate educational and professional standards.

(3) YOUR PRACTITIONER SHOULD BE A MEMBER OF A REPUTABLE PROFESSIONAL ASSOCIATION

I suggest that you only use a spinal health practitioner who is a member of his or her national professional association. These associations, which are listed in your telephone directory, provide many benefits to you, the consumer.

First, the associations only admit members who meet minimum educational standards. This criteria is of very tangible value for unregistered professions, as the association then assumes a 'watchdog' role over its members. If your spinal health practitioner is a member of an association, then you have some reassurance that they have met minimum educational standards, whether the profession is registered or not.

Second, professional associations provide a means of staying up-to-date with the latest technology, research and trends in the management of lower back pain. An isolated practitioner could never hope to develop as quickly as one who has the background support, combined knowledge and research resources of an entire profession. Furthermore, some professional organisations require their members to commit to ongoing education.

Finally, professional associations ensure that their members abide by a code of ethics and good practice. Any member who fails to practice to the required standard can be expelled from their association, although you should note that this does not stop him or her from practising.

If your practitioner is an association member, you at least have the knowledge that they meet acceptable standards of practice, ethics and education. As such, I advise you to use only practitioners who are members of their relevant group, particularly for non-registered professions.

(4) YOUR PRACTITIONER SHOULD THOROUGHLY EXAMINE YOU WHEN ASSESSING YOUR PROBLEM

This statement sounds so obvious as to be redundant. Yet many practitioners leap from 'hello' to dispensing their treatment in but a few seconds. Without a baseline level of examination, your spinal health practitioner has no way of knowing the underlying condition of your spine, and you will probably receive an inefficient or negligent treatment.

Back pain cannot reliably be diagnosed using any other method than a thorough clinical examination. The examination should include basic questions such as these:

- Where do you feel the pain?
- What does the pain feel like?

- Do you have any other symptoms associated with your problem, such as pins and needles or numbness?
- What causes and eases the pain?
- How long have you had the pain?
- How did the problem start?
- What is your general state of health?

The practitioner should also *look* at your spine—don't laugh, some practitioners don't even lift your shirt—and observe some basic spinal movements. He or she should also feel your spine, checking for tenderness, swelling, joint position and movement. Most back examinations should also include tests for nerve tightness.

If your practitioner does not perform these basic examinations, then you should pack your bags and go elsewhere.

Of course, many other aspects can be added into a spine examination. Your practitioner may test your muscle strength and flexibility, or check your movement patterns. He or she may use massage to evaluate your muscle tone, or to check for knots and trigger points. Postural evaluation is also frequently used, as are enquiries and observations about your lifestyle, job, or sporting technique. Blood tests may be necessary in some cases. Your practitioner may also use scans or X-rays to help confirm their diagnosis, although they should never rely upon them as a sole diagnostic tool.

In short, there are dozens of additional tests and examinations that your spinal health practitioner can perform to help gain a greater understanding of your problem. If you are attending a practitioner who is very dismissive, or performs only scant assessment before starting treatment, then please seek another opinion. After all, it's your spine, your time, and your hard-earned money.

(5) YOUR SPINE SHOULD IMPROVE WITH TREATMENT
You would be surprised how many times I have heard of patients who attended a spinal health practitioner for years without any noticeable improvement. This unethical treatment is simply overservicing, and is a breach of the trust that you place in your practitioner.

How much treatment is too much? Obviously, this is a very difficult question to answer, as circumstances vary so widely. However, for most ordinary back pain, I would suggest that an improvement level of five per cent per visit is a minimum standard for which to aim. Of course, the rate may vary; for example, some people feel slightly aggravated after their first visit, but then improve substantially thereafter. Nevertheless, if your overall improvement rate is any slower than five per cent per visit, then the treatment is probably ineffective.

Does this mean that if your spine has not improved by fifty per cent after ten visits that the practitioner is no good? Not necessarily.

However, if you have not improved at all after ten treatments, then you should expect that, in most cases, your practitioner will try a different approach. He or she should have many techniques and methods to treat back pain, and should consider trying another that may help you improve more quickly. In short, I would ask your health practitioner questions if they continue with unchanged treatment techniques, even though you are not improving.

Also, please remember that all treatment, no matter who administers it, is governed by the natural principle of *risk verses return*. As in finance, sport and almost every other sphere of life, faster or more dramatic returns can only be achieved if you are prepared to take higher risks. So if you want an instant, miracle cure for your back pain, the treatment may have to be more aggressive, and so may aggravate your condition. Conversely, if you don't wish to accept the risk of any exacerbation, then you may have to resign yourself to a longer, more controlled rehabilitation period.

Some people find that they benefit from maintenance visits to a spinal health practitioner. In some cases, regular sessions can be beneficial. However, if your spine is fixed properly, then you shouldn't require ongoing treatment. Usually there are other more relevant methods, such as exercise, to keep your spine healthy on an ongoing basis.

Chiropractors in particular argue that by having your spine regularly examined, problems can be detected and treated before they become painful. In this way, they are using preventative medicine, rather than reacting only when something is wrong. This argument is fine in theory. However, I feel that it overstates the case.

Consider the findings of the radiology studies as discussed in Chapter 27, in which MRI scans of people with healthy backs showed that generally about half of them had 'serious' defects, even though they had never experienced any pain. In other words, back problems are not always symptomatic. These 'defects' have never, and will never, cause any trouble in some people. Let sleeping dogs lie, I say.

Certainly, some patients will benefit from ongoing occasional treatment, and I am not wholly opposed to it. Usually, I wait for the injury to tell me that it needs regular maintenance treatment. However, those practitioners who routinely prescribe ongoing care for virtually every patient are, in my opinion, guilty of overservicing. Why undergo treatment for something that may never cause trouble again?

Is manipulation good for your spine?

Spinal manipulation occurs when a practitioner twists or thrusts your back with a short, sudden force. This creates an instant separation of the joint surfaces, which not only makes the vertebrae move, but results in the characteristic cracking sound.

Manipulation requires great skill to be effective. Suppose that your painful joint is very stiff, while the adjacent level moves normally. If the practitioner is not extremely careful when performing the manipulation, the loosest—i.e. uninjured—joint will be the one that moves and cracks. The stiff joint will remain locked in place. If this procedure is performed too vigorously or regularly, then the normal joint can be made unstable, meaning that you will have two problems!

For this reason, you should not deliberately crack your own spine with excessive force or frequency. If your back happens to click or crack while you are stretching it, fine. However, if you self-manipulate with too much enthusiasm you will simply create extra problems.

To circumvent this problem, many therapists use a technique called 'mobilisation', in which the hands are used to perform small, repeating oscillations on the joint. These movements have a similar effect to manipulation, but have the advantage of being more controlled and easier to localise.

These are days of evidence-based, insurance-driven medicine. Every form of treatment is justifiably being placed under the microscope. As such, there has been increasing debate in recent years about the benefits of spinal manipulation and mobilisation.

Many studies have shown that manipulation and mobilisation are effective methods to help some forms of lower back pain. In a recent wide-ranging U.S. government review, an eminent panel reviewed 112 research papers into the effectiveness of manipulation in treating lower back pain. Their lengthy, detailed report summarised their finding as such: 'The panel found manipulation to be a recommendable method of symptom control . . .' and '. . . evidence suggests spinal manipulation is effective in reducing pain and perhaps speeding recovery . . .'. For such a vast review to recommend manipulation puts it in a category of very high scientific justification—very few other treatment methods received such a recommendation.

Despite this, some doctors, and other representatives of the medical insurance industry, have recently cast doubt over the effectiveness of these types of passive treatments. While some of these reports imply that manipulation provides few long-term benefits, many of them miss the point. What these researchers often fail to accommodate is that different problems require different types of manipulation. Furthermore, and here is an even more important point, some types of spines will benefit from manipulation, while other spines will not.

Think about the four spine types, A, B, C and D, that we have used throughout this book. In my experience, people with unstable type A or B spines are sometimes worsened by manipulation. Conversely, manipulation often provides great benefits to those people with stiff or locked spines. So testing manipulation on a wide range of unclassified back problems is never going to prove fruitful. These studies are as silly as distributing the same set of spectacles to a group of people with poor vision, and then declaring that eye glasses are useless as they improve only a small percentage of patients.

In short, spinal manipulation and mobilisation have well-established place in the treatment of some, not all, types of back pain. However, the skill of the practitioner, as well as his or her clinical decision-making skills, are paramount to ensure a successful treatment. If the wrong technique is used, or if your back is unsuitable for mobilising, then these types of treatments may aggravate your problem. Most spine pain can at least be helped by passive treatment, such as mobilisation and manipulation, while many can be relieved altogether.

Summary

Many different options are available to you when choosing a spinal health practitioner. Besides being competent, trustworthy and affordable, you should look for a few other characteristics in a good practitioner.

Your practitioner should be highly educated, and support this by either government registration or membership of a reputable professional society. The practitioner should always thoroughly examine your spine, and his or her treatments should improve your pain at a reasonable rate. If you follow these guidelines, then you will hopefully find a caring practitioner who will assist you in your mission to banish your back pain for good.

34

Which spinal health practitioner is best for you?

Why physiotherapists are such lovely, wonderful people

Voltaire, the famous French philosopher, had an interesting definition of 'superstition': *someone else's religion*. He may have also been talking about a spinal health practitioner's version of superstition: someone else's methods. The waters of mistrust among the various professions run deep.

There is a weak excuse for this bias, as most health-care professionals are consulted only by the 'failed' patients of other practitioners. Because they rarely see patients who have been cured by other professions, spinal health practitioners can unintentionally develop a negative opinion of other approaches.

As a physiotherapist, I naturally incline towards the opinion that my profession is the best qualified to diagnose and treat back problems. Most of the contents of this book are based upon principles of care that I have learned as a physiotherapist, so I would be damning my profession with faint praise if I didn't talk it up at least a bit. Please bear with me if I get too exuberant.

Nevertheless, I am aware that many people have found relief from a wide range of treatment methods, so I will try to remain even-handed and objective during the following discussion. I have scant respect for some other self-help books that are nothing but advertisements for one profession or another, so I will try not to fall into this trap.

Having said that, some forms of treatment and pseudo-scientific therapies are generally unsound, and will do little if anything to help your problem. Here, I feel compelled to at least offer you my opinion, which you may take or leave as you wish.

To begin, we will look at *manual therapists* (professionals such as physiotherapists, chiropractors and osteopaths) who use their hands to work on your spine. Then we will look at the role of medical doctors in diagnosing and reviewing your back pain, and then examine the possibilities for natural and alternative therapies. Finally, you will learn of the advantages and disadvantages of spinal surgery and injection.

Physiotherapy

Physiotherapists use a variety of approaches and techniques to assess and treat back pain. First, a good physio will thoroughly examine your spine, and will feel the position and movements of the joints. Then, the treatment will often involve joint mobilisation, and perhaps muscle or nerve stretching. Many physiotherapists also use manipulation.

Often the session will involve teaching you exercises, and dispensing advice about how to avoid your problem in the future. Some physiotherapists also use deep massage or other muscular realignment techniques to help rebalance your joints.

Most physiotherapists also use electrotherapy, as outlined in Chapter 29, or various forms of heat or cryotherapy (a big word meaning 'ice'). Sometimes a physiotherapist may try spinal traction. In short, physiotherapists have a wide range of options with which to attack your problem, depending upon how it presents.

The main advantage of physiotherapy over other forms of treatment is that it does not rely on one strategy. Many alternatives are available to help your physiotherapist cure your problem. If a certain approach is slow or unsuccessful, then your physio can try a different method.

Another advantage of physiotherapy is its wide research base. Physiotherapists lead the professions in the practice of joint mobilisation, and have almost single-handedly developed techniques to improve nerve mobility. They are also specialists in movement analysis, while electrotherapy is also largely the domain of physiotherapists. The investigation of stability muscles, which I believe is the future direction of spinal health care, is also largely dependent upon the research and observation of physiotherapists.

In short, a good physiotherapist has a lot to offer you to help you to overcome your spinal pain.

Disadvantages? None. Physiotherapy is perfect. Problems simply do not exist . . .

OK, I'll try to be honest. Sometimes the treatments, particularly the joint mobilisation and the nerve stretches, can be painful. Just ask any one of my back pain patients how much fun they had while I pressed my thumbs into their sore joints, and, if you can ignore the curses and expletives, you'll get the idea. However, do not fear: if you're the type of person who is allergic to pain, then tell your physiotherapist in advance, as he or she doubtless has other less painful techniques that will help you overcome your problem.

Unfortunately, some physiotherapists have developed a dependence on electrotherapy and/or traction as the mainstay of their treatment program. While these machines have a worthwhile place as an adjunct to treatment, they do not replace the need for hands-on work and proper exercise instruction. If your physiotherapist seems to spend most of his or her time dashing from room to room just to change electrotherapy devices, then I suggest you try another practitioner who devotes a greater percentage of time to manual therapy.

Chiropractic

Chiropractic treatment, like all systems of manual therapy, is very complex. At the simplest level of description, a chiropractor assesses your condition by using X-rays and feeling your spine, looking for the presence of a *vertebral subluxation*. As defined by chiropractors, this is a spinal joint that is moving incorrectly (in other words, it is stiff or unstable) or is displaced.

A good chiropractor will usually assess your whole spine for problems, not just the area local to the pain. If the chiropractor finds a subluxed joint, then he or she will attempt to correct it by manipulation. By realigning and normalising the movement and position of the vertebra, health and function can hopefully be restored to your spine.

Chiropractors have had a long-running political battle with the medical profession. This antipathy still exists to some degree.

I am not sure why this hostility began. Perhaps it was due to chiropractors claiming that they could cure diseases through spinal manipulation. Although some renegade chiropractors still practise this philosophy, it is no longer part of recognised chiropractic doctrine.

Another possible reason for the mistrust is that chiropractors sometimes have different philosophies on medicine to a standard medical health care model. Or perhaps the resentment exists simply because chiropractors use the term 'doctor' for themselves. Whatever the reason, the reluctance of many medicos to refer to chiropractors is still apparent.

Chiropractors, as the lone wolves of the health-care field, have been subject over the years to a lot of criticism. Much of this criticism and 'chiropractor bashing' is no longer justified, as the excessive elements of the profession are slowly disappearing. A few of the objections are occasionally justified: some chiropractors *are* too rough; some chiropractors *do* overtreat; some chiropractors *still* have unscientific ideas about the role of the spine in disease processes. However, I'm sure you could apply these criticisms to some members of every profession, from physios to doctors to tasseographers.

I feel that you are most likely to gain benefit from chiropractic treatment if your spinal problem is due to stiffness, or if you have locked or seized joints. Conversely, chiropractic treatment may be of limited value if your problem is due to instability or weakness. The chiropractic reliance on manipulation, and comparatively minimal attention to retraining muscular stability, makes it less effective for unstable conditions.

Despite the above criticisms, a chiropractor who is highly skilled in spinal manipulation can provide benefits in the treatment and prevention of low back pain. As shown in the previous section, well-applied spinal manipulation has proven benefits, and chiropractors are one of the best placed professions to administer such treatments.

Osteopathy

Not much is known about osteopaths in Australia. Until recently most osteopathic training occurred overseas, so the number of local practitioners was small. However, osteopathic training is now available at Australian universities, so the profession is gradually entering the health-care fold.

On the surface, osteopathic treatment appears similar to chiropractic. At a clinical level, the differences between the two professions become more apparent to an educated eye, as some treatment philosophies and techniques are unique to osteopathy.

Osteopaths use various manual techniques for achieving their goals, including manipulation. They also use other 'joint positioning' techniques, which rely on slow movements that allow abnormal muscle tone to abate. Because these movements are gentle, they are useful when forceful manipulation is undesirable. Osteopaths, like most manual therapists, take a holistic view of a problem, and so may offer advice on exercise and posture as well, and examine and treat other parts of your body.

One of the problems with osteopathy in this country is its varied origins. As many osteopaths trained overseas, the approaches can vary markedly from one practitioner to the next. However, these differences should contract as time passes, and the training becomes more uniform. A phone call to your osteopath before you attend for treatment is probably the best way to ensure that his or her treatment philosophy is commensurate with yours.

Medical doctors—General practitioners

Your local doctor is a good place to start if you are unsure about your back pain. Your doctor's wide-ranging medical knowledge ensures that he or she is less likely to confuse your back symptoms for other maladies. Furthermore, your doctor can refer you for blood tests, which can detect rare abnormalities that can lead to lower back pain, and can order most types of radiology if necessary. A doctor can also assess whether your problem is serious enough to warrant referral to a surgeon.

For treating back pain, a medical doctor can prescribe drugs, although, as discussed in Chapter 24, this all-to-easy avenue of treatment is sometimes overdone. Your doctor can also provide reassurance—a precious commodity—and advice on how to best cope with your pain. A really, really good practitioner might also advise you to read a copy of this book!

Please be realistic about how much treatment your doctor can provide in his or her consulting rooms. Your local GP is probably a very hard-working person, who consults patients with all manner of problems and diseases, from the flu to depression to lacerations to cancer. Commonsense will tell you that your doctor cannot be a specialist in every area, so while your doctor's wide medical knowledge confers advantages, it can also be a disadvantage when it comes to specific, hands-on help.

Further to this point, a good general practitioner should recognise his or her limitations. Hopefully, he or she has a network of other local spinal health practitioners to refer to, who have the specialised knowledge and techniques to deal with your problem. Your doctor should remain in contact with this practitioner, intervening with further suggestions or investigations if your problem does not progress as expected.

Some doctors are now turning to other methods, such as spinal mobilisation, manipulation or electrotherapy, in order to help their patients recover from their problems. A similar development is occurring with acupuncture. This provides advantages for geographically isolated or financially destitute patients who rely on their GP for all of their health care. However, for the general population, I feel that other health professionals are better qualified for the task of administering specific treatment to your spine.

Other professionals such as physiotherapists, chiropractors and osteopaths have studied for many years, concentrating primarily on musculoskeletal medicine. Unfortunately, some general practitioners are attempting similar work after attending short courses of sometimes only a few weeks' duration. The negative consequences are predictable.

You may, of course, find a doctor who has completed significant further study and training in the art and science of back mobilisation, manipulation, muscle balance, neural tension, movement analysis and so on. This doctor will probably nominate that he or she has a 'special interest in manual therapy', and will note the extra training on his or her business card. In this case, where the doctor has completed considerable further training, then he or she has obviously taken the time to properly develop the necessary skills before using them on you. Some of the world's foremost manual therapists began their professional lives in medical practice.

However, in my humble opinion, most doctors' skills lie in the art of general practice, not hands-on spinal treatment or electrotherapy. Even though your doctor is doubtlessly doing his or her utmost to help you recover, I feel that they would serve you better by using a referral pad, not attempting a session of quasi-electrotherapy/manipulation in their consulting rooms.

In short, your local doctor is an excellent place to start your consulting. He or she has the widest range of medical tests available, and a broad general knowledge. However, don't be afraid to ask for a referral if you would like some extra help.

Acupuncture

Acupuncture is a health-care system developed in China over 2000 years ago. The practitioner uses fine needles that he or she inserts into various spots, known as *acupoints*. Other traditional methods to stimulate these points include using fingers, known as acupressure, and the burning of material in small cups, known as *moxibustion*. Modern acupuncture also uses technology such as laser and electrotherapy to stimulate acupoints.

Traditional Chinese medical theory says that the acupoints sit along lines, or channels, known as *meridians*. Your body's natural energy, known as *ch'i*, circulates around the meridians. Pain or other problems develop when this natural energy circulation is blocked. The acupuncturist, by needling or otherwise stimulating these points, is said to be able to unblock the flow of energy, which allows the body to heal the problem itself.

Attempts to reconcile acupuncture theory with modern medicine have provided few answers. No substance that represents ch'i has been identified, and the meridian channels have no physical basis.

Other researchers have attempted to define the effect that acupuncture has upon the body, and have put forward various theories. Some say that acupuncture works on the nervous system, creating an effect similar to the gate theory (see Chapter 20). Others feel that acupuncture may somehow cause the body to release endorphins (discussed in Chapter 26), while others have postulated that it somehow regulates the flow of the body's natural chemical electricity. However, when all the evidence has been sifted and examined, we still do not have any clear understanding of how acupuncture works.

Nevertheless, in the end, the most important question to you is 'does it work'? Numerous studies have been undertaken to answer this question, and they are united on only one point: they are contradictory. Some studies show that acupuncture borders on miraculous, while other research shows that acupuncture does nothing at all. Although it is widely used, the medico-scientific jury is still out on the true effectiveness of acupuncture.

In the same USA government review that examined manipulation (as mentioned in the last chapter), a panel examined twenty-four studies that looked at the effect of acupuncture on lower back pain. Let me share the results with you.

Many of these studies found that patients who received acupuncture treatment for lower back pain fared better than those who did not. For some people, this finding is the end of the argument. Acupuncture works. Period.

However, the panel reviewed other studies that cast doubt over these findings. For example, some researchers compared patients who had correctly applied acupuncture to a control group who received 'placebo' acupuncture, where the needles were deliberately placed in the wrong spot. Of course, neither group was aware of whether their treatment was correct or not. In these studies, no significant difference was found in the recovery rates or pain levels of either group, suggesting that much of the power of acupuncture is due to the placebo effect.

So as far as acupuncture as a treatment for back pain goes, nothing is certain. Even if you find that it helps to temporarily relieve your pain, you would be foolish to rely on acupuncture alone. Other techniques, such as exercise, relaxation, or joint mobilisation, may still be necessary or useful for you to make a full and permanent recovery.

I'd like to briefly revisit an issue that I mentioned in the last chapter. Many practitioners of acupuncture, including medical doctors and other health practitioners, have very minimal training in acupuncture. Some of them may have simply studied a book on the subject, before proudly erecting a sign in their waiting room. Since no regulations currently exist to control the administration of acupuncture, you should ensure that your therapist is accredited with a relevant *acupuncture* association.

In the end, much of the decision about whether to try acupuncture or not is up to you. Sorry to sit on the fence, but the studies are too contradictory to draw any strong conclusions. Try acupuncture treatment if you wish, as its side effects are minimal. You can then assess for yourself if you feel any benefits. I've met many people who say that they've benefited from acupuncture, and you may well be another.

Massage

There are many different types of massage. They include such exotically named styles as Shiatsu, Swedish, Lymphatic Drainage, Deep Tissue, Remedial, Trigger Point Therapy, Soft Tissue Manipulation, Bowen and Sports Massage.

What are the differences between these various methods? Not much. However, there are subtle deviations. Shiatsu, of Japanese origins, uses deep local pressure over muscle knots, as does trigger point therapy. Swedish and lymphatic drainage tend to be long flowing and relaxing, while deep tissue and remedial are more vigorous and painful. Soft tissue manipulation may encompass short arc friction-type massage, Bowen includes some 'pinching' methods, while sports massage blends deep muscular work with percussive 'slapping' techniques.

In general, most types of massage achieve the same effects: they help to loosen tight muscles, 'deactivate' trigger points or knots, and promote an overall sense of relaxation. For these reasons, a good, deep massage may help relieve your pain.

However, please be aware that massage should be only a small part of your rehabilitation, not the whole program. Massage works primarily on muscles, and does not effect discs, bones or joints, and so cannot effectively treat the vast majority of back pain. While massage may help you to feel better, it rarely cures the underlying cause of a problem when used in isolation.

For this reason, I suggest that a masseur should *not* be your first professional contact if you have back pain. Even a highly skilled, experienced masseur may not have the training to effectively diagnose your problem, and may inadvertently miss a more sinister cause. By all means have a massage if it helps you to feel better—and it probably will—but please ensure that your back is receiving other necessary treatment.

Reflexology

Reflexology, a specialised type of foot massage, works on the theory that certain zones within the foot correspond to body parts. The reflexology doctrine continues that by massaging and stimulating these zones, relief can be obtained in distant areas.

Reflexologists do not claim to diagnose problems, but instead promote their craft as an overall health booster. Obviously, reflexology is easy to apply, is more pleasurable than many other forms of treatment, and has very few, if any, side effects.

Here, dear reader, is where I would like to share with you the extreme lengths of research to which I subjected myself, in order to bring you accurate information. My hard-edged study and in-depth investigation knew no bounds the day that I, without fear of the consequences, subjected myself to a one-hour long aromatic foot massage. This extra effort was all in order to provide you with a more accurate picture of the benefits of reflexology. I hope you appreciate it.

Did I feel wonderfully relaxed after the session? Yes.

Was the foot rub calming and soothing? Yes.

Do I think that reflexology can directly cure back pain? No.

In my opinion, the body zones are a load of rubbish. However, even if you share this belief, you may still find that the relaxation afforded by the massage helps you to temporarily manage your pain.

Natural medicine: Naturopathy and homeopathy

Natural medicine attempts to harness the power of the human body to heal itself. The principal of 'the healing power of nature' underlies all natural medicine treatments; if you improve your body's health and balance, it will heal itself. Like much of medicine, naturopaths often quote this principle in Latin—*vix medicatrix naturae*—which I suppose they do to make it sound cleverer.

Naturopathy takes a holistic approach to health, rather than attempting to identify and treat specific diseases or processes. To encourage this process, natural medicine uses many related strategies.

HERBAL MEDICINE makes use of plants as a source of remedies, whether they are fresh, dried, or ingested as teas, tablets or extracts.

HOMEOPATHY is based on a theory called the 'law of similars', meaning that if a substance can cause a disease, then a minute dose of that substance can also cure it. Hence a homeopath will study your symptoms, and will prescribe you a natural remedy that, if given to a healthy person, would produce signs and symptoms resembling yours.

AROMATHERAPY makes use of sweet-smelling oils, which are used via methods such as massage or inhalation. Aromatherapists believe that certain smells can stimulate various responses within the body, and by combining the right oils, they can enhance your wellbeing.

IRIDOLOGISTS believe that by studying the iris, the coloured part of the eye, they can identify areas of the body in which a problem may exist.

Many natural therapists also incorporate other techniques such as acupuncture, massage, nutritional advice, counselling and stress management into their programs.

Some facets of natural medicine may help your lower back pain, particularly as an adjunct to other forms of treatment such as manual therapy or exercise. Perhaps, by helping you to decrease your stress levels—whether by counselling, massage, aromatherapy, reflexology, whatever—a naturopath may assist you in overcoming this common cause of back problems.

A detailed analysis of your diet may reveal problem areas, which you can then correct by changing your diet, or taking occasional supplementation. These steps may help improve the healing capabilities of your body, and increase your physical tolerance to stress. Of course, a naturopathic massage will help to relax tight muscles, while acupuncture may help to relieve your pain.

For reasons already outlined in Chapter 25, I do not believe that herbal or homoeopathic remedies have accrued enough hard evidence to prove that they help you to get rid of your back pain forever.

Of course, some of these preparations may have mild anti-inflammatory properties. However, there are not enough rigorous trials to show that these remedies do what they claim. I see little point in taking a preparation that has not been adequately tested, particularly for a problem so localised and specific as lower back pain.

This situation may change, with natural medicine courses now being offered as four-year degree courses at university-accredited colleges. However, until proper scientific study replaces conjecture, and until government regulations force all herbal and homoeopathic claims to be proven through clinical trials, then I suggest that you let other people play 'health lottery' with these preparations. Ditto for aromatherapy and iridology.

In short, some aspects of natural medicine can provide pain relief, and may help to fortify your body and relax your mind. However, naturopaths are not trained in the science of spinal diagnosis, so I suggest that you use natural medicine as an adjunct, rather than a front-line treatment option.

Other techniques: Pilates, Feldenkrais, Alexander, Yoga

Occasionally through human history, a few dedicated people have devoted their lives to the destruction of piracy, greed and injustice from within society.

Er ... sorry, that's the Phantom ...

I meant to say 'devoted their lives to the elimination of injury, pain and arthritis from within their bodies'. These people, through careful observation of their own musculo-skeletal problems, gradually developed their own system of rehabilitative exercises. By then teaching their methods to others, their methods slowly gained popularity, and some now enjoy worldwide recognition. The most noted of these techniques are:

(1) *Pilates* (pi-LAH-tees)
(2) *Feldenkrais* (FEL-den-crise; the 'crise' is pronounced as in 'crisis')
(3) *Alexander* (I'm sure you know how to pronounce 'Alexander')
(4) *Yoga* falls into a similar category, although to my knowledge it was not developed by a single practitioner.

Some of these techniques are very abstract, making them difficult to describe in a few paragraphs. I will do my best.

PILATES

Pilates is an exercise-based rehabilitation program. Using a series of 500 exercises, Pilates training aims to restore strength and balance to the entire muscular system. The exercises are designed to be performed in a variety of postures and positions, and using different apparatus, many of which slide, glide or rock.

The emphasis of the program is on the abdominal, lower back and buttock muscles, which the founder of the movement, Joseph Pilates, felt were the 'power centre' of the body. The instructors emphasise the control of body alignment, a correct breathing pattern, and careful concentration as the keys to a successful work-out.

Pilates instructors become qualified through a certificate course of two to three weeks. However, full certification is not granted until the instructor has completed a 600-hour apprenticeship, during which he or she will observe, then assist, and finally instruct clients in the method.

Joseph Pilates was very astute when, just after World War I, he noted that the stomach, back and buttock muscles were the centres of the body's strength and control. The slow, controlled nature of the exercises means that the gains would, for most people, outweigh any potential disadvantages.

Many people with lower back pain, particularly those with weak or unstable spines, would benefit from regular Pilates sessions. If you are reasonably fit, and enjoy gymnasium-type work-outs, and can commit to regular sessions, then the extra movement, strength and balance that the sessions provide would probably be beneficial.

FELDENKRAIS

The Feldenkrais method, developed by a Russian doctor in the mid 1900s, is based on self-exploration of how your body moves. A 'teacher' will help you to observe and learn the nuances of how your muscles and joints move, and to explore how your body reacts when performing basic functions.

By increasing your movement awareness, you can learn how to avoid certain actions that may cause pain, or create other problems such as stiffness. By learning more about your actions, you can establish new patterns of movement that do not cause dysfunction. The result is a more flexible and balanced neuromuscular system.

Feldenkrais treatment is no simple matter. To benefit from Feldenkrais may take months, even years, of careful self-observation and training. This technique is not a quick fix, and requires great motivation and self-responsibility.

The advantage of Feldenkrais is that it empowers you to be the master of your own problem. The skills of movement awareness that you learn through Feldenkrais provide a framework for you to self-manage most musculo-skeletal problems. The results may therefore be more permanent than other types of treatments.

Feldenkrais practitioners must complete an accredited training program of eight months, which is interspersed with work, self-learning and practice over four years.

Obviously, the Feldenkrais system is not for everyone. However, if you've had chronic pain, and are frustrated with your lack of progress with conventional treatment, then you may reap great benefits, as the principles behind this system of rehabilitation appear to be sound. Just make sure that you're motivated to stay for the long haul, and can spare the time and effort to practise regularly.

ALEXANDER

F.M. Alexander was a young Shakespearian actor who developed voice coarseness while touring Australia at the turn of the century. Unable to find a medical cure, he discovered through self-observation that he could lessen his problem by correcting his head and neck posture. Spurred on by this discovery, he continued a gradual process of self-awareness, and found that by altering his postures and habits, many of his other problems disappeared.

Noticing his wellbeing, other actors asked for his help. Alexander gradually developed a system of touch and instruction that he used to correct the postures and habits of his students, which became the basis for his technique.

A doctrine of the Alexander technique is that 'the very fact of our existence involves us in habitual misuse of ourselves'. In other words, to put it in terms of this book, we naturally develop poor movement patterns and postures. Good thinking, Mr Alexander.

An Alexander teacher, through touch and instruction, will help a student to become more aware of, and ultimately to correct, any poor habits or postures. This 'recoordinating' will ultimately help you to avoid the movement patterns that cause the constant misuse of your body, leading to increased flexibility, better control, and less pain.

On paper, this technique appears philosophically similar to the Feldenkrais method. One difference is that Feldenkrais uses a series of exercises and self-exploration to help you develop self-awareness, while Alexander uses touch and instruction. Like Feldenkrais, the Alexander technique may provide you with lasting benefits for your spine and body, provided you commit the time, effort and concentration to this demanding form of rehabilitation.

YOGA
Most people are aware of the body-contorting positions that constitute an advanced yoga course. You doubtlessly already know that yoga will help to increase the flexibility of your muscles, joints and nerves. However, yoga goes deeper than simply stretching exercises. It combines relaxation with meditation, and uses a philosophy that the mind and body are one, and that peace can be achieved by uniting them with the universe.

While this may sound like heady stuff, yoga is, in principle, a healthy hobby for your spine. The benefits of mobility, relaxation and peaceful thinking are all likely to have a positive impact on your spinal health.

Your new-found knowledge of spinal mechanics should tell you that the stretching and flexibility components of yoga are more likely to help people with stiff spines, types C and D, rather than the unstable joints of types A or B. If you have a stiff spine, or if anxiety and mental tension are a big component of your problem, then yoga may be a useful addition to your back care program.

Surgery

Some conditions, such as cancer, fracture or dislocation, require immediate surgery. Other 'red flag' indicators that surgery may be immediately necessary include sudden or progressive muscular weakness in the legs, or bladder/rectal pins and needles and weakness.

However, for most cases of lower back pain, I feel that you should fulfil the following five criteria before you even begin to consider spinal surgery:

1. Your pain should be severe and/or disabling.
2. In most cases, you should have waited for at least six weeks to see if your condition improves naturally.

3. You should have seriously attempted other less-invasive forms of therapy and exercise first.
4. You should be comfortable with the idea of surgery.
5. Your pain should be predominantly in your leg, not in your back. Localised back pain responds poorly to surgical intervention. Only patients with nerve-related pain (severe sciatica, for example) can expect to benefit from surgery. If you have localised back pain but no leg pain, then you can virtually disregard surgery as a treatment option.

If you do not fulfil *all* of these five criteria, then I suggest that you should pursue other forms of treatment at this stage.

First, the bad news. Spinal surgery is complex and expensive. Like all surgery, it can be dangerous. Specifically, your risk of death is about one in 20,000, and of infection about one in a hundred. Furthermore, spinal surgery has potential side effects of nerve damage. One per cent of patients are left with residual foot weakness, and a tiny number (less than one in 20,000) become paralysed from the waist down. If you are considering surgery and are worried about any of these statistics, then please discuss them carefully with your doctor.

Furthermore, if you have surgery that fails, repeat surgery is rarely effective, and other forms of treatment such as manual therapy are then disadvantaged.

Now the good news: if you have severe, chronic, nerve-related pain, then surgery may be your quickest option for a pain-free spine. It is a proven form of treatment, and when used wisely on appropriate candidates it can be very successful.

There are three basic categories of spinal surgery, as outlined below.

(1) DISCECTOMY AND LAMINECTOMY
The 'ect' part of these complex-sounding words simply means 'out' while the 'tomy' bit means 'cut'. By putting these bits together, you can see that a discectomy is a procedure in which the surgeon 'cuts out your disc'. The same principle apples to a laminectomy, in which the lamina (the short arm of bone that forms the side of the intervertebral canal) is removed.

This type of surgery is most effective for pain that arises from compressed nerves. In this case, the surgery can be ninety per cent effective in relieving leg pain.

Originally, these operations were performed as open procedures, which meant that the surgeon had to cut your spine to access the problem area. Now, with the advent of the arthroscope, the surgery can often be completed using tiny wire-like instruments, meaning that side effects and complications are considerably lessened.

(2) FUSION
Two vertebra can be fused, or grafted together, using a variety of techniques. First, a piece of bone, usually harvested from your pelvis, can be used to hold the bones together. Second, the surgeon can fix your spine using metallic plates, rods, wire or screws. Sometimes these techniques are used in combination. Fusion operations are, as commonsense dictates, most useful for unstable spines.

(3) DISC-HARDENING INJECTIONS
A chemical called 'chymopapain', which is derived from paw-paw, can be injected into a disc. It reacts with the nucleus, causing it to shrink. This lessens the chance that a prolapsed disc will push onto a nerve.

This procedure was once recommended for patients with prolapsing or herniating discs. Although studies have shown that the chemical is more effective than a placebo, chymopapain injections are not as effective as normal surgical procedures. They also cause occasional severe allergic reactions, sometimes even death. Most surgeons now prefer other procedures.

If you feel that you are a candidate for surgery, please discuss the options carefully with your doctor *and* your surgeon. Remember, a good rule of thumb is that your pain should be severe, chronic and nerve-related. You should have already attempted other types of treatment before you submit to the surgeon's knife. While you should never undertake surgery lightly, in some cases it is the best and most rapid cure.

Spinal injections

Two types of injections can be used in an attempt to relieve severe spinal pain. The first is called an *epidural*, in which medication is injected into the area around your nerve roots. This procedure aims to numb the leg pain associated with a compressed nerve. The second type of procedure is when medications are injected directly into your spinal joints in an effort to decrease the local inflammation.

Different medications have been tried with these procedures, including anaesthetics (that make you go numb), analgesics (pain relievers) and cortico-steroids. Corticosteroids are not, as some people mistakenly believe, the same types of drugs that cheating athletes and body builders use to gain a strength advantage. Rather, these types of steroids are powerful anti-inflammatory agents.

I feel that spinal injection is best left as a second-last resort in the options queue, just ahead of surgery. The relief is usually only temporary—a couple of weeks perhaps—although some people experience decreased pain levels for a few months. However, if your pain is severe and persistent, then an injection may provide you with some temporary relief of your pain, and may allow you to perform an exercise program with greater efficiency. Perhaps an injection may help you to avoid further surgery.

Below are some side considerations upon which you should reflect before agreeing to spinal injection as a front-line therapy.

1. Both types of injection have limitations as to which conditions they will help. Epidurals are most useful against nerve-related pain, rather than localised back pain.

    Conversely, joint injections are useful only for local facet joint or sacro-iliac joint problems. Unfortunately, the deep, diffuse nature of the intervertebral discs renders the injection ineffective. Therefore, bulging, herniating or degenerating discs cannot be satisfactorily treated with joint injection therapy.

2. Spinal injection is useful only for a single injury. Multiple sites of inflammation or wear and tear (a very common finding in degenerating spines) require multiple injections, which is neither practical nor efficient.

3. Injections are invasive, and so carry a minor risk of infection. They have other occasional complications, ranging from transient headaches to meningitis. OK, meningitis is extremely rare, but it *is* potentially fatal. Sometimes the medication itself also has local side effects, including weakening of the local ligaments and tendons.

4. Spinal injection procedures are difficult, and require a highly trained doctor to ensure their safety and success. They are not as simple as a vaccine jab, but require careful guided placement of the needles. Sometimes a device called a 'fluoroscope' is used that allows the doctor to visualise your spinal joints.

5. And of course, there is my favourite objection to many forms of spinal treatment: spinal injections do not cure the real cause of your problem. They simply decrease the local pain response and/or the inflammatory process. In due course, the vicious cycles of microtrauma continue to produce more problems, so the pain returns, sometimes worse than before.

If you are considering having a spinal injection, I feel that you should attempt other more conservative treatment procedures first, such as exercise. However, if you are desperate, and have a localised, non-responsive joint or nerve problem, then spinal injection may provide you with some temporary relief.

Summary

Many types of treatment are available to you. Manual therapists, such as chiropractors, osteopaths and physiotherapists, are trained in the art and science of spinal treatment. Your doctor can assist with other investigations and referrals, and is an excellent place to start if you are unsure.

Other therapies such as acupuncture, massage, natural medicine and reflexology can form a valuable adjunct to your treatment plan, although you should not depend on these disciplines as front-line therapies. Various other methods have differing benefits for your spine, and may be worth your consideration. Finally, surgery is a proven option for those with severe, long-lasting, nerve-related pain.

35

Putting it all together

Over to you!

Congratulations! You're almost there. Apart from a few of the obligatory appendices that I've tacked onto the back, this is the last chapter in this book.

So far, you've learned a lot about back pain. Believe it or not, you now know the rudiments of anatomy, evolution, kinesiology, myology, ergonomics, physiology, radiology, nutrition, pharmacology and psychology. You must be a genius!

In short, you've learned an awful lot about back pain over the last thirty-four chapters. Now, one question remains to be answered: *How do you get started?*

First, realise that the solution to your back pain is unique. As I've indicated repeatedly in this book, what helps one person's problem may hinder another's. So before you undertake any rehabilitation, you must perform some self-assessment to determine where the heart of your problem lies. In this way, you won't make any unnecessary alterations. Similarly, you won't forget to correct an area that desperately requires adjustment.

Obviously, your back pain type is a good place to start. I trust that you have already completed the quiz in Chapter 11.

Armed with the knowledge and principles that you have learned in this book, some careful self-examination will help you to decide which factors are contributing to your problem. This process is not simple, but is essential. As you know, any treatment program that is not preceded by a thorough assessment is doomed to failure.

How many areas should you pinpoint? Generally, the longer you have had your pain, and the more disabling it is, then the more things you should change.

If you've suffered a single bout of minor back pain, then altering a couple of areas should be sufficient. You probably don't wish to buy a new bed, change your job, set up your study room with ergonomic furniture, and embark upon a whole new fitness and exercise routine in response to one minor twinge. Conversely, if you've been suffering with frequent or continuous pain for years, then multiple, far-reaching changes such as these may be in order.

As you read through this book, you probably encountered some situations that made you think '*Aha!* That sounds like me.' These areas are a good place to begin your changes. In Chapter 19, you made a provisional list of situations that sometimes hurt your spine. You've learned a lot since then, so below is an expanded list of questions to help you decide which areas need attention. These questions are by no means exhaustive, but should help to stimulate your thinking.

Are all of your spinal joints loose and mobile?	Yes	No
Are your nerves and muscles flexible?	Yes	No
Are your abdominal, back and hip stability muscles balanced and toned?	Yes	No
Are you sure?	Yes	No
Is your sitting posture usually correct?	Yes	No
Do you have a supportive chair?	Yes	No
Do you use appropriate lumbar support when sitting?	Yes	No
Do you use a correct lifting technique, which includes contracting your stability muscles?	Yes	No
Can you perform all of your normal household tasks without pain?	Yes	No
Is your mattress correct for your back type?	Yes	No
Do you sleep with an appropriate posture?	Yes	No
Do you perform aerobic exercise at least four times per week?	Yes	No
Every week?	Yes	No
Is your diet usually healthy and balanced?	Yes	No
Is your body mass index between twenty and twenty-five?	Yes	No
Do you have positive thoughts about your pain, focusing on what you *can* do to help it, rather than what you *can't* do because of it?	Yes	No
Have you considered orthotics, footwear or postural taping as an adjunct to your treatment?	Yes	No
Do you sometimes use heat or ice to help your pain?	Yes	No
Have you consulted a good spinal health practitioner, who examined your spine carefully before performing any treatment?	Yes	No

If you answered 'No' to any of the above questions, then it is an area that may require further thought, and possibly some changes.

Continue the questionnaire below. However this time, any questions to which you answer 'yes' probably require attention.

Do you sometimes stand with a poor, unsupported posture?	Yes	No
Are there any work duties that often make your back hurt?	Yes	No
Do you regularly perform any prolonged or difficult activities (e.g. sitting or bending) that may cause microtrauma to accumulate in your spine?	Yes	No
Do you ever perform activities that are dangerous (e.g. twisting while lifting)?	Yes	No
Do you ever perform activities that are unsuitable for your spinal type?	Yes	No
Are you sometimes anxious or stressed?	Yes	No
Do you suffer from other stress-related problems, such as headaches, skin rashes, irritability, etc?	Yes	No
Does your back pain sometimes worsen during times of high stress?	Yes	No
Do you have negative thoughts, such as frustration, blaming or anger, about your pain?	Yes	No
Do you lack motivation to fix your problem? *If so, why?*	Yes	No
Do you frequently depend on medication for pain relief?	Yes	No
Do you often rely on bracing for pain relief?	Yes	No
Do you ever rely on rest as a treatment option?	Yes	No
Have you ever used treatments that are unproven, or that have been ineffective?	Yes	No
Are there any other activities or situations that cause your back to hurt?	Yes	No

Well done. You're getting there. Now that you have demarcated your problem areas, you can create your own personalised rehabilitation program. I suggest that you use a pen and paper to plan your approach.

First, write down your problem areas, roughly in order of relative importance. Then, by reviewing the principles and suggestions in this book, incorporate solutions to each of the problem areas, and approximate dates by which you hope to have achieved them. By writing these goals down, you commit yourself to achieving them. No wishy-washy excuses—the exact strategies, as well as their commencement or achievement dates, are there in black and white.

If you have a specific activity that is causing your pain, then most of your efforts should go into either (a) modifying the activity, or (b) changing your spine so that it can cope with that activity. Commonsense is your best guide in this regard.

Of course, you should employ front-line strategies first. Rehabilitation techniques such as stretching and stability exercises, a daily fitness program, relaxation techniques or using a decent chair are proven, reliable tools to help cure your problem. Other types of treatment, such as new shoes, nutritional supplements and reflexology foot massages are second-line options. Use these treatments as an adjunct if you wish, but please ensure that you are not using them as an easy way out, instead of putting effort where it is required.

Of course, your goals can be short-term plans, or long-term visions. Simply, just picture how you want your spine to be, envisage the steps that will get you there, then write them down. It's that simple!

Let's look at three case studies, to illustrate how you might undertake the extremely important task of building a rehabilitation strategy.

CASE ONE
The problem
Luke was a twenty-two-year-old cricketer who opened the bowling for his local A-grade team. After the second game of the previous cricket season, Luke noticed pain in his lower back. As the season progressed, each game affected his spine with increasing severity. His pain after each game gradually worsened, and his movements became extremely stiff on the morning following each game. By the end of the season, Luke's pain forced him to bowl at a reduced pace, and he could barely complete ten overs without spending the next three days in agony.

Now, in the off-season, Luke had comparatively little pain. He could perform most other activities without restriction, except his back sometimes ached if he stood in one place for more than thirty minutes. However, after bowling a few balls in the back yard to his brother, Luke again felt a spasm of pain. He realised that the problem, which he had simply hoped would disappear, required intervention if he were to complete his dream of playing cricket for his State side. He had four months to rehabilitate himself before the first game of the next season.

The program
Obviously, the main factor in Luke's problem was his cricket bowling. This diagnosis is straightforward, as he experienced significant pain after performing this activity, yet very little pain at other times. Therefore, Luke directed most of his efforts at this component of the problem.

He developed two broad goals. First, to change his spine so that it could cope with the rigours of bowling, and second, to change his bowling style so that it better suited his spine.

To begin, Luke performed the spinal assessment in Chapter 11, and determined that he was back type AC. Using this category as a guide, he commenced a strengthening program for his lower back stability muscles, with emphasis on his abdominals. He gradually added exercises to his program, and consulted a physiotherapist occasionally to check on his progress and advance his exercises.

PUTTING IT ALL TOGETHER

Luke took note of the advice in Chapter 17 regarding standing and walking, and made a concerted effort to carry himself with a better posture, and to use his ever-strengthening stability muscles. As he has also experienced occasional knee problems, Luke consulted a podiatrist, who prescribed orthotics to correct his flattened arches, and recommended a more appropriate pair of sports shoes.

He started on a fitness program of rowing, which he completed six times per week, with an easy day always following a harder day. Initially his spine ached, and he fatigued very quickly. Nevertheless, Luke persisted and gradually improved, and by the first game of the next season he could row for forty minutes at a good pace without any spinal discomfort.

Luke felt justified in scanning briefly over the advice for sitting, bending, lifting and lying, as his problem was not related to these areas. Luke also considered that his diet was acceptable, and decided against wearing a brace or taping.

As Luke was normally a confident and laid-back type of fellow, he also dismissed relaxation and positive thinking as irrelevant to his problem. However, at the first training session of the new season, he started work with a bowling coach to alter his technique. Initially he found this change very difficult, as he had practised his old action for many years. Two weeks later, frustrated by his lack of progress, Luke tried some visualisation techniques.

Before each training session, Luke sat quietly for twenty minutes and worked through the relaxation exercises. Then, when his mind was relaxed, he visualised himself bowling with his new action. Repeatedly he practised his new perfect action in his mind's eye.

He was pleasantly surprised, and so was his coach, when his technique suddenly improved. He mastered the new action within a few weeks, and found that not only was his spine more comfortable, but his accuracy and pace improved as well.

Luke was nervous before the first game of the new season. Would all his hard work pay off? Before the game he relaxed, and again visualised himself bowling perfectly with his modified action. This procedure took only ten minutes, as he was adept after two months of practice. He also performed his exercise routine as a warm-up, which consisted of not only stretches, but stability exercises as well. He repeated the exercises during the lunch break.

After the game, Luke was delighted to discover that he had very little stiffness. He noticed a slight pain, and applied some ice for thirty minutes as insurance.

As the season developed, Luke found that his spine improved, rather than deteriorating as it had in the previous season. He gradually progressed his stability exercises, and continued to row, although his cricket commitments forced him to decrease to three sessions per week.

Except for one exacerbation that required four visits to his spinal health practitioner, Luke completed his season without further incident. He received the top bowling award at the club dinner, and heard a rumour that the State selectors would be keeping a close eye on his progress during the ensuing year.

CASE TWO
The problem
Maria was a thirty-five-year-old legal secretary. She spent most of her days in the typing pool at work, and loved to go out to dinner or to the movies on the weekends. She had never experienced any previous back troubles, not even a twinge.

One Sunday morning, Maria went outside to fetch the morning paper. As she bent to retrieve the newspaper from a garden bed, she felt a twinge in her back. Ten minutes later, as she sat having coffee, the pain began to worsen. It continued to bother her intermittently for the rest of the day, and she felt very stiff as she dressed for work the next morning.

She didn't last very long at work. By ten o'clock her spine was aching so much that she went to the local medical centre for a check-up. The doctor, on hearing her history and viewing an X-ray, told her that she had torn a disc. He told her to rest for a week, and gave her a pamphlet on correct lifting methods. It was her incorrect bending technique when she picked up the newspaper, her doctor assured her, that had caused the trouble.

Maria went home, and lay in bed reading magazines for the next two days. For the rest of the week, she continued to rest. She sat in front of television watching video movies, and wrote letters to friends. However, her back pain did not improve—in fact, it seemed to be worsening. She decided to do something about it herself.

The program
Maria's case is not as simple as it first seems. Although she injured her back when bending to lift the newspaper, experience tells us that a normal, healthy spine would have managed this simple action without problems. Rather than blame this single, unobtrusive incident for all her troubles, Maria realised that her spine had accumulated micro-trauma, and had simply chosen this moment to let her know that it was degenerating. Instead of focusing on her lifting technique, she attempted to determine the underlying cause of the accumulated weakness in her spine.

After reading through the list near the beginning of this chapter, Maria realised she had many possible causes for her condition. Her muscles were weak, and she didn't always bend properly. She acknowledged that she sometimes felt over-stressed, and that her diet was often poor. In fact, she had problems with most items on the list to one degree or another. However, as this was her first bout of pain, she decided to concentrate on the two factors that she felt were most at fault: her poor, prolonged sitting posture, and her lack of general fitness and flexibility.

Rather than lounge around on the sofa waiting for her back to heal itself, Maria decided that an active approach was more likely to help. The next morning she went for a twenty-minute swim at the local pool, which she followed with a gentle ten-minute walk that afternoon. After discovering from the quiz that her spine was type B, she completed a set of the appropriate stability exercises both morning and night.

She avoided sitting as much as possible for the next two days. In the meantime she purchased a lumbar support device for work, and rolled an old towel for the same purpose at home.

Within two days, Maria was feeling much better. The extra exercise and movement, combined with better postural awareness while sitting, had been the key elements to her recovery. She returned to work for half a day without incident, and the next day recommenced her normal shift.

Maria had no further pain. She continued to swim for fun and fitness. She also went on using the lumbar roll both at work and at home, as she found that her spine felt far more supported with it.

With just a few simple changes, Maria converted a potentially chronic problem into a transient pain. The right advice, followed by some basic changes to her habits, were all that she required to rid herself of her problem for good.

CASE THREE
The problem
Daniel was a fifty-two-year-old bank manager. Over the last eight years, Daniel had worked his way up from teller to manager, with his back pain exhibiting a similar meteoric rise. What had begun as a mild gnawing pain had gradually worsened, and his lower back now ached continually.

Daniel's general condition was not good. He was fifteen kilograms overweight. He was also very unfit as he did not have time to exercise, and he was so inflexible that he could bend forward only as far as his knees. He often felt stressed, but he figured that a bit of tension helped him to perform at a higher intensity at work.

A year previously he had visited a doctor for his pain, who had told him that he had arthritic changes in his spine—quite a shock for a youngish man of fifty-two. The doctor had written him a prescription for some anti-inflammatory tablets, and referred him to a local manual therapist. However, Daniel was far too busy at work to attend the remedial sessions, so he had relied on the medication to control his pain. Although his stomach was starting to exhibit signs of dyspepsia, he felt that he had no other choice but to keep taking the medication, so he took some antacid tablets twice a day as well.

Over the last three months, Daniel's pain had considerably worsened. Whereas he used to have occasional good days, he now had pain almost all of the time. In particular, his spine ached when he sat, which unfortunately constituted a large percentage of his working day. He was so stiff when he arose from bed each morning that he could barely walk until he had stood under a hot shower for ten minutes.

Daniel's constant pain was now affecting his concentration at work. It made him irritable and tired. He spent his weekends resting in front of the television, as he felt his spine was now too sore for gardening, which was his only other hobby.

Daniel realised that his back pain was controlling and dominating his entire life. Finally, after eight years, he decided to do something about his problem. After reading this book and contemplating the lists at the beginning of this chapter, Daniel was horrified to discover that almost every area required attention.

The program
As Daniel was doing virtually everything 'wrong', and he had long-standing, severe pain, he had to make major changes to his lifestyle and attitude if he were to cure his problem.

On completing the back pain quiz, Daniel found that his spine was type D, and that he had severe neural tension. His major initial strategy involved a short program of exercises to loosen his tight joints and nerves, which he dutifully completed twice per day.

Daniel assessed that his work chair (an old wobbly typist's chair, with a low, unsupportive backrest) was also a major contributing factor. He applied to head office for a new chair, which they initially refused. However, after some careful negotiating, his employers agreed to pay half the cost. Daniel purchased a new, full-backrested chair, and picked up three lumbar support devices: one for work, one for home, and one for his car. He used them religiously from that day forward.

He took careful note of the advice for lifting and bending, and applied many of the hints to his hobby of gardening. He replaced a few tools with a more suitable long-handled version. Daniel also threw away his saggy, twenty-year-old innerspring mattress. He replaced it with a firm six-inch foam mattress, which he underpinned with a plywood base. If this strategy helped, he planned to buy a new bed in a few months' time.

Daniel then turned his attention to his stress level. At first, he simply could not manage the relaxation exercises properly. He tried for two weeks, but failed to improve. In desperation he bought a cassette tape that guided him through the relaxation process. After using the tape for a few weeks, he finally achieved a deeply relaxed, peaceful state of mind.

After further practice, Daniel was able to attain a deeply relaxed state without the aid of the cassette, and with further practice he became adept. He soon started noticing that his everyday demeanour was more composed, and surprised himself, and his secretary, by actually saying good morning to her!

After doing some further research into stress management, Daniel also adjusted his work approach in order to make it less mentally taxing. He refused to tackle other people's problems, and delegated more responsibility to his staff. Initially they were resentful, but soon the branch was operating more efficiently than ever before. Not only that, but Daniel now had half the worries and responsibilities that he had shouldered before, and consequently more spare time.

Daniel used this extra time well: he joined a gymnasium in an effort to lose some weight, which was something that he wouldn't have contemplated a month before. Initially he performed a gentle cardiovascular program of stationary rowing, riding and treadmill walking, and was horrified to find that his heart rate shot up alarmingly with even the slightest exertion. However, Daniel persisted, and three weeks later he discovered to his own amusement that he was enjoying his gym sessions.

Initially, Daniel chose not to include any positive thinking in his program, as he thought that the concept was a bit too 'alternative' for his tastes. However, a few weeks later he had a presentation to deliver at head office, and was feeling nervous and uncertain. After reviewing his notes in his office before the presentation, Daniel decided to try some visualisation techniques, as he had twenty minutes to spare anyway. He completed a cycle of relaxation exercises—he was now adept at these—and then started repeating thoughts to himself such as 'I am confident, calm and relaxed'. He then repeatedly pictured himself giving a perfect presentation.

Daniel was so surprised at his own confidence during the presentation that he decided to give the positive thinking techniques another try. That night, he used some phrases for better spinal health. He was again amazed to discover that his pain lessened almost immediately. From that day forward, Daniel's attitude toward his back pain changed completely. Of course, his pain levels permanently dropped, too.

Daniel stopped taking the anti-inflammatory medication, with no adverse reaction. During subsequent occasional flare-ups, he used a hot-water bottle to ease the aches and stiffness, rather than handfuls of anti-inflammatory tablets. Soon his stomach dyspepsia disappeared as well.

After reading a nutrition guide that was recommended by a dietician friend, Daniel made some simple changes to his eating habits. No third helpings of dessert for a start! Initially he didn't notice any major weight loss, but two months later, he realised with a wry smile that his belt buckle had moved in a couple of notches.

Three months after starting his program, Daniel's spine was well and truly improving. His pain was only half as intense as previously, and only hurt during stressful periods or after prolonged sitting, rather than continuously.

Instead of waking up in the morning with a stiff, aching back, then rushing off to a stress-filled and pain-racked day at the office, Daniel now had a whole new approach. He would wake up in the mornings and stretch for eight minutes, then complete some relaxation and positive thinking exercises for five minutes, before heading off to a productive day at work. He then worked off any accumulated stiffness and tension, as well as a few calories, at the gymnasium on the way home.

Six months later, with his pain down to only ten per cent of its original intensity, Daniel was a changed man. His back pain, which had once dominated his life, had been a catalyst for a remarkable turn-around. It took a lot of personal effort, but Daniel was now fitter, more relaxed, had greater productivity and suffered far less pain than he had for twenty years.

He had only one wish: that he'd started sooner.

Have you got the idea? I know it's not simple, but I'm sure you can do it.

Just one final point before I sign all effort over to you.

Human nature means that we tend to concentrate on jobs that are *urgent*—filing a report, catching a bus, or getting to the bottle shop before closing time—rather than doing the things that are truly *important*.

This focus on the present-day, urgent tasks means that we have no time for the important jobs. Those vital, small changes that would make a huge difference to our lives are swamped by thousands of far less important tasks that must be done immediately.

Research has shown that people who effectively manage their time are those who first do the *important* things, before allowing themselves time for the *urgent* but less important tasks. If you copy this method, you will steadily achieve the things that are most important to you, rather than filling your days with hectic but unproductive duties.

If your back pain is decreasing your quality of life, then it is obviously important. However, it is rarely urgent. Getting rid of your

PUTTING IT ALL TOGETHER

back pain has no deadline, no cut-off point, and you won't lose your deposit if it's not achieved by a certain date. So it is often ignored, or swamped under an ever-expanding pile of urgent but less vital jobs.

If this sounds like you, then I suggest you place your rehabilitation plans at the top of your 'to do' list every day, rather than waiting for a spare five minutes to arrive into which you can cram some exercises. If you schedule the time every day—in other words, if you make it a habit—then changes will come naturally and steadily.

Your lifestyle won't be attacking your spine, it will be helping it.

You'll soon find that your muscles strengthen and your spine becomes more flexible. Your mental tension will abate, and your attitude toward your problems will brighten. Good posture will become automatic, and your whole approach to getting rid of your back problem will be second nature. Your discomfort will decrease, and before you know it, your back pain will disappear.

Because you've treated the deep-down causes of your problem, rather than just covering over the symptoms, your back pain will disappear *forever*.

At the start of this book, I mentioned that about five billion people in the world currently have, or will soon experience, back pain. Well, I reckon that number just dropped to 4,999,999,999. Guess who the fortunate person is?

You.

Epilogue

Spinal pain, as you now know, is a complex science. Even though spinal health practitioners have come a long way in their understanding of spinal pain, I'm sure that there is still much to learn. I'm still learning, too, so I'd be interested to hear of your experiences in implementing your program. Please write to me at any of the following addresses, and let me know how you go.

E-mail: johnperrier@hotmail.com

Website: www.ecn.net.au/~jp/index.html

Bulimba Physiotherapy Centre
Shop 3
114 Oxford St
Bulimba
Brisbane 4171
Australia

Mansfield Physiotherapy Centre
Suite 9
Wishart Square
corner Newnham and Wishart Roads
Wishart 4122
Australia

Your story would be even more interesting if you also included your test scores from Chapter 11 (your F-E, S-U and neural tension scores) as well as your back pain type—A, B, C or D.

Of course, I am also interested in the experiences and opinions of other spinal health practitioners—whether or not you agree with all of my ideas.

JP

Appendices

Preventing osteoporosis

Seven factors affect the density of your bones:

(1) Exercise
Regular *weight-bearing* exercise will dramatically increase the strength of your bones. Studies have shown that otherwise healthy people lose an incredible amount of bone mass if they are forced to rest in bed for prolonged periods, even though their diets and hormone levels are maintained at perfect levels.

Always remember that regular weight-bearing exercise is your best defence against brittle bones. Walking is the simplest, and probably best, form of defence. See Chapter 26 on fitness for more details and guidelines.

One small point to note for female athletes and their coaches: extreme exercise, such as marathon running, can cause hormonal imbalances that not only destroy your menstrual cycle, but can ultimately cause severe osteoporosis in even very young athletes. Please exercise in moderation.

(2) Hormone replacement therapy
Many doctors are now prescribing HRT for post-menopausal women, with good results. This type of treatment is simple to apply, although it does have side effects. See your doctor if you feel that you are at risk of developing osteoporosis.

(3) Other drugs
Many other drugs are now entering the aged-care market which are specifically designed to target osteoporosis. These drugs may be useful for both men and women. See your doctor for further details.

(4) Sunlight
Your body requires Vitamin D to metabolise calcium. A regular walk in the sun will do the job.

(5) Smoking
Studies have linked the habit of cigarette smoking to a higher incidence of osteoporosis. You already know that smoking is horrific for your

health, so if you're still doing it, I doubt that this extra morsel of evidence is going to make you change your ways.

Go ahead, keep smoking ... I'll see you in hospital when you are old, lying in traction with a fractured hip, and wheezing through an oxygen mask.

(6) Diet
Researchers have had trouble in gauging the effect that increasing calcium intake has upon your bones. However, commonsense dictates that extra calcium, which is most easily obtained from milk and milk products, may help to fortify your body's stores of this mineral. In short, your diet forms one part of a sensible osteoporosis prevention program.

(7) Relax!
Stressologists tell us that the hormones of the fight-or-flight response suppress your body's long-term maintenance programs. Bone-building falls into this category.

Therefore, if you are constantly or frequently stressed then your bones will gradually weaken. The moral of the story is that relaxed people have stronger bones. Hard to believe, but true.

Some common anti-inflammatory medications
Prescription-only drugs

Name of medication This is what's inside the capsule	Common brand names This is what's written on the outside of the box
Diflunisal	Dolobid
Diclofenac	Voltaren
Ibuprofen	Brufen
Indomethacin	Indocid, Arthrexin
Ketoprofen	Orudis
Mefanamic acid	Mefic
Piroxicam	Feldene
Naproxen	Naprosyn, Flexin
Sulindac	Clinoril

Over-the-counter drugs

Name of medication This is what's inside the capsule	Common brand names This is what's written on the outside of the box
Aspirin	Aspirin, Disprin
Ibuprofen	Triprofen, Act 3, Nurofen, Actiprofen
Naproxen	Naprogesic